J T WILSON AND THE FRATERNITY
OF DUCKMALOI

For Simon
With many best wishes

Pat, Morison

THE WELLCOME INSTITUTE SERIES IN THE HISTORY OF MEDICINE

Forthcoming Titles

Social Medicine and Medical Sociology in the Twentieth Century
Edited by Dorothy Porter

Operative Chymist
Anthony Morson

Ashes to Ashes: The History of Smoking and Health
Edited by Stephen Lock

Academic inquiries regarding the series should be addressed
to the editors W. F. Bynum, V. Nutton and Roy Porter at
the Wellcome Institute for the History of Medicine,
183 Euston Road, London NW1 2BE, UK

J T WILSON AND THE FRATERNITY OF DUCKMALOI

Patricia Morison

Amsterdam – Atlanta, GA 1997

First published in 1997
by Editions Rodopi B. V., Amsterdam – Atlanta, GA 1997.

© 1997 Patricia Morison

Design and Typesetting by Christine Buckley, the Wellcome Trust.
Printed and bound in The Netherlands by Editions Rodopi B. V.,
Amsterdam – Atlanta, GA 1997.

British Library Cataloguing in Publication Data
A catalogue record for this book is available from the British Library
ISBN: 90-420-0232-8 (Bound)
ISBN: 90-420-0246-8 (Paper)

Morison, Patricia
J T Wilson and the Fraternity of Duckmaloi
– Amsterdam – Atlanta, GA:
Rodopi. – ill.
(Clio Medica 42 / ISSN 0045-7183;
The Wellcome Institute Series in the History of Medicine)

Front cover:
Duckmaloi Camp, September 1895

© Editions Rodopi B. V. Amsterdam – Atlanta, GA 1997

Printed in The Netherlands

In memory of Katherine and Louise

Contents

Introduction

The history of medicine and the history of science need biographies to dig beneath the strictly professional contributions of individuals to their field and to explore what they did, and perhaps why, in the context of their personal outlook and the values and beliefs of their times. All too often doctors and scientists do not keep their papers, or not enough to yoke their personal story to their professional career.

James Thomas Wilson (1861 to 1945) is an ideal subject for such an exploration. He was the first Challis Professor of Anatomy at the University of Sydney from 1890 to 1920, and then took the chair of anatomy at Cambridge University until 1934. He left a fair-sized volume of papers both professional and personal, and had wide interests and activities including philosophy and university ideals, medical science and education, biology and the Darwinian debate, empire and military affairs. His 33 years in Sydney were a time of transition for Australia from colonies to nationhood, and Sydney University's transition from a small classics-dominated teaching institution to a large vocation-dominated one. He was an important university leader; a leading scientist at the centre of significant scientific work on Australian fauna and part of an international network spanning the various disciplines of biologists.

This 'life and times' treatment of Wilson attempts to describe his professional work in sufficient detail to be of use to scientists and medical educationists, while painting in enough of the personal and cultural background to interest general readers. The endeavours of Wilson and his colleagues are primarily of historical interest, but their underlying preoccupations remain topical: pure versus applied science; competition among scientific disciplines; the struggle to interpret Darwin's theory without placing *homo sapiens* at the top of an evolutionary tree; the international community of science; Australia's place in the world.

Acknowledgements

This story of James Thomas Wilson could not have been told without the assistance and encouragement of Wilson family members: daughters Katharine Reid and Louise Hutchinson in Sydney and Dorette Cuthbert in Scotland, sons Douglas, John (and his wife Anne) and Maxwell in Britain, Amy Milligan (née Lorrain Smith) and grandson Patrick de Burgh in Sydney, who provided personal recollections and private papers, now lodged in the archives of Sydney University. Katharine and Maxwell generously supported the research work needed to collect other source material on Wilson, in Australia and Scotland.

Personal recollections by others are also essential to the story: from friends of the Wilson family including Mary Edgeworth David, Maisie Gibbs (née Martin), Mary Haswell, Lady Marnie Bassett (née Masson), Lady Constance Murray, Nancy Osborne and Mungo MacCallum III; from medical people among Wilson's former students including Grace Cuthbert Brown, A G S Cooper, Raymond Dart, M Britnell Fraser, Arthur Fell, Howard Green, Frank Goldby, H Leaver, Ian Mackerras, Sir Douglas Miller, R A Money, Sir Kenneth Noad, J Swift Joly, B M Willmott Dobbie; from Sir Marcus Oliphant who, as a student, knew Wilson in Cambridge, and from A J E Cave. Thanks for their memories are also owed to the sons of two of Wilson's colleagues: Louis Schaeffer Jr whose father was Wilson's legendary assistant, and Frank Hinder whose father H V C Hinder was one of the Fraternity of Duckmaloi.

Assistance with library and archival material was provided by Naomi Mitchison (née Haldane); Collum Smith-Burnett of the Aberdeen College of Education; Rosanne Clayton of the Australian Academy of Science Basser Library; Gerald Fischer, Kenneth Smith and Tim Robinson of the Sydney University Archive; Brenda Heagney of the Australian Medical Association Library; Gwendoline Baker of the Australian Museum in Sydney; Walter Makey of the City of Edinburgh; Ruby Davies of the Anatomical Society of Great Britain; E H R Ford of the Anatomy School at Cambridge University; M J Atkin of the Old Schools, Cambridge; I C

Cunningham of the National Library of Scotland; Desmond Donaldson of the Dumfries and Galloway Regional Council; Dr E C Boterenbrood, Curator of the Hubrecht Embryological Collection. Archival assistance was also given by staff of the Australian War Museum, the Medical Archives of Johns Hopkins Medical Institutions, and the Australian Archives in Canberra and Melbourne.

Reproduction of illustrations is acknowledged, courtesy of the following published sources: William Epps' *Life of Sir T P Anderson Stuart*; Warren Dawson's *Sir Grafton Elliot Smith*; *Sydney University Medical Journal*; *Hermes*; *Australia's First – A History of the University of Sydney Volume 1 1850–1939*; *Centenary Book of the University of Sydney Faculty of Medicine*; *Obituaries of Fellows of the Royal Society*; and the Journal of Anatomy. Other sources include the Archives of the University of Sydney; Medical Archives of the University of Edinburgh; Mitchell Library, Sydney.

Helpful comment and suggestions for various draft chapters, from the perspectives of their expertise respectively in medicine, science, history, or just plain writing, was given by Professor Michael Blunt, Dr John Calaby, Professor M A Kaufman, Dr Geoffrey Kenny, Emeritus Professor Oliver Lancaster, Dr Reg Passmore, Professor Jack Still, and Dr J M G Wilson; by Leonie Foster (Round Table), Steve Sturdy (Scottish Idealists); by Dr Barry Smith, Dr Jim Gibbney and Professor John Ritchie of the Australian National University; and by Michael Page.

Illustrations

Abbreviations

Wilson and Family

AW	Anne Wilson (daughter-in-law)
DC	Dorette Cuthbert (daughter)
TDGW	Douglas Wilson (son)
HW	Helen Wilson (sister)
JCR, or J	Jane Clunies Ross, (formerly de Burgh) 'Jeanie' (daughter)
JES	Jane Elizabeth Smith, 'Jeanie' (first wife)
JLS	James Lorrain Smith (brother-in-law)
JTW	James Thomas Wilson
JJGW	John Wilson (son)
KR	Katharine Reid (daughter)
LH	Louise Hutchinson (daughter)
MMW	Mabel Millicent Wilson (second wife)
JMGW	Maxwell Wilson (son)
P de B	Patrick de Burgh (grandson)

Wilson's Colleagues and Correspondents

AEM	Arthur Edward Mills
AMacC	Alexander MacCormick
CJM	Charles James Martin
CSS	Charles Scott Sherrington
GES	Grafton Elliot Smith
HJW	Herbert John Wilkinson
JIH	John Irvine Hunter
JPH	James Peter Hill
JSH	John Scott Haldane
MH	Marion Hines-Loeb
MWM	Mungo William MacCallum
RBH	Richard Burdon Haldane
SAS	Stewart Arthur Smith
TPAS	Thomas Peter Anderson Stuart
TWED	T W Edgeworth David
WAH	William A Haswell

Bibliographic Sources

AA	Australian Archives
AAAS	Australasian Association for Advancement of Science (later ANZAAS)
ADB	*Australian Dictionary of Biography*
AM	Australian Museum (Sydney)
AMG	*Australasian Medical Gazette*
ANL	Australian National Library (Canberra)
AWM	Australian War Memorial (Canberra)
British Ass	British Association for the Advancement of Science
BMJ	*British Medical Journal*
BL	Basser Library (Canberra)
Calendar	*Calendar of the University of Sydney*
CUR	*Cambridge University Reporter*
DNB	*Dictionary of National Biography*
DT	*Daily Telegraph* (Sydney)
J of A	*Journal of Anatomy*
MJA	*Medical Journal of Australia*
N&R	Notes and Reminiscences (by JTW)
PLS	*Proceedings of the Linnean Society of NSP*
QJMS	*Quarterly Journal of Microscopical Science*
RBP	Rosemary Bigwood Papers
RSO	*Royal Society Obituaries* (*Biographical Memoirs of Fellows of the Royal Society*)
SMH	*Sydney Morning Herald*
SSM	Scot Skirving Memoirs
SUA	*Sydney University Archives*
SUMJ	*Sydney University Medical Journal*
U of S	University of Sydney (SM) – Senate Minutes (PBM) – Professorial Board Minutes
WP	Wilson Papers

1

A Border Scot

'Though Kentish by birth, I am Scotch to the core', said Thomas Wilson as he was about to leave Scotland forever in January 1888,[1] at the age of 63, to join his son James Thomas Wilson, a demonstrator in anatomy at the new Medical School in Sydney, New South Wales.

Thomas was born in Kent because his father James, like many another Scot harassed by economic difficulty, had migrated there in 1822 with his bride Henrietta Glover of Dumfries to make his way as an orchardist. Two children were born there: a daughter who died in infancy and then Thomas on 28 January 1825. The Kentish venture must have failed or the pull of Dumfriesshire proved stronger for their four younger children were born there between 1826 and 1834. James found work as a gardener and sawyer and all his children, except James who trained as a coachbuilder and migrated to Australia, eventually settled in the district: John a blacksmith in Dumfries, Robert a photographer in Dumfries, Marion married to a local farmer, and Thomas a schoolmaster in Moniaive.

Thomas had approached adulthood as an apprentice tailor, then he managed somehow to qualify as a teacher, spending a number of itinerant years on both sides of the Border before being appointed on 14 January 1856 to the Free Church School in Moniaive in the rural parish of Glencairn. He was back, with his bride Helen of fifteen months, in the home of his paternal ancestors. Helen's family roots were in Border country too. Born on 11 November 1824 in the neighbouring rural parish of Kirkmichael she was the youngest of the eleven children of David and Grace Brown. David, a stonemason, claimed family connections with Sir Walter Scott and Thomas Carlyle, and Grace was of the Johnstone clan, renowned in Border history for their long feud with the clan of Maxwell.

1

Bonds of Scottish kinship are strong. Thomas and Helen Wilson were among clusters of their kin around Moniaive and Dumfries, and at the seaside resort of Gatehouse-of-Fleet, the home base of Thomas's Edinburgh cousins the Glovers. Some of Helen's family had moved further afield: in North America were two sisters and a third, Jessie, in Australia. In her mid-twenties Helen had gone alone by sailing ship to the United States to help look after the young family of her dying sister Grace. So when she married Thomas Wilson, on 11 October 1854 in the Free Church at Ruthwell in Dumfriesshire, Helen was an independent-minded, widely-travelled woman of 30, earning her living as an infants' teacher.[2]

In early February 1856 Helen and Thomas Wilson moved into Mill Cottage in Ayr Street, or 'Mill Raw' as it was called. Sited picturesquely near the junction of three streams feeding the river Cairn, Moniaive was then a village of 500 people serving an agricultural community of about 2,000. As well as farming, droving and shepherding, there was employment for masons, weavers, carpenters, clog- boot- and shoe-makers; also for dykers, since the river flats were prone to flooding.[3]

Geography made Glencairn a green and pleasant corner of the earth, but history's influence was sterner. The stone cross in the centre of the village, erected in 1638 in the time of the Covenanters, symbolized the spirit of its people. Almost two centuries later, and a quarter of a mile away, another and larger monument to this tradition was raised by public subscription. Of hewn stone and 25 feet high, it is a memorial to the Reverend James Renwick the native son who was the last covenanting martyr to be executed in Edinburgh in 1688. Renwick, a militant student of extreme views, excommunicated all other ministers in the belief that his band of zealots, the Society Folk, was the only true church. For a Glencairn historian however, writing in 1893, he was 'the gentle youth who put courage in the heart and backbone in the body of the speedily diminishing band of Covenanters'. A strolling player, Charlotte Deans, who lodged there in 1826, described Moniaive as a place 'abounding in fierce Cameronians with little money and plenty of pride'.[4]

The Browns and the Wilsons were strong supporters of the Free Church created by a great upheaval of conscience in the Established Church of Scotland, the 'Disruption' of 1843. Protesting against 'moderation and evils of patronage' nearly one-third of its ministers followed Dr David Welsh and Dr Thomas Chalmers out of its General Assembly at Edinburgh, taking with them many elders and dominies and most overseas missionaries. Nearly half of the Church of Scotland's communicants left to establish another national rival ecclesiastical and educational organization, the Free Church of Scotland. A complex affair affecting all areas of Scottish life, at the heart of the Disruption lay the issue of control over the spiritual and community responsibilities of the Kirk. Lord Cockburn deemed it the 'most honourable feat for Scotland that its whole history supplies'. For Thomas and Helen Wilson it was all of a piece with their turbulent regional heritage.[5]

The parish of Glencairn was a conspicuous success for the Free Glencairn
Kirk. Under the leadership of the young Reverend Patrick Borrowman practically all communicants of the Established Church 'came out' with him in June 1843 and scarcely six months later he conducted the first service in Moniaive's newly built Free Church. 'A kind of omnipresence would attach to his person', wrote his successor of Borrowman, who served his community indefatigably for nearly 50 years:

> A keen rider on horseback, and a quick, he would push from Presbytery meeting to some congregation in its bounds without a Free Church minister. Virginhall, Closeburn, Durrisdeer, Balmaclellan, and Wallacetown were all worked by him for a time. He passed from place to place here addressing a prayer meeting, there organising a Kirk-Session, then, having lit the small lamp bound round his chest, he mounted his horse and rode off somewhere else to repeat the business.[6]

When Thomas Wilson started as schoolmaster, on 3 March 1856, the Reverend Borrowman was in his prime, serving a congregation zealously building church, manse and schools, promoting their new covenant with God for the spiritual good of Scotland. Thomas Wilson took up his post with enthusiasm, being admitted as a teacher by the Presbytery; then Treasurer of the Church Court, and subsequently session clerk, church elder and superintendent of the Sabbath School. In 1865 the Wilsons moved into a new house built by the Church on school grounds for the schoolmaster.[7]

Thomas and Helen's three children were born in Mill Cottage in Ayr Street: Helen Brown on 25 April 1857, Henrietta Glover on 15 June 1859 and James Thomas on 14 April 1861. But the young family was soon diminished by one, for three-year-old Henrietta died on 19 August 1862 of 'bronchitis 1 week' according to her death certificate. 'Wee Jamie' at sixteen months did not remember Henrietta, but her death did make a difference to his life by emptying the space of four years that lay between him and Helen who became a motherly companion as they grew up. At age 10 she wrote to her mother, who was away recuperating from an illness, with news centred on her six-year-old brother:

> James still has the cough he had on Saturday morning but we are taking good care of him and hope he will soon get better ... We were all at Church yesterday ... and in his sermon Mr B. [spoke of Jesus] as the shadow of a great rock in a weary land and at night when James was sitting on Papa's knee he said Papa I was thinking about the shadow of a great rock in a weary land and then Papa explained it all to him and asked him if you had a long journey to go would [you] not like if it was a hot day to have the shadow of a tree. So Jesus is the shadow from sin.

Her father added a note that 'James has scarcely at all coughed this morning so I think you may keep your mind quite free in regard to him'. He was glad she had arrived safely and was as well as could be expected, but 'I am sorry to see the Cab-man disappointed you & so that is two shillings dead lost which I exceedingly grudge. Had it served your purpose I would not at all have minded it. But I must see & get the one back from the fellow when I am down'. Fair dealing was a basic principle with Thomas and economy a basic necessity.

Two months later Helen wrote again, a little out of patience, that Jim 'was petted because he could not get a boy to play... I am sorry to say that he is become a naughty boy since you went away, and am afraid you will have to come home soon again'. 'Wrastlin' Jamie' was never still and difficult to restrain, but Helen was also wishing her mother home on her own account, 'that I might get to school'. Her father added a note of reassurance to his wife: 'I have just taken a look over Nell's letter & albeit it is true that Jim has displayed some little naughtiness yet she is going a little too far in making such a grievous complaint about him. I have no fear but he will keep all right yet'.[8]

In late May 1869, and now aged 12, Helen accompanied her father to Edinburgh where as an elder he attended the General Assembly of the Free Church. While her father attended meetings and lectures, Helen visited the Glover relations and was shown the sights of Edinburgh: the castle, the guards and guns that signalled one o'clock Greenwich time, Princes Street gardens, Calton Hill, Sir Walter Scott's Monument, the grand shops in Princes and Nicholson Streets and 'all the hospitals but one'. A letter from Jim told her that 'Doctor Grierson said that the curious beasts with stiks for shells the name was caddisbait'; and another piece of information: 'I have been sorting up the store room for my Museum and I have got a lot of curious stones'.[9]

Like most Scottish children of his day, Jim Wilson was raised on porridge and the Bible. His mother taught him his letters by the time-honoured method of committing long passages of the Bible to memory, absorbing as he did so its art and wisdom: the foundation of a high, wide and sober Scottish education. Both parents being teachers and committed to the fervent Free Kirk, it might have been predicted that young Jim was set for a dour upbringing. But this God-fearing home emphasized the New Testament rather than the Old, with an awareness more of God in his Heaven than the Calvinist devil and his works. They were thinking folk who, as Carlyle taught, are the worst enemies of the prince of darkness. They had secular interests like botany which the mother's love of flowers engendered, and the father's interest in astronomy. And let not the porridge be overlooked among the blessings of the Wilson household: Scottish oats, freshly ground and carefully cooked was a different dish from the 'infeerior soort o' pooding' generally known to the rest of the world.

Then there was Dr Grierson of Thornhill, a market town eight miles east of Moniaive. A local oddity, Dumfriesshire-born and bred, Edinburgh-trained, Grierson practised medicine and peddled natural history. Revered by the poor for his compassion, trusted by mothers as 'safe', gifted in winning the confidence of children, he had a place in the immediate homelife of many families in the district. He was more widely known as a 'forby queer man', whose enthusiasm was collecting things animate and inanimate, also knowledge, wide, various and indiscriminate. He was a familiar figure out of doors, negligently dressed in shabby trousers, an old coat too short for him, a shepherd's plaid on his rounded shoulders, a felt hat green with age on his long dark hair. Elastic sided boots, battered but always in a state of practical repair, completed the costume. In the summer he usually had a bunch of young companions combining nature studies and recreation in their playground of hills, woods and streams. There were also a ruined tower, an old fort, a moat, hillside graves, an ancient cairn, and Maxwelton, the tall white house where Annie Laurie once lived.

Like Walter Scott's character Old Mortality, in whose tradition he stood, Grierson was frugal in his personal habits, unworldly in his dedication to his self-appointed task. But where Old Mortality was devoted to the sacred duty of restoring the inscriptions of the scattered hillside tombstones of the Covenanters, Dr Grierson's devotion was to collecting things and fostering talent in the studious young. To this end he advanced his educational views at meetings of learned societies like the British Association and the Social Science Congress held at Glasgow in 1874, gave public lectures, supported various local educational, scientific, literary and political societies, opened his museum and library to the public and formed the Society of Enquiry for local youths to read and discuss their papers on natural history and kindred subjects. His knowledge was cumulative rather than deep, and as a teacher he rather liked the role of the oracle. His religion was undefined, though he did maintain a connection with the Virginhall Free Kirk.[10]

When eight-year-old Jim Wilson was beginning his first museum Dr Grierson was outgrowing his, and on 22 June 1869 the foundation stone of a handsome two-storeyed building was laid. Dr Grierson's driving enterprise, assisted by his friend the Duke of Buccleuch and community interest, opened this new museum in July 1872. It held a wealth of wonder, of local origin and from far corners of the earth, for by this time Dr Grierson had won wide renown. He had been collecting for 30 years. Many youngsters owed their first impulse as naturalists to Dr Grierson's inspiration. A few were to achieve fame on their own account. His museum contained flints, shells, rocks, an antique jug, an even older cross, fossils, coins, botanical specimens, snakes, monkeys, birds, butterflies, harpoons, spears and swords, a letter written by Walter Scott, an autographed poem by Robert Burns. A marvellous jumble it was, and perhaps, according to one's view of the world, a true reflection of the state of nature. For the doctor loved chaos, or the 'law of higgledy-piggledy' as a prominent American biologist later facetiously defined Darwin's theory of evolution.[11] Jim Wilson was later to be remarked upon for the breadth of his interests, and for that he owed something to Dr Grierson. Another quality, meticulous order, he must have got elsewhere.

The brisk authority of Mrs Wilson ensured a well-ordered household, but she spent much of her time out and about on church and school affairs. Besides being the able partner of the schoolmaster, Mrs Wilson was best remembered in Glencairn for 'her appreciation of the works of nature', especially flowers, which was something she would have had in common with Dr Grierson. But the doctor's slack theology aroused in her a spirited antagonism such as to preclude a relationship built on any other interest, as an episode reported by Helen to Jim indicates:

Dr Grierson came over to see Mrs Proudfoot ... and of course he called. He told Mamma much to her horror (as you may imagine) that he had been down at Dfs. [Dumfries] preaching ? to about two hundred monks and nuns on 'natural religion'. And he threatened in fun but Ma thinks half in earnest too, to bring some of them over with him sometime to call upon her. She says she'll say 'There's the door we want no "osiers" here' if he does; and when Papa laughed at it and said he could do no harm even if he did so she said 'He might set them on the track of my poor son'.[12]

Her anxieties flowed over her family in 'reasonable and unreasonable surmises', remonstrances, forebodings and bewailings, which added some fun to family lore. Her familiarity with the local dialect, in which she wrote some poetry, privately printed, surprised even at times her family, who stayed more within the confines of cultivated Scots. A bustling Scotch body of decided opinions who gave generously of herself and lived in tune with the community and 'auld custom', her directness of manner and expression had considerable charm.[13]

Thomas Wilson stood foursquare for tradition too, but *Thomas W.* intellectual curiosity and enjoyment of study and controversy took him to a higher and wider plane. A deliberate act of self-assertion had made him a schoolmaster with no ambition for a life of ease, for while the Scots put education above most things they paid their teachers poorly. When first appointed to the Glencairn Free Church School in 1856, Thomas Wilson's salary was sixteen pounds ten *£16/10/- per* shillings a year plus a house at an annual rental of five pounds paid *year* by Church collection. Pupils' school fees substantially augmented this income. In addition there were 'perquisites' for clerking, precenting, administering the poor fund; his services as Session Clerk and Treasurer for the Free Church carried some small fees. All told, in the first years of his appointment, Thomas Wilson's total income was about sixty pounds per year, but as a result of State aid it had risen by 1867 to around eighty-five pounds per year and in 1876, after the State had assumed full responsibility for education, one hundred and thirty-six pounds. This was still well below the salary of the local minister though above that of a skilled artisan. Schoolmastering allowed Thomas time and opportunity to pursue *£136* 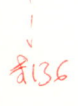 his interests: astronomy, cabinet making, gardening, bowls, politics (he was a Gladstonian liberal of course), music, books, church affairs. Though restricted by hard economic facts and the national code of values, his life was not narrow.[14]

Thomas enjoyed hearty good health. Even after buses and trains became available he preferred to walk, because of the expense; an aversion to timetables may also have had some effect. He thought nothing of walking nearly 20 miles to Dumfries to visit a sick relative or attend a lecture at the Mechanics Institute. In 1881, aged 56, he walked all over the parish to 'number the people' for the Census. On this expedition he accepted the company of Jim, on vacation from University, to allay his wife's fears of going 'alone all the way up to Concrach'. Thomas was of medium height and solid build, his stance as much as his dress suggesting vigour. His face had a heavy look, due to a fleshy knob of a nose and a prominent brow which became more pronounced as his hairline receded. His deep-set eyes were shrewd and sensitive. He spoke forcefully: 'I absolutely and entirely deny…', or 'I absolutely and entirely affirm…' were characteristic phrases. But the influence of his counsel was for temperance, moderation and justice all round, as a school episode recounted by daughter Helen illustrates. A pupil Maggie McCulloch, in trouble with her mother, falsely blamed her teacher Helen, and 'her mother wrote me a very impertinent note at night, and I just sat down and wrote a very sharp reply and Ma was to take it up at once, but Pa would not let it go and told me to wait till morning. When morning came he wrote a cooler note for me stating what happened exactly as it did and I sent it up'.[15]

Thomas's interests occupied centre stage, as in most middle class households of the time, and the family indulged his buoyant spirits. 'Pa has been quite miserable and out of his element all the evg. because he had not the papers', wrote Helen to Jim on 21 November 1881. 'They did not come till the late-bus and so he had to do without them but now he has got them and is quite happy again. He made up for it as well as he could by reading Greek, and praising himself greatly and dinning our ears therewith'. A little later on: 'Papa is in grief just now over the loss of the Stafford Election'. Still later: 'Papa is busy reading a report of Principal Rainy's speech lecture last evg. in St. George's (Free) …'. He could be brusque, for instance when he found his wife and daughter miserable over Jim's departure for Edinburgh:

> Papa got quite angry at Ma and me for weeping at tea. I daresay he
> felt it rather dull, and so to enliven us a little he treated us to a few
> words of consolation – commonly called scolding. By-and-bye, in
> consequence I suppose of his comforting words we brightened up a
> little … Pa laughs at Ma and me but then you see 'He haint got no
> sentiments, he's in the show bizness'.

Just so. He had sentiments but they were not for show.[16]

As the schoolmaster Thomas had to organize the teaching of religious knowledge, the three R's, English grammar plus geography and history for his 80 pupils, at levels to suit ages from four to fourteen years. If required he taught mathematics, Latin and Greek, and might also have introduced some pupils to his own special interests of astronomy, music and carpentry. Mrs Wilson, who returned to teaching in October 1863, taught sewing and later the popular subject of natural history. The school year was in three parts, the long summer term from May to October being broken by a harvest vacation of six to eight weeks around July. School attendance was affected by seasonal demands for labour, and sickness or absence of the mother often kept girls at home. To organize a teaching programme around these eternal impediments required ingenuity and 'the beauty of patience' which Thomas Wilson was wont to extol; that and the 'whiteness of truth'.[17]

[margin note: beauty of patience, the whiteness of truth]

Discipline was firm. Mr Wilson employed 'the master's restraint that disciplined the head', recalled one ex-pupil; 'the curb, the words of rebuke [were] tempered by love'. Another remarked that Mrs Wilson 'bulked fully as much in the recollections of his schooldays as Mr Wilson; and that, while his memories of the latter were of a somewhat mixed character ... those associated with Mrs Wilson were invariably of an agreeable character'. The cooler observation of a visiting American teacher was that 'the highest tension of authority which I anywhere witnessed was in the Scottish schools'. But the same American was impressed by Scottish thoroughness in teaching the 'intellectual part of reading' and the vigorous mental interaction of teachers and pupils, such as to make the most lively schools in the United States 'almost like dormitories'. What the dominies lacked in gentleness, he concluded, they made up for in a prodigious expenditure of energy and vivacity. One of Thomas Wilson's former pupils remembered him not merely 'for the manner in which he taught them the abc, the three R's, or even their Latin, Greek and mathematics; but still more for the better and higher education which he imparted by precept and example, which trained them to become good citizens, good men and women, good Christians'. Both of his children, being also his pupils, were doubly exposed to their father's values. In his son's mature judgment 'he was one of the salt of the earth'.[18]

[margin note: school disciplined but lively]

During Thomas Wilson's teaching career a new order came into being. Scottish educational traditions were democratic, comprehensive and religious: education should be available to everyone to the level of ability; it should be broad as well as vocational and give training in faith, character and citizenship. But in the chaos wrought by a century of industrialism on the parish system of education, Scotland's high rate of literacy fell steadily. After 1843 the divided Church added wasteful duplication to the problems of parish schools. English values came with State aid (government inspections and the coding of teaching and learning for payment by results) and added to sectarian tensions between the Church of Scotland and the Free Church. The old Scottish system came to an end when the State in 1872 assumed direct responsibility for the education of the whole people of Scotland, and vested financial control in a new department at Whitehall; all other administration was vested in local School Boards, elected by ratepayers. The first noticeable effect was a dramatic decline in schools under church authority. The Free Church at the height of its spread in 1851 owned 712 schools, and after some consolidation still had 523 in 1872, but three years later had only 151.[19]

The Glencairn Free Church School was one of those lost to the church. It transferred to the School Board 'after some discussion and dissension' in November 1874. Thomas Wilson probably opposed the move: religion was for him the dynamic centre of all education. Formal religious instruction was moved to the beginning or end of the daily timetable so that parents, if conscience dictated, could remove their children without interrupting the school programme. The Sunday School became the main instrument for delivering religious education to the community. Thomas Wilson played a leading role in the running of the Free Church Sabbath School in Moniaive and while he was its Superintendent it increased in vitality and size.[20]

'Remember the Sabbath Day to keep it holy.' Of all the Presbyterian Churches the Free Church observed the fourth Commandment most strictly; and that, allied with its strong support for Temperance and its frown on dancing, theatre and gambling gave it a reputation for rigid moralism at odds with its doctrinal position. Fundamentally the Free Church stood for the Gospel of forgiveness and redemption, but within Scotland it was seen as the voice of Puritanism and elsewhere it gave all Scots that reputation. For the Wilsons the Sabbath was a different day, unrelieved by frivolity but also untroubled by temporal vexations. Its rituals included a quiet breakfast, the donning of clean 'best' clothes for morning church with its lengthy sermon, a ceremonious midday meal, a quiet afternoon for reading 'good books' and

Sabbath school, then a light supper and church again for the adults. The Free Church was fond of rotund oratory, the probable reason for its ban on the reading of sermons. It could also be intellectually sharp. At all events the congregation, whose rights in church government the Free Church had vehemently reasserted, required to be satisfied. Though Jim Wilson later became an unorthodox Christian he regularly attended church and listened to the sermon with a keenly critical ear.[21]

Throughout Jim Wilson's youth Sabbatarianism was a controversial issue. In 1863 a proposal to open the Edinburgh Botanic Gardens on Sunday was defeated by religious opinion led by the Free Church. It was not till 1889 that the gardens opened, and then followed Museums and Galleries, Sunday train services and the playing of military bands in royal parks, marking the end of evangelical supremacy. Thomas and Helen Wilson did not go as far in Sabbath observance as those who denied walks in the countryside, and were unlikely to have supported Sunday closure of the Edinburgh Botanic Gardens. They approved of theatre but not dancing, which caused some soul-searching in their daughter. Helen reported to Jim that at a party she attended:

dancing

> I sat and enjoyed the fun of seeing them dance and would have been quite happy if it had not been for the consciousness that *they* would not like to have me sit and take no part in it. Do you know Jamie, if I had *learned* to dance I am quite sure I should not have been able to resist the temptation for not only would I have *liked* it, but I should not have wished to look unsocial. I wish I knew what I *ought* to do in such cases. I felt as if it would be wrong to do it and I felt as if it were wrong also *not* to join. I could not break up their party either or I would much rather have left when they began ... I wish I could have a talk with you on this subject, for it seems to me too, that the principal objections raised against dancing have equal weight against any other amusement, viz. a waste of time.

Jim probably had similar feelings at the time, but throughout his adult life he endorsed bans on dancing, and golf, on Sundays. Years later in Sydney his daughters occasionally found themselves in the predicament of his sister.[22]

Helen and Jim grew close in their teens. Intelligent, sensitive and vulnerable, they gave each other support through the ups and downs of romantic vicissitudes. On equal terms they discussed love and marriage, parental authority, religion, education, and local gossip for which Jim developed an aversion. Jim was more earnest than his sister, perhaps from an early awareness that family responsibilities would fall on his shoulders. He could be impatient and sometimes prim: for one of her more intractable difficulties he responded with 'soothing words' and 'useful advice' to apply for 'help from above'. With thanks she replied with a subtle allusion to the four years difference in their age: 'I have got many an answer to prayer already that I know of and I expect to get many more yet'. Helen was inclined to chide, for instance in the use of language, but her disposition was more playful than her brother's and she was endearingly candid about her own shortcomings: 'I fear I must confess that I am very indolent indeed when I can be so. There's not one thing that I know of that I would like – except study and I doubt I am too lazy for that even.' That was consoling for Jim who suspected the same of himself. Many years later, when Wilson was asked his opinion on extra-sensory perception, he replied: 'I don't know about that, but I do know that you can be so close to someone that you know what the other is thinking. It was like that between Helen and me'.[23]

As adulthood dawned, so did separation for Jim and Helen, a development more keenly apprehended by the elder of the two. She could bear anything she once wrote 'Only and this "only" always comes up I want to keep you and some way "cant" or as you would say *don't* trust God for that'. She kept his letters – the earliest ones as much from amusement as sentiment – and teased him with 'I think I shall bequeath them to my nephews and nieces!!!? Shall I?' She did.[24]

Helen decided to become a teacher. Following the usual custom she started as a pupil teacher in her father's school, three to six hours a week for two years, receiving about fifteen pounds in the first year, eighteen pounds fifteen shillings in the second, and finally her Pupil Teacher's Certificate. In January 1877 she entered the recently established Free Church Training College at Aberdeen, then open only to women. It was not a residential college. She found lodgings at 53 Huntly Street in that old congested city of grey granite and fickle climate. Aberdeen then had an exceptionally high incidence of pulmonary tuberculosis. She encountered a heavy programme of studies with daily lectures, daily practice teaching and homework most evenings. Little joy, much anxiety and indifferent health was the common student experience. By late October 1877 she was in the midst of 'multitudinous exams' and on the 27th Jim wrote her a note of encouragement: '"A'm glad a'm no' you." But fight them out and come home victorious'. Victorious she was. In December 1878 she graduated with a First Class Certificate, taking 13th place in a class of 36.[25]

In October 1877 Jamie sent Helen the good news of his own success:

> I have passed in five subjects. So I am delighted but of course I have
> still certain extra subjects that I must pass in, & which I will study
> this winter viz Greek and the Higher Mathematics. So I'll be 'right'
> busy this winter still besides a dip into Botany and Anatomy. If I
> get on well I think I'll begin German.[26]

The clever son of the Free Church dominie had embarked, under
the tuition of his father and Dr Grierson, on the long road of
medicine and had passed the first stage for the Edinburgh University
Entrance. Medicine had the advantage of delivering the professional
equipment for a living as well as a sound training in science. Dr
Grierson was such a model. Wilson's favourite subject was natural
history, an interest that led many another young naturalist into
medicine, given the ability and the means. Charles Darwin began a
medical course at Edinburgh University in the 1820s but he was so
outraged by the state of hospitals and the crudity of surgery that he
abandoned it. Nor could he tolerate anatomy as it was taught then
by Professor Monro tertius. Things had improved somewhat by the
1870s.

Science in Scotland had yet to achieve high university recognition
but it did have wide popular appeal, especially among the self-
educated. That appeal was not tainted by unbelief, though
contemporary religious scepticism built its house on the same natural-
history foundation. It was common for clergymen to be geologists.
Unlike England and America, Scottish religious opinion was not
unduly disturbed by theories of evolution. The Free Church
numbered among its congregations many who were self-educated and
self-reliant, and who for their faith had stood up against comfortable
establishment opinion. They well knew the hazards of adversity, so the
idea of 'the survival of the fittest' declared a truth which their own
experience affirmed. The Reverend R S Candlish of St George's Free
Church in Edinburgh may have feared Darwinian theory but argued
that it did not threaten 'any very terrible results to the theologians'.
On the other hand Hugh Miller, the most prominent Free Church
publicist and a geologist of standing, did foresee a threat to religion if
'the clergy as a class suffer themselves to linger far in the rear of an
intelligent and accomplished laity ... Let them not shut their eyes to
the danger which is obviously coming. The battle of the Evidences
will have as certainly to be fought on the field of physical science, as it

[handwritten margin note: Free Church not disturbed by Darwin, comfortable with science.]

13

was contested in the last age on that of metaphysics.'[27]

Earlier work of Scottish geologists had prepared the way for Charles Darwin's definitive exposition of the theory of evolution by natural selection, in the *Origin of Species*, published in 1859. Another Scot, Robert Chambers, a self-taught publisher and writer, had retired for three years from public life to write *Vestiges of the Natural History of Creation*, published in 1844. Charles Darwin read it carefully and was not impressed, but it had so great an appeal to the man in the street as to constitute 'a landmark in the popular thought of the nineteenth century and especially in the land of its author'.[28]

Debate about creation and the natural order were common when Jim Wilson's parents grew to maturity, so it is not surprising that both of them developed an interest in science as naturally as they accepted the tenets of their Calvinist religious faith. They were happy and proud of their son for his scholastic achievement and choice of profession. They could not afford to put him through university, but that difficulty was surmounted by a loan from Mrs Wilson's better circumstanced sisters in Dumfries and from a local man, Mr Barber of Tererran, a substantial landowner in Glencairn and an elder of the Free Church.[29]

On 23 October 1878 Jim wrote again to Helen, now nearing the end of her course in Aberdeen, to tell her that he had passed 'all the prelim. subs. necessary for the degree of MB. and CM. & I only require Greek for MD.' Greek he was never to get. On that subject his father was ever to be his master. But that was a very small cloud in a wide blue sky. At that moment he was exhilarated: 'Rejoice with me', he wrote, 'for I feel now free'.[30]

Notes

1. Quoted in *D&GS&A*, 11.1.1888.
2. Family background: Late in life JTW drew up family trees for the Wilsons and the Browns, later expanded by his granddaughter Mary Hutchinson. Further genealogical work was done by Rosemary Bigwood (RBP) on public records in Scotland: *Census 1851, 1861*; Official Public Records of Glencairn, Dumfries, Troqueer; and records of the Free Church. On Thomas Wilson and Helen Brown: *ibid.*, and information from DC and KR. Scottish Border: Muir, Ch. II; Ferguson, 279; Binding, 45.
3. Village of Moniaive: Monteith, 62.
4. History of Moniaive: Prebble, 267; Fyffe, 6; Charlotte Deans, quoted in Corrie, 'the gentle youth': Barber.

5. Formation of Free Church: McLaren, Ch. 8; Drummond and
   Bulloch, 'most honourable feat': quoted Prebble, 325.
6. 'A kind of omnipresence': Fyffe, 13.
7. Thomas Wilson, Schoolmaster: Records of Free Church of
   Glencairn, entries for 14.1.1856, 3.3.1856, 2.3.1857, 6.4.1857,
   14.2.1865, and November 1865. RBP.
8. See Note 2. Letters: HBW to HW, 18.9.1867 and 21.11.1867;
   'wrastlin' Jamie': DW to author, 15.11.1980.
9. Helen's visit to Edin. with her father: letters HBW to HW, 22.5.1869
   and 28.5.1869, JTW to HBW, 25.5.1869.
10. Dr Grierson of Thornhill: Waugh, Ch. 11; *D&GS&A* obit., 28.9.1889.
11. 'law of higgledy-piggledy': E B Wilson, quoted in Mayr, 518.
12. 'her appreciation of the works of nature': *D&GS&A* of 11.1.1888.
    'Dr Grierson came over': HBW to JTW, 21.3.81.
13. 'reasonable and unreasonable': HBW to JTW, 21.11.1881.
14. Thomas Wilson's appointment: Records, Free Church of Glencairn,
    14.1.1856; Scotland, 194 and part 3; BPP *Annual Report*; Barber
    1893, 23. Background to school teaching: James Scotland;
    Committee of the Privy Council on Education in Scotland (*HMSO
    1876/7*); Board of Education for Scotland (*British Parl. Papers* GD
    342/7845); HM Inspector's Report for Glencairn Free Church
    School (*BPP, H of C, 1854 Vol 52*); David Fyffe; William Barber.
15. walking to 'number the people' and 'alone all the way': HBW to
    JTW, 21.3.1881. 'I absolutely and entirely' and 'her mother wrote to
    me': HBW to JTW, 18.10.1881.
16. 'Pa has been quite miserable', 'Papa is in grief' and 'Papa is busy':
    HBW to JTW, 21.11.1881. 'Papa got quite angry': HBW to JTW,
    4.10.81.
17. Free Ch School Moniaive: BPP, HM Insp Reports, 1004. School
    year: Vol. 1 Scotland, 24, 203, 214; *HMSO Minutes and Reports*,
    143; 'the beauty of patience' and 'whiteness of truth': Brownridge,
    D&GS&A, 11.1.1888. Daily routine: Scotland, 200; Records, Free
    Church of Glencairn, 12.10.1863.
18. 'the master's restraint': Brownridge, *D&GS&A*, 1.1.1888. 'bulked
    fully as much': Corrie, *D&GS&A*, 11.1.1888. 'the highest tension'
    and 'intellectual part': Horace Mann, quoted Vol. 1 Scotland, 201–3.
    'for the manner in which': Brownridge, *D&GS&A*, 11.1.1888. 'he
    was one': JTW to LH, 12.3.1930.
19. Education administration: Drummond and Bulloch, Ch. 4.
    Government aid, loss of Church powers: *ibid.*, 93–9. Decline in Free
    Church Schools: *ibid.*, 100; Vol. 2 Scotland, 43.
20. 'after some discussion': Records, Free Church of Glencairn, Nov.

1874. RBP. Drummond and Bulloch, 100. Sunday School: Fyffe, 15.

21. Wilson Sabbath: J, *Notes for Biog Sketch of JTW.*

22. 'I sat and enjoyed': HBW to JTW, 18.10.1881. Later observance by JTW: Notes, LH and KR.

23. HBW to JTW, 18.10.1881, 31.10.1881. 'I don't know about': KR notes.

24. 'Only and this "only" always' and 'I think I shall': HBW to JTW, 18.10.1881.

25. Helen's teaching training in Aberdeen: Scotland Vol. 1, 105 and Vol. 2, Ch. 7. Helen's lodgings: letter HW to JTW 8.10.77. 'Multitudinous exams' and '"A'm glad a'm no you"': JTW to HBW, 27.10.1877. Helen's results: James Scotland, via Callum Smith-Burnett, Principal Librarian to author, 18.2.1981.

26. 'I have passed': JTW to HBW, 27.10.1877.

27. Scottish view of Darwin's theory: Drummond and Bulloch, Ch. 8. 'any very terrible results' and 'The clergy as a class': quoted *ibid.*, 231, 232.

28. Earlier Scottish geologists: James Hutton in the eighteenth century, and Sir Roderick Murchison and Sir Charles Lyell in the nineteenth. 'a landmark in the popular thought': Drummond and Bulloch, 225, 226.

29. Financial help for JTW: DC Notes.

30. 'all the prelim. subs', and 'Rejoice with me': JTW to HBW, 23.10.1878.

2

Edinburgh

The following spring, on Wednesday 30 April 1879, Jim Wilson arrived in Edinburgh to begin his medical studies. Just 18 years old, tall, spare and plainly clad, he was a fair-haired country boy whose most remarkable feature was a pair of sharp blue eyes. Dutifully his first concern was to send a postcard home: 'Arrd all right, will write at length soon',[1] which he chose to address from 'Dunedin', Edinburgh's Gaelic name.

Dunedin is gaelic

As a capital Edinburgh was of some consequence. Though never of great commercial importance she rivalled London as a cultural and intellectual centre. Ancient links with Holland and France, and more recently Germany, gave Edinburgh a European outlook, and her philosophers and medical school brought her to intellectual prominence long before London won prestige in these fields. Indeed from the Scottish point of view the English intellectual tradition was provincial, empirical in spirit and aristocratic in character. Scottish tradition combined a metaphysical outlook of an anti-empirical sort with a democratic system. 'Broad and shallow' it was called, as against 'narrow and deep' for the English. Unfairly, by the test of civil service examinations introduced in the 1870s, Scottish education became stigmatized as inferior. Whether Scottish medical education was inferior depends on one's view of medicine as primarily a craft or primarily a science. English medical education evolved out of medical practice in hospitals, whereas Scotland from the beginning housed medicine as a legitimate academic calling in its universities and gave honour and encouragement to research in the medical sciences.[2]

The University was much more a part of Edinburgh's civic life than Oxford and Cambridge. Affectionately known as 'The Old

17

Quad', the University began as 'The Tounis' College' and for 300 years, until it became independent in 1858, was financed and administered by the Town Council. Students surged in and out of its archways on the signal of an hourly bell, a familiar sound in the streets of the city. The Student Union met in rooms over Maclachlan and Stewart's bookshop opposite the University. There were no residential colleges and students like Wilson who came from the country lived in digs scattered throughout Edinburgh. Wilson found lodgings on the top floor of 13 Claremont Place, Edinburgh 6, now at the western end of Henderson Row, not far from the water of Leith where it passes the Royal Botanic Garden: a pleasant spot, with the green grounds of the Edinburgh Academy opposite, and a distant view of the Forth with the Fife coast beyond. Convenient too: a little over a mile's walk through the orderly streets of the new town to the Old Quad on the other side of High Street. His landlady Mrs Jane Maxwell, was a widow who came from Middlebie, Dumfriesshire. She was probably also a member of the Free Church. One of her daughters taught music, so it was here perhaps that he learned to play the flute.[3]

Wilson began his university studies on 1 May 1879, 'a proud and happy youth' he recalled 50 years later. 'It is comic to remember the feelings of awe with which I looked up to persons of my present standing. But I am bound to say that a professor in Edinburgh in those days was much more of a somebody than his present nominal compeers. "There were giants in those days".'[4] Mellowing time may have increased their stature in Wilson's mind but a review of Edinburgh's professors of the time suggests that indeed there were giants then.

In the chair of rhetoric and English literature was David Masson, friend of Dickens, Carlyle and Thackeray, a Milton scholar and literary critic, also prominent in the cause for higher education for women. In classics William Sellar built a high standard in Latin and in mathematics George Chrystal strengthened the University's research reputation. In the divinity chair was Dumfriesshire-born Robert Flint, who taught theology in the manner of a philosopher. Flint and three others were staunch defenders of Scotland's intellectual heritage: John Stuart Blackie in the Greek chair whom Gladstone called 'the most outstanding living Scotsman'; Alexander Campbell Fraser the professor of metaphysics and author of an important work on Berkeley; and Professor Henry Calderwood who taught moral philosophy.[5]

In science, the chair of natural philosophy was occupied by the

18

burly figure of P. G. Tait, mathematician and experimental physicist who, with Lord Kelvin, was joint author of the famous textbook, *Treatise on Natural Philosophy*. Alexander Crum Brown in the chair of chemistry 'had an important influence on chemical speculation'. Archibald Geikie, the first occupant of the geology chair was, in 1879, only 43 years old but already had international standing as a scientist. Sir Charles Wyville Thomson, professor of natural history, was a major contributor to oceanography as the leading scientist on the *Challenger* Expedition of 1872–6. During Thomson's absence on the *Challenger* one of his locums was T H Huxley, Darwin's bulldog. But the giant that most impressed Wilson was William Turner, anatomy professor and Dean of Medicine, later to become Principal of the University, the first Englishman to be so honoured. To him Wilson years afterwards paid this tribute:

> A native of Lancaster, a graduate of London and student at Bart's, he came to Edinburgh as assistant to Professor Goodsir, whom he succeeded. Notwithstanding his English antecedents, he eventually became even more Scottish in academic sentiment than the Scots themselves. The numerically large Medical School necessarily involved a large Anatomy Department with a relatively large staff of graduate demonstrators. Partly owing to this and largely also to the inspiration of the Chief, the Anatomy School of Edinburgh became the nursery of teachers of Anatomy for the whole British Empire.[6]

The most impressive feature of the University's history in the last half of the nineteenth century was the resurgence of the Medical School. From the doldrums in the 1820s it had risen through the influence of such men as Robert Christison, Britain's leading toxicologist, James Young Simpson who introduced chloroform as an anaesthetic, the surgeon James Syme, and his son-in-law Joseph Lister who revolutionized surgical practice with antisepsis. John Hughes Bennett developed a comprehensive course in physiology and pioneered the use of the microscope as a teaching instrument. The teaching of anatomy in the broad framework of comparative anatomy was restored to its classic eminence by the genius of John Goodsir (who also, in the 1840s, took Edinburgh to the forefront of biological research with his work on the cell) and his successor William Turner.[7]

If the commanding figure of William Turner impinged on Wilson's thoughts at all in the first session it was from a considerable distance, for he was but one of 376 new medical students. However he had an early opportunity to observe the leaders of the medical

19

faculty in full academic regalia. At four o'clock on 5 May the newly appointed professor of botany, Alexander Dickson gave his inaugural lecture in the chemical classroom. He was accompanied to the reading desk by the Principal, Sir Alexander Grant, Bart., who was preceded by the mace bearer, by Professors Maclagan, T R Fraser, Crum Brown, Turner, Grainger Stewart, and by Sir Wyville Thomson, and Sir Robert Christison, Bart., and a number of other gentlemen. But this heavy academic convoy did not overawe the student audience. 'So soon as Dr Dickson began his address, a number of the students present entered upon a series of interruptions, which, with here and there a brief interval of quiet, was kept up throughout the whole course of the proceedings', reported *The Scotsman* next day. It was an occasion 'evidently viewed... as an exceptionally favourable one for getting rid of exuberance of animal spirits'. Scottish students were an unruly breed, for they had no collegiate traditions as in Oxford and Cambridge and little civilizing personal contact with their teachers, who seemed more like their natural enemies.[8]

[margin note:] rowdy students

[margin note:] little contact with teachers

The first session covered Wilson's favourite subjects, botany and natural history. Professor Dickson, though trained for medicine, was fully engrossed in botany, and paid little heed to the purely professional departments of the medical curriculum. 'The medical man', he said in 1881, 'while he performs his duties to his suffering fellow creatures, ought never to forget at the same time what he owes to medical science and to posterity'. Professor Sir Wyville Thomson similarly had abandoned his medical training at the bidding of a stronger interest in natural science and had made his mark in botany, geology and natural history before his appointment in 1870 to the natural history chair at Edinburgh. He was occupied with writing up the work of the *Challenger* oceanographic expedition, a task which overtaxed his strength. In the summer of 1879 he was struck down by illness and died in 1882, aged 52. Wilson's class of 1879 was the last he taught. In his examinations Wilson achieved creditable results with first class honours and the bronze medal in botany and second class honours in natural history.[9]

On Saturdays, field excursions in botany took the students to remote districts. Scientifically these expeditions were more sophisticated than Dr Grierson's but like them they were also recreation. With no residential colleges to confer *esprit de corps,* traditions fostered by such excursions, along with university ceremonies and student societies, assumed great importance. Competitive team sports were becoming established in the University by Wilson's time but volunteering was more popular than the sporting clubs. The University Company of Volunteers for Home Defence was formed by a medical professor, Robert Christison, in 1859 when France was in a belligerent mood. The medical school was prominently represented by both staff and students, among them Wilson and his future senior colleague in Sydney, T P Anderson Stuart. Professor Turner, an enthusiast from the beginning, had succeeded Christison as captain in 1876, and Dr John Duncan, Wilson's future chief in surgery was an original member also. The Company could frequently be seen on Saturday afternoons drilling in the Old Quad or skirmishing over Arthur's Seat.[10]

It was still possible in Edinburgh to be simply a student, making no other commitment to university life. The 'meal sack man' like Carlyle who arrived with his food on his back, 'spurned delights and lived laborious days' till it was time to walk home again or find work to pay for the next session's fees, was still around. Wilson lived frugally – he was sometimes hungry – but better-off than the 'meal sack man', and trained to an interest in community affairs. He joined the Dumfries and Galloway Literary Association 'the smallest society in the University and the longest winded' according to J M Barrie whom Wilson as treasurer once dunned for his membership subscription. It debated questions like 'Is the policy of the Government worthy of the confidence of this Society?' and 'Beauty of Mind versus Beauty of Body', and they read about six essays a year on 'The Genius of Robert Burns'. It was in this chauvinist fraternity that Wilson met Jim Smith, or James Lorrain Smith to give him his full name, then an Arts student reading philosophy, who became an intimate friend and in the fullness of time his brother-in-law.[11]

Lorrain Smith

Another social bond was the kirk. The cleft in the Church of Scotland exhibited itself every Sunday. The clang of church bells across the streets of Edinburgh called the faithful, each to his own, a little before or a little later than the rival. The singing of hymns could be heard from both, but brethren they were not, and annually the two ecclesiastical assemblies celebrated their differences. Wilson usually attended Free St George's in Maitland Street where the Gladstonian Dr Alexander Whyte, 'always ready to go on fire', could be relied on to preach a vigorous sermon, and Wilson became an active member of that church's Literary Association. Occasionally he attended the Free High at the Head of the Mound, to hear Dr Walter Smith who couched his sacred fire in shrewd, more homely accents. Membership of the Free Church was another thing Wilson had in common with Jim Smith, whose father, another Walter Smith, was the Free Church minister in the border parish of Half Morton, Dumfriesshire.[12]

After the three month vacation, the long winter session began in the last week of October 1879. Wilson settled down to the study of chemistry and anatomy. Wilson had no great enthusiasm for chemistry, though he registered a sound pass at the level of second class honours. With the three basic sciences of botany, natural history and chemistry under his belt he passed the 'first professional' stage of the course, and custom conferred on him the privilege of wearing a high-crowned silk hat though it is unlikely he did so. Now he moved to the periphery of William Turner's personal orbit. The academically heavy 'second professional' stage encompassed four subjects: anatomy, physiology, materia medica and pathology.

Turner was Britain's leading anatomist, a man of great strength, enthusiasm and authority. In 1880 he was 48 years old and had been in the chair for 13 years, after 13 years as senior demonstrator to John Goodsir. Turner had a ready aptitude for Goodsir's teaching and research ideals and quickly became a comparative anatomist like all Scottish anatomists. But on Darwin's theory of evolution the two men differed: Goodsir's Calvinist backbone stiffened against it, while Turner embraced it. In the 1860s Turner had advised Darwin on rudimentary structures and variations in man and the higher mammals, questions which he developed as research interests, along with nerve histology (microscopical structure of nerve fibres), the placentation of mammals, the comparative anatomy of sea mammals, human craniology and the anatomy of the brain. His industry was extraordinary. Over 60 years he published four or five papers annually.[13]

Turner's anatomy, in keeping with Scottish traditions, was based on morphology (comparative anatomy), an autonomous science containing 'the very soul' of natural history in the opinion of Charles Darwin who revolutionized it with his theory of descent from a common ancestor. Prior to Darwin, morphologists like the celebrated Richard Owen of the British Museum had been occupied with classifying organisms into theoretical 'morphological types' or 'archetypes'. After Darwin, morphologists busied themselves in the search for anatomical evidence of evolution from common ancestry in all phyla of the animal kingdom, including man. Turner's introductory lecture dramatized this theory, sketching the evolution of organic life from its simplest forms through the development of the vertebral column with its changes in shape and curves, the formation of limbs and so on, concluding with the resounding

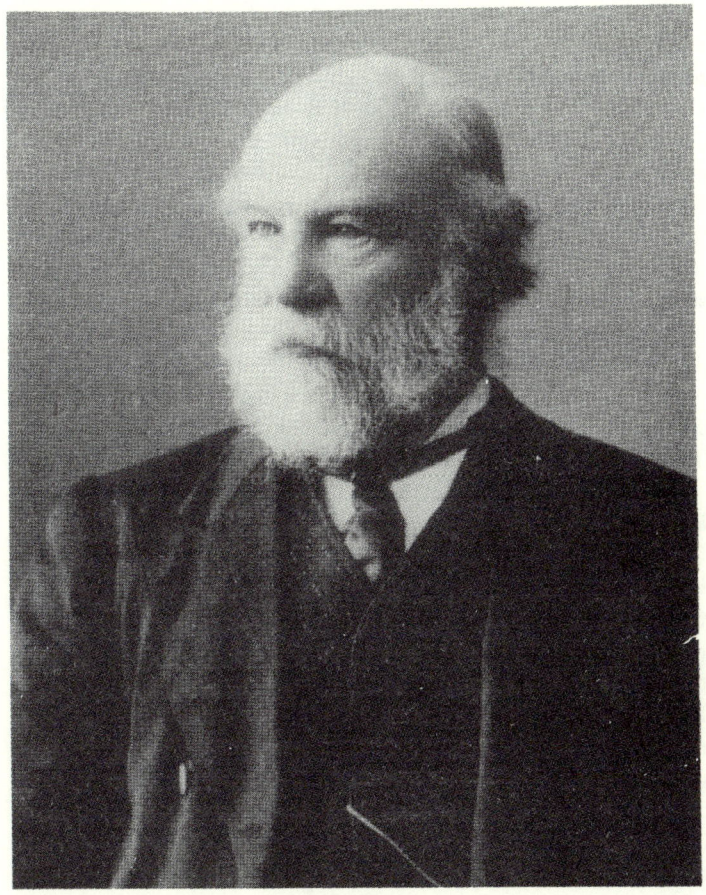

Sir William Turner (Courtesy Edinburgh University Medical Archives)

words: 'Man alone stands and walks erect.' This was the broad, captivating context. The hallmark of Turner's teaching was his emphasis, as a matter of principle, on accurate detail. 'Depend on it', he argued, against those who contended that the minutiae of topographical anatomy was wasted labour for medical students,

> whether you learn or do not learn, in the minute details of the more important subjects of study lies the difference between slipshod information and the kind of knowledge, the possession of which makes a man feel that he is treading on firm ground and not on shifting sand.[14]

The lecture, which has the advantage of being cheap, was the traditional Scottish teaching method. Given the huge student numbers enrolled at the Edinburgh medical school there was no alternative. But to redress the sense of inequality instilled by the authority of the lecturer on the rostrum, there was for anatomy students in the winter sessions the informality of the dissecting rooms – for hygienic reasons dissection was reserved for the winter session – where a team of graduate demonstrators assisted Turner in more personal teaching. Turner's vigour and enthusiasm fired his students. He held a series of practical examinations which became very popular. Classes of about 200 were divided into teams of 15 to 20 and each student was examined orally on a given specimen, scoring points for or against his team, a system which led to intense competition by the end of the session and made heavy demands on Turner. But he was built like a bull and seemed to thrive on it.[15]

Turner was a prominent figure in medical politics. A Fellow of both Royal Societies (London and Edinburgh), also both Royal Colleges of Surgeons from 1873 till 1905, a representative of Edinburgh and Aberdeen Universities on the General Medical Council, he was appointed in 1881 to a Royal Commission on medical training. Seeking to establish one examining authority for the whole of the British Isles or, failing that, Divisional Boards in England, Scotland and Ireland, the Commission in 1882 recommended a system of standardized examinations independent of all teaching authorities. But Turner effectively scotched this proposal with a minority report arguing that local licensing powers be preserved and that teachers be also examiners. The Medical Act of 1886 embodied Turner's argument. He thus preserved the principle of variety in medical education and protected the autonomy of the Scottish system.[16]

In the winter session of 1879–80, while working for an exam, Wilson met a fellow medical student who was to play a significant part in his life. John Scott Haldane, already an arts graduate and just a year older than Wilson, belonged to an old and respected land-owning family to whose reputation this branch, the Haldanes of Cloan, contributed some lustre in the fields of politics, philosophy and science. Wilson and Haldane were Lowlanders with a developed interest in natural science and evangelical Christianity. Haldane's parents were Baptists, but after his father's death in 1877 John was influenced by his elder brother Richard who in his mid-teens had experienced a religious crisis, resolved by several months of study of philosophy and theology at Göttingen. Moving away from all

24

established religious creeds, Richard's lifelong passion became philosophy, to which he made a notable contribution, though he became better known for his distinguished career in law and politics.[17]

Wilson's friendship with John Haldane grew through an interest in philosophy. They and Jim Smith became associated with a group of young philosophers led by Richard Haldane and his friends James and Andrew Seth, Robert Barbour and W R Sorley. A religious temperament, a receptiveness to German thought, a distaste for both materialism and the dogma of institutionalized religion took them into the Idealist school of philosophy led by T H Green of Oxford and Edward Caird of Glasgow. This philosophy combined an anti-ecclesiastical pantheism with a commitment to social reform in the spirit of the 'new liberalism', then a growing political force opposed to the economic values of traditional Liberal politics.[18]

Scottish idealists perceived the inability of either a materialist political philosophy upholding *laissez-faire* or a divided church squabbling about dogma to deal with the enormous social problems of the rapidly industrializing Lowlands. They saw themselves as social, political, and philosophical radicals, addressing the essential problems of human need amid dehumanizing social conditions. The State, they argued, should promote the conditions for individuals to achieve their full potential while the individual should strive for self-realization and the development of the human personality as a whole. And it asserted the dominion of the spiritual over the material: 'the more experience is spiritual the more it is real'.[19]

Materialism in science was a matter of great concern among biologists. Darwinian theory had found a relatively easy acceptance in Scotland, though its mechanistic implications bothered some. More controversial were the strident mechanistic doctrines of the '1847 Group' of physiologists in Germany – Hermann Helmholtz, Emil du Bois-Reymond, Ernst Brücke and Carl Ludwig – who held that all aspects of living phenomena could be reduced, by laboratory analysis, to the laws of physics and chemistry. Brilliant research by these men seemed to establish the validity of this claim and it was taken up with great enthusiasm by young physiologists and by none more keenly than William Rutherford under whom Wilson and John Haldane began the study of physiology in 1880.[20]

Professor Rutherford had behind him impressive research experience under du Bois-Reymond in Berlin and Carl Ludwig in Leipzig. Also, as one of T H Huxley's lieutenants at the Royal College of Mines, South Kensington in the early 1870s he had taught the revolutionary elementary biology course which, by associating cell theory with evolution and stressing laboratory techniques, dissection and microscopy, stimulated the development of histology (microscopical anatomy) teaching in British universities where it was absorbed by physiology departments as part of the 'new' or 'experimental' physiology. Rutherford returned to Edinburgh in 1874 to teach it there to large classes of 400 to 500 students. Despite a penchant for 'playful sarcasm' he was a popular lecturer and many students attended his classes for two years in a row. Haldane however was antagonized by Rutherford's mechanistic opinions and a few years later, but still aged only 23, in a dissertation 'Body and Soul', read before the (undergraduate) Royal Medical Society of Edinburgh on 9 March 1883, publicly challenged them.

> Professor Rutherford, in his lectures on Physiology, says that sensation, ideation and, other psychical phenomena, are produced in the brain by nerve cells or groups of nerve cells. It is not creditable to science that it should be necessary to point out the contradiction, evident though it be, which is involved in all such statements as this.

Haldane did not say why this statement was not creditable to science, or if he did it was not reported. But he was in good company. The distinguished physicist Professor P G Tait spoke for many Scottish scientists in deeming the application of materialist principles to physiology 'pernicious nonsense'.[21]

In another essay 'The Relation of Philosophy to Science' in collaboration with his brother Richard published later the same year, John Haldane sought to demonstrate 'that the phenomena of life were unintelligible unless there entered into the constitution of biological experience relations of a highly different order from those of mechanism'. Mechanism he argued dealt with cause and effect which had only limited application to physiology, for physiology was more concerned with the concept of reciprocity between the parts of an organism (and between an organism and its surroundings) in a coordinated system, dominated by the determining influence of the whole on the parts. The activity of a living organism is directed by the *purpose* of self-maintenance or self-preservation. Machines could only be repaired, changed or improved by outside agency whereas living systems were invested with the power of self-repair – a newt could regenerate a severed limb – the power of adaptation as demonstrated by hypertrophy

[margin note: Haldane: teleology not mechanistic]

26

(growth through enlargement of cells) and by the power of development. In these innate capacities of living things Haldane postulated no mysterious force; the vitalist argument was as radically unsound as the mechanists' he believed, introducing as it did the supernatural into the operation of natural processes. Such capacities were simply 'a more concrete and comprehensive view of the forces with which physiology familiarly deals', and in which teleology (ultimate purpose), not mechanism, was the distinguishing feature. That, he believed, was the only intelligible concept of biology.[22]

There is no record of Wilson's view of this question at that time, but as he progressed through the physiology course and read more of T H Green's Idealist teachings which inspired Haldane's anti-mechanist stance he made himself familiar with the arguments. Wilson was not given to hasty opinions; his instincts were wary. No doubt the Haldanes were impressive and persuasive but he maintained his independence. He did not for example abandon religious practice like the Haldanes. Throughout his life he was strict in church observance despite his rejection of the dogma of orthodox theology, including the divinity of Christ and everything else which contradicts the natural order. To avoid misrepresentation he did not advertise his religious views but on grounds of conscience several times in later years he declined nomination for election as a church elder. He took communion 'as a toast to the Almighty', and he followed as a disciple Jesus Christ the man.[23]

Mechanism was everywhere in the ascendant. Materia medica, the third subject of the second professional stage, was taught by Professor T R Fraser who made pioneering contributions to the connection between chemical constitution and physiological action. And pathology, the fourth subject, was dramatically expanded by new experimental methods when two new brooms swept into the pathology department in 1881: the Londoner W S Greenfield in the chair, and his young Scottish assistant German Sims Woodhead who conducted a new course in practical morbid histology. An inspiring teacher, Woodhead's main research was on tuberculosis. The fact that Wilson's family had a history of tuberculosis – his uncle Robert Wilson died of it in March of that year – may explain why Wilson had a particular interest in this subject, though pathology was in any case gathering more interest. The discoveries of Louis Pasteur and Robert Koch establishing the germ theory of disease were bringing into being the new science of bacteriology under the wing of pathology. Sims Woodhead was impressed by Wilson's natural ability and industry, and the extent of his knowledge in pathological histology; Greenfield recruited him as a clinical clerk and as an assistant demonstrator, noticing in particular Wilson's 'zeal and thoroughness in his work ... great kindliness of disposition and courtesy of manner'.[24]

In the late 1870s and early 1880s medicine in Edinburgh was visibly on the move. In October 1879 the new Royal Infirmary was completed and 'the great flitting' from the dank old septic buildings in Infirmary Street to the new 'many-windowed shining sort of pavilion' in Lauriston Place was completed. By this time also the new medical school in Teviot Place, across the Middle Meadow Walk from the new Infirmary, was nearing completion. The traditional proximity of school and hospital was thus preserved. Turner, assisted by his senior demonstrator, D J Cunningham, superintended the transfer of the Anatomy Department to the new premises which he proudly opened in the winter session of 1880–1 as accommodation unsurpassed in the British Empire. Nevertheless a 50 per cent increase in student numbers since 1874 when the buildings were designed meant the new accommodation required all sorts of adjustments. Turner emphasized the cosmopolitan character of the student body, especially the high proportion of Colonials, including many Australians. One of these, Theo Barker from New South Wales, was Wilson's particular friend.[25]

Assisting Professor Rutherford in the removal of the Physiology Department to the new building was his recently appointed assistant, Thomas Peter Anderson Stuart, who in two years time would be busy with the foundation of a new medical school in Sydney, New South Wales. In 1880 Anderson Stuart had crowned a brilliant medical course with the Ettles Scholarship, awarded annually to the best medical student in the final year. To his fellow students he was 'the greatest man ever known at passing examinations', taking no fewer than ten medals during his course. He then qualified for the MRCS in London, and sat the first examination for the FRCS in which he scored the highest marks ever won up to that time. His appointment in October 1882 as professor of anatomy and physiology in Sydney prevented his completing the FRCS.[26]

But he was not a popular student. Tall, gauche, and unfavoured in looks – nicknamed 'coracoid' on account of his large nose – his best assets were a first-class brain and a strong combative instinct. Born in Dumfries in 1856, he was the only child of a strong-willed mother who was the dominant influence in his early life. His father Alexander Stuart, a tailor, town councillor and magistrate was 'a very able man' wrote his son, 'who would have done better in life if he had attended to his own affairs instead of the affairs of the town'. He was less than encouraging to his son's ambitions but that proved more of a spur than a hindrance.[27]

Anderson Stuart's childhood was dour. His favourite reading was Chambers' *Encyclopaedia* and neither religion nor anything else sparked any spiritual inquiry. The family attended the Established Church of Scotland but he was not required to attend Sunday school, where he found the teachers 'inept', and the conduct of the scholars 'exceedingly bad'. The sermons he could not understand: 'Religion', he later asserted, 'is of the heart and not of the head'. In food for the heart Anderson Stuart was not well served. He was a solitary boy, haunted all his life by loneliness and fear of failure. In vacations Anderson Stuart seems usually to have holidayed alone, twice on the Continent, and when in his third year he suffered a nervous breakdown he took a change of scene, again alone, in a farm grieve's cottage in Braemar, doing his own provisioning and cooking, walking the long days away on the hillsides.[28]

The summer of 1881 was a happy one for the Wilsons. After an acute attack of tonsilitis in mid-July Jim recuperated in Moniaive in time to enjoy a visit by his American cousins, Harriet Jane Brown and her eldest brother, the Reverend Walter Scott Brown, a graduate of Princeton University. Jim and Walter set out on a tour of Wilson and Brown country, reconnoitring family history in Dumfriesshire and Galloway, including of course Ecclefechan, the birthplace of Thomas Carlyle in whom they had a proprietary interest, and a few days at Gatehouse-of-Fleet with the Glovers. The American Browns – particularly Harriet – took a hold on the affections of Helen and James and a lifelong friendship resulted, sustained mainly by letters. 'Dear Hattie' became a bright and familiar personality among her Scottish kin. It was probably this connection that prompted Wilson's notion a few years later of going to the United States. But he never did.[29]

On 13 September 1881, Wilson made his first visit to the home of his friend Jim Smith, at the Free Church Manse, Half Morton, Dumfriesshire. He stayed a week. The Reverend Walter Smith, minister of the parish for 25 years, had been a teacher until he was dismissed in 1843 for his adherence to the Free Church. Ordained at Half Morton in 1844, he returned as minister in 1856 after an eight-year term in Liverpool, having in 1847 married Margaret Lorrain Brown, of an old border family. They raised four sons and four daughters who all pursued intellectual and cultural interests: John became a medical missionary; Walter a Professor of Philosophy at

Lake Forest University, Illinois; Annie a mycologist at the British Museum and one of the first women to be a fellow of the Linnean Society of London and to receive an OBE for services to science; William the first head of the Department of Psychology in the University of Edinburgh; and Jim, Wilson's particular friend, was to have a distinguished academic career in medical science concluding with the chair of pathology in Edinburgh University. The youngest daughter, Jane Elizabeth, or Jeanie, close to her brother Jim in age and sympathy, became Wilson's wife in 1890. The black sheep was Joseph, who went a-roving and finally settled in Melbourne, Australia.[30]

In September 1881 Jeanie was 17, slim, attractive and golden-haired, and had that summer qualified for the Junior Certificate of the University of Edinburgh. She was preparing to study music in Leipzig. Of his week at Half Morton, Wilson recorded only four brief diary entries:[31]

13.9.81 Went to Half Morton for first time

15.9.81 Kirkconnell

16.9.81 Marsh House Canonbie

20.9.81 Left H.M.

His vacation ended on 3 October, leaving his mother and sister bereft in Moniaive, as Helen with forced wit reported that evening:

> I refrained from looking out of the school window at you as you went off for I felt sure that I should be quite upset if I did, and that would never have done, I was giving a geog. lesson & just went on looking very grim and scolding all the while as usual, ie. 'whistling to keep my courage up'. Poor Mamma felt it worse than ever before I think…. [Later] we brightened up a little and thereafter proceeded to finish packing your hamper by stuffing in your brush & padlock, which two important articles you had left behind.

And then an interruption to her letter:

> Rap! – rap!! – rap!!! What can it be? A letter from Jim. Oh delicious! My *ownest* brother. We are so glad to see it and that you are all right. What a pity that you put yourself so much about. That's the first of the 'good' letters again. You see if there is a loss there's always some gain. If you did not go, we should not get 'good' letters, nor should we have happy meetings if we had not sorrowful partings. 'Chords that vibrate sweetest pleasures, thrill the deepest notes of woe'.[32]

30

A trying winter was in store for Helen. There were two marriages in the district, one of them wounding. Hardest to bear was the anxiety that these events excited in her mother about Helen's marriage prospects. Illness beset the family too. Helen had barely recovered from a bout of neuralgia, sore teeth and a cold when her mother was confined to bed for a month with something similar. Helen shouldered the burdens of nursing and housekeeping as well as teaching. She wrote lengthy letters to Jim, often apologizing for her meagre progress in German or 'scribing', a task she undertook for him. Evidently her brother was now the senior partner, which must have seemed natural to Wilson who had always been the focus of family interest. She was desolate with weariness at the end of October but by late November both mother and daughter seemed restored in health and Helen's interests and ambitions revived:

> There's nothing like hard work for keeping one from grumbling and fretting ... I wish I could have been in Edinh when Moody and Sankey are there. and I also wish that I could have been when you are there, but as both are out of the question I must just be contented. You will see by that that I am not *quite* contented yet. I want to learn, and I want to read and I want to do a great deal more of work than is at all possible, so I have plenty of unsatisfied wishes after all – but on the whole I am wonderful *for me*. I don't think my face wd *sour* your milk just now.[33]

That excerpt is from Helen's last surviving letter. She died the following spring of 'congestion of the lungs', probably tuberculosis, just one month short of her twenty-fifth birthday. Her death was a devastating blow that Wilson recorded in his diary with stark brevity: '25/3/82 Nellie died'. The previous day in Berlin, Robert Koch had made his dramatic announcement to the Physiological Society that he had isolated the tubercle bacillus.[34]

Because of Helen's death, Wilson did not take all the examinations for the second professional at the same time. Materia Medica was deferred. Nevertheless, he had an anxious time of it in July 1882 when he sat the examinations for Anatomy, Physiology and Pathology. He reported to his parents on 25 July 1882,

> I do not yet quite realise that as far as exams are concerned I have done with Anatomy, Physiology & Pathology. I was awfully afraid of Physiol. in wh. I have already told you I found I had made several mistakes. Well in that subject curiously enough I made a 'B'

(80% or over) in both the written & oral. My paper had otherwise
been good. I was awfully afraid of my oral in Anatomy but got thro'
all right. Pathology written I must have made nearly full marks in I
think & the oral in it was almost a farce. So I am another stage on
for which I am very thankful indeed. But I would not like soon to
have another fortnight like the last and I intend to be home as soon
as I possibly can... I am wearying for the garden & the fields.

According to this account of his 'second professional' examinations
Wilson would seem to have distinguished himself most in pathology
and least in anatomy. During the autumn vacation he paid visits to
friends again, more than likely the Smiths at Half Morton.[35]

Wilson had by now entered his clinical years, a nomadic style of
learning as he attended outpatient clinics, observed in the operating
theatres, walked the wards of the new Royal Infirmary, attended
midwifery cases in their homes and dispensed in district clinics. He
was now more fully appreciating the medical life and had advanced
to more familiar relations with some of Edinburgh's medical bigwigs.
After the pathology oral examination he relaxed at Dr Byrom
Bramwell's for supper. Dr Bramwell was an extra-mural lecturer in
clinical medicine, whose outpatient clinics were a memorable part of
Edinburgh's medical training. For 30 years hardly a student failed to
attend them. Wilson made a distinct impression on Bramwell:
'[Wilson] is extremely clever, both with his hands and with his head,
and is, amongst other things, a most excellent microscopist.'[36]

The University's clinical teachers were generally well regarded.
Professor Grainger Stewart, a big flabby man, taught good plain
medicine, both in the classroom and at the bedside and conducted a
large private practice. Alexander Russell Simpson, nephew of James
Young Simpson, was an earnest, zealous and painstaking teacher of
midwifery, a skilful operator and a voluminous contributor to
medical journals. Medical jurisprudence was taught by the debonair
Douglas MacLagan, the complete old world physician, a former
President of both colleges and well-known as an adviser to the
Crown in many *causes celebres*. Professor Thomas Annandale who
taught clinical surgery was 'a capable, bold neat-handed surgeon' but
not scientific and not a good teacher. For clinical surgery Wilson
enrolled with John Duncan, an extra-mural teacher.[37]

The Royal Edinburgh Infirmary was quite independent of the
Medical School with regard to its staff appointments. It conferred
the right of clinical instruction on physicians and surgeons
(provided they were Fellows of one or the other Edinburgh

Colleges) regardless of whether they held the correlated university teaching positions. So there developed two distinct schools of clinical instruction: one officially part of the school and the other extra-mural. Competition between them was intense, for in those days students' fees went straight into the teachers' pockets. This rivalry gave students an awkward choice: the better teacher was sometimes extra-mural, but for good examination results it was better to stick with university teachers. Anderson Stuart chose the latter course and struck discord: his professor of clinical surgery was Joseph Lister whose great antiseptic message was caustically repudiated by James Spence the professor of systematic surgery, for whom Stuart dressed, who took great pride in his old grey operation coat stiff with coagulated blood and other discharges.[38]

[handwritten margin note: Lister vs Spence]

John Duncan was a disciple of Lister. An imposing grey-bearded gentleman who drove about in a yellow dog-cart drawn by a pair of high-stepping horses, he was recognized as an accomplished scientific teacher with an attractively subdued style in lecturing, like thinking aloud; he was also a cool operator whose favourite expression in trying circumstances was 'quite'. For Wilson he was 'one of the finest clinical teachers I have ever known' and Wilson was one of Duncan's best students. Having noticed Wilson from his early student days, Duncan recognized him as 'one who, by natural ability and patient industry, was certain to attain success in his professional career'. In the midst of exams on 19 January 1883, Wilson dashed off a brief note to his parents:

> I must tell you the result of J.D.'s class exam. I find I'm only *second* not first but I have 97 per cent so couldn't have been much better. One is 98. I'm 97 another 96 another 95 another 93. Close run isnt it? They are all seniors. I shall work hard to cut out the other man next time. Won't be easy either. I don't know who he is as we have all mottoes. He dont know me either.

He must have worked hard for he did cut out the other man and was awarded Duncan's prize 'with an unusually high percentage of marks'. For a time as an undergraduate Wilson was Duncan's class assistant, as well as clerk and dresser in the wards; he so distinguished himself in these duties that after graduation Duncan appointed Wilson as his Resident or House Surgeon at the Infirmary for the winter session 1883–4.[39]

The last six months of Wilson's course were heavy weather. In February 1883 he recorded in his diary that he was 'knocked up with bronchitis', an episode that lost him a month and in April he had the deferred examination in Materia Medica. It was 'a tussle to pull thro' but he passed with a comfortable margin. 'I must confess I feel no little pride this day' he wrote to his parents on 19 July, announcing his results. He graduated MB, CM, with second class honours on 1 August 1883. Apart from a bronze medal for botany in his first year and John Duncan's prize for clinical surgery, Wilson's academic performance was not remarkably distinguished. He did not have a precocious mind like Anderson Stuart; his needed time to mature.[40]

John Haldane however had failed the MB and was angry about it. On 30 July 1883 he wrote to Wilson: 'I dare say you may have heard that the Faculty simply ratified the decision of the examiners in my case. I sent them a long letter on the subject of their lecturing and examining and told them that I should not come up for their Examinations again so long as things are as they are'. So he cast around restlessly, looking for an alternative to subjecting himself again to the Edinburgh authorities. In 1885 he sat again for the MB. in Edinburgh, and passed. But he got his grievances off his chest by writing a criticism of the medical school, published in the form of anonymous letters to the editor of the *Scotsman* in 1885 and finally in 1890 as a pamphlet. Wilson supplied some of the material.[41]

While allowing that some departments were better than others and the teachers generally speaking 'kindly', 'of some philosophic attainment' and 'faithfully endeavouring to teach', Haldane maintained that the standard was bad, produced by a system 'utterly unworthy of a School with such traditions as ours'. The course was a heavy burden of miscellaneous knowledge unconnected to principles or theories, and giving no coherent understanding of the healing art. So it did not satisfy the scientifically inclined student, nor did it guide the future practitioner. No student, he concluded, except perhaps the professional prize-taker could enjoy this system. He recommended a closer alignment of theory to practice, honours awarded on the basis of theses, teaching loads reduced by incorporating the extra-mural teachers within the university system, a ban placed on private practice for teachers, and provision made for teachers to pursue scientific research so encouraging them 'to live the lives of men of science, and not of overpaid drill-sergeants'.[42]

Though expressed with the passion of idealistic youth, Haldane's criticisms were fair. Huge student numbers were adversely affecting the quality of the medical course. As teaching took first priority the research effort declined and that led to stereotyped courses. Student numbers levelled off in the nineties, mainly due to the rise of new universities in England, Ireland, the Empire and the United States. Meanwhile Germany had become the centre of scientific medicine and post-graduate students were flocking there. Edinburgh's pre-eminence was beginning to wane.[43]

Haldane was confronting a bigger problem than he knew, one which still confounds medical educators. Under the pressure of large student numbers and accelerating scientific and technological advances, it seemed less and less possible in the space of four or five years to turn out the 'safe' general practitioner, launch the specialist and the scientist equipped with appropriate skills, endowed with a liberal education and imbued with the spirit of inquiry. Haldane himself never had to come to grips with these problems, for he found his niche in physiological research. But for Wilson medical education was to become a lifelong preoccupation.

In July 1883 John Haldane and Jim Wilson were reading T H Green and considering their futures. In Half Morton Jim Smith and his family were in mourning. Mrs Smith had died in June. Jeanie cut short her musical studies in Leipzig, leaving at Easter 1883 with a 'Directorial Certificate' testifying that she had made 'very estimable progress'. The Reverend Walter Smith wrote to Mr Thomas Wilson at Moniaive in July thanking him for his letter of condolence:

> We are also under great obligations to your son for the interest he
> has taken in us and for his unprecedented kindness to Mrs Smith.
> There are others that have reason to remember his visits to Half
> Morton. I trust we shall have the pleasure of seeing him here again.

Wilson did visit Half Morton again that autumn, as well as Gatehouse-of-Fleet. By October he was back in Edinburgh, now at the Royal Infirmary as John Duncan's Resident House Surgeon; and Jeanie was back in Leipzig, not re-enrolled at the Conservatorium but assiduously attending concerts.[44]

In Moniaive, Wilson's parents were cherishing the hope of his becoming a general practitioner and before his final examinations had informed him of a possible position assisting a doctor in Buxton, to which he responded:

> I must say I felt gratified to know that anybody wanted me as
> assistant. I suppose I'll be good for something after all. But I must
> certainly stay with John Duncan this winter if all is well it will
> make me worth more both to myself & whoever employs me. I
> shouldn't mind going to Buxton after that of course if I got a decent
> 'screw'.

Between July and the winter with John Duncan he had hopes of a sea trip as ship's surgeon, for he concluded that letter of 19 July 1883 with, 'I believe that I shall *probably* get a ship about the end of Augt or beginning of Sept'. He was a year out. It wasn't until August 1884 that this opportunity presented itself.[45]

Wilson had six satisfying months at the Royal Infirmary as John Duncan's House Surgeon, in which capacity, said Duncan, 'he had large opportunity of studying disease, not only in the surgical cases under his own charge, but also in other wards of our Infirmary. As House Surgeon he discharged his duties thoroughly and well.' Wilson had an aptitude for surgery and Duncan recommended it to him as a career. He worked with another surgeon, P H MacLaren, 'a great man at strictures and stone and all sorts of things' who also thought well of him. As a student, wrote MacLaren, Wilson

> was always engaged in work over and above that enjoined in the curriculum ...[which included] scientific investigations both in Physiology and Pathology and has made himself an adept in demonstrating normal and morbid Histology.

MacLaren noted that Wilson, as Duncan's House Surgeon, had 'an excellent knowledge of the theory and practice of Surgery, that the wards under his charge were administered carefully [and] that his manner is gentle and full of tact'. Another surgeon, C Watson MacGillivray, observed 'the careful and able way' he did his work in John Duncan's wards and the 'various improvements' he introduced in 'the method of dressing'. Wilson had, said MacGillivray, 'high character and great abilities', 'wide professional knowledge, admirable tact, combined with pleasant and gentlemanly manners'.[46]

Experimental work with Duncan on 'aseptic atmosphere' occupied him a good deal. Duncan acknowledged that his 'thorough attention to detail and acquaintance with modern methods in the various departments of medical investigation have been of great use to me'. Haldane reported to him from Oxford in February that the work there in this area 'has been mostly chemical, as to antiseptic substances produced by putrefaction ... very difficult to investigate for various reasons'. German work, including Robert Koch's, was more useful. But Wilson's chances of studying in Germany were nil. By the end of April hospital life was bleak: 'I wish Duncan were back ... Nurse Turnbull has not been quite well and has gone for a holiday and that greatly adds to the desolate feeling about the wards just now'. He was stale. He did however enormously enjoy his time

36

as a resident, and valued ir ever after. Over 50 years later he reflected on it:

> ... I know of no more delightful & exhilarating experience than that of house surgeon or physician with all its human & professional interest – with just sufficient responsibility to make one feel that one matters and yet that that responsibility is shared & not all on ones own shoulders. I nearly wept in the cab that carried me away from the hospital at the end of my period of residence![47]

In their letters Jim and Thomas Wilson exchanged reports on similar interests. They both followed the fortunes of Gladstone and Home Rule for Ireland. The father reported on a paper he was writing on the theory of music, the son on chairing a meeting of 'The Society' which was drawing up a 'very good syllabus for next winter', opening with a lecture by Professor Masson. A highlight of social news was the celebration of the University's tercentenary in April 1884 which brought distinguished visitors in medicine, science, law, arts and literature from Britain, Europe, the United States and the Empire. Professor Turner hosted a medical luncheon for 450 guests in his new 'bright and airy theatres and laboratories... where the dissecting room shows like a conservatory and where morbid pathology is pursued as a fine art'. Turner in toasting the 'sister Medical Schools' emphasized again – he never lost an opportunity – the cosmopolitan character of the Edinburgh school, stamped on it by the genius of his predecessors, and he paid a special tribute to the University of Leyden as Edinburgh's 'nursing mother'. Wilson was kept busy as a steward at this gathering, and enjoyed seeing at close quarters 'most of those world renowned European swells ... I actually shook hands with Robert Browning & helped him on with his coat ... Then on Friday Haldane introduced me to his uncle Prof. Burdon-Sanderson of Oxford'.[48]

But 'the festivities got rather tiresome near the end'. He had decisions to make about his future. Was he to become a country doctor as his parents wished, a surgeon as John Duncan advocated, or pursue science as Haldane recommended? Under the wing of his distinguished uncle, John Burdon Sanderson the Waynflete Professor of Physiology of Oxford, Haldane had begun work in a little clinical laboratory at the Infirmary on the 'elimination of aromatic products in disease'. With the idea of making the project 'decently large' he suggested to Wilson that the two of them collaborate on it in Oxford and London for six weeks.

37

If you would do the clinical part and assist in the chemical part I would do most of the chemical part. The results would be published in the Local Government Board *Reports*. The L.G.B. are to supply the reagents and chemicals which I haven't got & which would be needed, but of course there would be no pay of any kind.[49]

Haldane seemed unaware that Wilson was in no position to entertain the prospect of an unpaid collaborative venture, however attractive scientifically. Now fully trained he had to think of his obligations. He had debts and a responsibility for his parents, now beginning to age. He managed to get a locum tenens to a general practitioner at Dunscore for a time in the summer of 1884. Competition for medical appointments was intense among the streams of Edinburgh graduates. For his immediate needs – a rest and time to think – Wilson pinned his hopes on a posting as a ship's surgeon, telling his parents in April:

I must now probably be more dependant on circumstances than ever, and may have to trot off on a ship at a few hours' notice. My only fear is – and it is a fear, that such notice may not come at all. But I have good hopes of it.[50]

Notice came at the beginning of August 1884.

Notes

1. 'Arrd all right': JTW postcard, 30.4.1879.
2. Scottish intellectual traditions and the English: Davie, *passim*.
3. 'The Tounis College': Horn. University's two sessions left a long summer vacation when poorer students could earn funds for another year's tuition. JTW's lodgings: City Archivist, to author, 21.1.1981. Landlady: *1881 Census* RPB. Learning flute: KR.
4. 'a proud and': JTW to KR, 1.5.1929.
5. Main sources on university teachers: Horn, Barrie, Davie. 'the most outstanding': Barrie, 29.
6. 'had an important': Comrie, 707. Geikie: *International Dictionary of Scientists*. Wyville Thompson: *DNB*. 'A native of Lancaster': JTW, quoted JPH, *RSO* on JTW, 644–5.
7. Medical School: Horn, 197–200; Comrie, *passim*; Turner, Ch. 3. Goodsir's interest in the cell anticipated the work of German pathologist Rudolf Virchow, who dedicated his *Cellular Pathologie* (1858) to Goodsir: Comrie, 621.

8. Medical students 1879/80: research by JMGW on Uni of Edin
   Archives shows 376 new students for that year. Total medical
   students: Turner, 146 shows rapid rise in late 1870s to nearly 1600
   by 1880–1, peaking at 2000 by end of 1880s. 'So soon as' and
   'evidently viewed': *Scotsman,* May 1879.
9. 'The medical man': quoted in Gray, 227. Results: WP.
10. Excursions: Alisma, 32. Volunteers: Horn, 206; Turner, 98–104;
    Epps, 30.
11. Meal sack man: Scot Skirving, *SSM* Vol. 1, 178. Dumfries and
    Galloway Literary Assoc.: Barrie, 58–9.
12. Free High and Free St Georges: the latter was moved from west end
    of Princes Street in 1869 to make way for the railway. The new
    building attended by JTW was at east end of Shandwick Place:
    JMGW to author, 16.3.1983.
13. Turner's reputation: Newman, 237. Influence of Goodsir: Obit. of
    Turner in *BMJ,* 26.2.1916, 326–31; Gray, 282.
14. Turner's lectures, 'Depend on it': and 'Man alone stands': Turner,
    124–8; Keith, *BMJ,* 26.2.1916, 328.
15. Demonstration classes: Turner, 130–1.
16. Royal Comm. of 1881 and Turner's report: Turner, 289–95;
    Newman, 239.
17. The Haldanes: Mitchison, 17; RBH 1928b. Richard was created
    Viscount Haldane of Cloan in 1911 for services to the State.
18. Appeal of Idealism: Sturdy; Passmore, 60; Muirhead, 174;
    Copleston, 173, 191; Richter, 19; JTW 1903b. Idealism suited the
    cast of mind of the Lowlanders, according to RBH 1928b, 164.
    The range and scope of the Idealist movement in Britain was first
    publicized when a group of its younger men, mainly Scots, issued
    their manifesto in 1883, edited by Andrew Seth and Richard
    Haldane.
19. Andrew Seth: later Professor Seth Pringle–Pattison. 'the more
    experience': RBH 1928b, 30.
20. The '1847 Group': Geison 1978, 14. Rutherford: Geison, 130–49,
    332–3; Comrie Vol. 2, 608–10; Gray, 242–4. Rutherford's tribute in
    1875 to his Continental teachers: 'Physiology is indebted to these
    and many others, principally because they have brought a profound
    knowledge of physics to bear on the phenomena of life.'
21. 'playful sarcasm': Comrie Vol. 2, 694–5. 'Professor Rutherford': JSH,
    quoted Gray, 297. 'pernicious nonsense': Tait, 24–5. The Haldanes'
    essay of 1883: in Seth and Haldane, *Essays in Philosophical Criticism.*
22. 'that the phenomena': RBH 1928b, 28. Most of John Haldane's 1883
    lecture is in his 'Life and Mechanism', in *Mind,* 9 (1884), 27–47.

23. as a toast': DC to author.
24. Ascendance of mechanism: Gray, 296. Professor Fraser: Comrie, Vol. 2, 701–2. Greenfield and Woodhead: Comrie, 697; Guthrie, 288. Opinions on JTW: Testimonial in JTW letter of application to Prince Alfred Hospital, 1888, for position of Hon. Pathologist.
25. 'the great flitting' and 'many windowed': Scot Skirving, *SSM* Vol. 2, p. 3. Student increase and cosmopolitan character: Turner, 152, 286 (Colonial students increased from 16 per cent in 1868 to 30 per cent of medical school by 1913).
26. Epps, 36–7.
27. TPAS: *ADB*. 'coracoid': Scot Skirving, 204, *SSM*. 'a very able': quoted Epps, 13.
28. TPAS' childhood and youth: Epps, Chs 1 & 2. 'Religion is': quoted Epps, 24.
29. Wilson's American cousins: JTW, Notes, MS sheet for 1881–3.
30. Lorrain Smiths: Ewing, 322. Rev. Walter; J Clunies Ross, 'Biographical Sketch of James Thomas Wilson (1861–1945)', typescript, 4–5. Careers, family members: James Lorrain Smith, *Reminiscences*.
31. JTW diary entries: Notes for 1881–3.
32. 'I refrained' and 'Rap! – rap!! – rap!!!': HBW to JTW, 4.10.1881.
33. Troubles at home: HBW to JTW, 18.10.1881, 31.10.1881. JTW the senior partner: JTW to LH on birth of her son Ted, 1930. 'There's nothing like': HBW to JTW, 21.11.81.
34. '25.3.82 Nellie died': JTW Notes. Robert Koch's announcement: Sourkes, 26.
35. 'I do not yet': JTW to parents, 25.7.1882. Visits to friends: JTW, Notes.
36. Supper at Dr Byrom Bramwell's: JTW to parents, 23.7.1882. Opinion of JTW: letter of application to PAH, 1888.
37. Comments on teachers: Scot Skirving, Vol. 1, 181–5. *SSM*.
38. Extra-mural school: Turner, Ch. xvii and 385. Spence's coat: Epps, 33.
39. John Duncan: Comrie, 677; Scot Skirving, 199, *SSM*. 'one of the finest': JTW quoted by Hill, *RSO* (1945), 644. 'one who, by natural' and 'with an unusual': JTW testimonials from Duncan, 3.5.86 and 2.5.1884. 'I must tell': JTW to parents, 19.1.1883.
40. 'knocked up with': JTW, Notes. 'a tussle' and 'I must confess': JTW to parents, 19.7.1883. Entry to Royal Infirmary: JTW, Notes.
41. 'I dare say': JSH to JTW, 30.7.1883. Haldane's MB: Mitchison, 4. Haldane's criticism: begun in Feb. 1884 (letters to JTW 15.2. and 19.2.). JSH wrote to JTW about anonymous letters to *The*

Scotsman,(1885), and his pamphlet *A Letter to Edinburgh Professors By a Medical Student* (1890). Naomi Mitchison, to author..

42. Quotes: Haldane, *ibid.*, vi, 33, 40, 46.
43. Student numbers: Turner, 147–55.
44. Jeanie's studies: Certificate in WP. 'We are also': Rev. Walter Smith to Thomas Wilson, 2.7.1883. Concert programmes and newspaper clippings suggest Jeanie was in Leipzig Oct. 1883 to Jan. 1884, and Hanover in March.
45. 'I must say I felt' and 'I believe that': JTW to parents, 19.7.1883.
46. JTW and surgery: Hill in *RSO* 1949, 644. 'a great man': JSH to JTW, 15.2.1884. Opinions on JTW: application in 1888 for position of pathologist at PAH.
47. 'has been mostly': JSH *ibid.* 'I wish Duncan': JTW to parents, 21.4.1884. '... I know of': JTW to J, 13.12.1939.
48. 'The Society': either D'fries and Galloway Literary Assoc. or the Free St George's Literary Assoc. 'very good syllabus': JTW to parents, 27.3.1884. Medical Luncheon and 'bright and airy' and 'nursing mother': Turner, 414–16. 'most of those': JTW to parents, 21.4.1884.
49. 'the festivities': JTW to parents, 21.4.1884. 'the elimination' and 'decently large' and 'If you would': JSH to JTW (n.d.) 1884.
50. JTW's locum tenens at Dunscore: inferred from JSH letter (n.d.)1884. 'I must now probably': JTW to parents, 21.4.1884.

3

The Sea and Philosophy

For the well-to-do, sea voyages were a popular recreation and a way of recuperating from illness or exhaustion, an indulgence which medical men of narrower means could also exploit as ship's surgeons. New medical graduates often did so, the usual condition of the shipping line being a contract for two voyages.

Wilson was offered a ship's surgeon post by the 'Blue Funnel Line' (the Ocean Steamship Company) and he joined the SS *Telemachus* leaving Liverpool on 2 August 1884. His first trip abroad was not the professionally desirable tour of the Continent enjoyed by his more fortunate colleagues, but a round trip of about four months on one of the Empire's busiest commercial sea lanes to the Far East. To equip himself he bought a large stock of dress shirts, having been told he would be required to dress for dinner every evening. It was a costly mistake, but they did good service for many years.[1]

Aboard the SS *Telemachus* Wilson found his medical duties light till the ship reached Penang when 150 Chinese passengers were taken on and then another 202 at Singapore, but they were mainly healthy, ulcers being the commonest malady. He also did 'the ship's writing ... ie. at the cargo books' but that was not an onerous duty either. He turned to his studies: a lesson a day in German, Ganot's books on Physics, Light and Electricity, Blackwood's manuals on Kant and Hegel, T H Green's *Introductions to Hume's Treatise on Human Nature*, Carlyle's *French Revolution*, Dicken's *Barnaby Rudge*, and some poetry. He was now in company that did not 'admit of thinking conversation' but it afforded him an interesting reflection:

I have realised the difference to me between a Scotchman & Englishman. Mr Moss the Chief Engineer is a 'Fifer' & we can

42

generally find something to talk about. The difference is not only that of subject but of the very mode of thought.[2]

By early September he had settled into his new regime, eating well and with relish, putting on weight, muscle-toned by 'the perpetual gymnastic exercise' of walking on deck. Shipboard life was refreshing:

> being thus continually in the open air is a splendid change to a student ... I enjoy it every day still. What a relief to feel that you dont need to be doing anything at all. Sh!

After years of austerity, indifferent health and the stress of learning, he was at last able to relax and enjoy the novelty of wide horizons. His letters to his parents exhibited a heightened sensitivity, an immediate, uncomplicated verve. From Ceylon, as they passed the Point de Galle, he caught a breath of perfume and 'sense of *promise*', he was wonder struck by the tropical skies and was even 'glad of the experience' of a monsoon wave which almost swept him overboard in the Indian Ocean.

Penang harbour confirmed exactly his preconceived picture, 'the same rigging the same Chinamen with the same pigtails & parasol hats, & umbrellas & slippers & garb generally', and in the motley town itself his interest focused on the social contrasts. The 'Chinese Aristocracy' driving in 'garries' were 'quite as stuck up as any gigman at home could possibly be', while the Chinese coolies pulling rickshaws usually with two occupants, scampered along as if it were no trouble. Bodily physique varied from 'miserably developed' to 'great stout lordly looking fellows' among the Chinese, and the 'black fellows' were 'splendidly made, fine big muscular fellows, who are certainly not kept down by their tailor's bills'. He looked approvingly on the mixture of European and Eastern customs, the state of the roads and municipal facilities, reflecting the influence of British rule, and pounced on a Scot in the shape of a policeman who helped him converse with the Chinese shopkeepers. Hong Kong by night with its tiers of lamps on the hillside reminded him of the old town of Edinburgh and sailing up the Min at Foochow prompted thoughts of Loch Lomond: pleasant homing thoughts which were in contrast with the evidence of war all around. Only weeks before the French had attacked the Pagoda anchorage at Foochow, completely destroying the Chinese fleet.

A typhoon which lashed them for two days and two nights approaching Shanghai was in keeping with the threatening political climate. The whole area was then a dangerous place for Europeans;

even in British Hong Kong there were forts and rifle pits everywhere and stone-laden junks ready for sinking to close the channel to Shanghai if the French attempted access. Foochow was a very melancholy sight, its harbour littered with the remnants of the Chinese fleet. There Wilson met another Scot, Dr Underwood, whose beautiful house had been destroyed by Chinese looting of European areas following the French attack and the pair of them discussed these events and 'Glencairn & its inhabitants & Edinh & its academic life'. These conditions prevented much sightseeing, but the Chinese excited Wilson's interest. They were a warm-hearted, cheerful, charming people and some of them very good-looking though their malodorous gardening methods and habits like opium smoking drew his censure. Their history, their customs and their outlook on life intrigued him.

The journey home was uneventful. Fewer passengers, mostly English, only one 'unhealthy looking prospect', a dipsomaniac, who boarded at Shanghai and died before reaching Singapore. Thereafter, smooth seas, congenial company, the occasional greeting of a passing ship, beautiful sunsets, cooler nights, arrival at Gravesend on 4 December, and then home. There was no place like it, yet he felt the winter cold more keenly this time, 'shivering & cowering indoors in bleak Scotland. It needs all the attraction that homeliness & social life can give it to make it outbalance the soft climate of the south'.

Jeanie at this time was studying English Literature under David Masson in Edinburgh, taking first class honours, the fourth prize and a certificate from the Edinburgh Association for the University Education of Women, at the end of the Winter Session.[3] But Wilson could not have seen much of her. According to the usual practice he had signed up for two voyages and he left Gravesend again on the SS *Telemachus* on Christmas day 1884. Four days later, off Cape Finisterre, he had found his sea legs and was rejoicing in his escape from the 'murky climate and leaden skies' of Scotland to the 'loveliest of moonlight nights'. On this trip he made careful observations of the fascinating tropical skies and reported them to his father. He drew up another programme of systematic study which included P G Tait's *Recent Advances in Physical Science* (1876) and *Heat* (1884) a recent paper by Haldane (probably 'Life and Mechanism' published in *Mind* in 1884), more Ganot, Green's *Introductions to Hume* for the second time, Berkeley and some poetry by Milton and Tennyson. First priority went to 'an hour per morning of Greek ... Mind I dont want *anyone* to know that I'm going at Greek'. It was an indication that he had ambitions for the Edinburgh MD.[4]

44

The vigorous scientific debate between the vitalists and the mechanists preoccupied him. He was disposed, like Haldane, to pitch his tent with neither camp, though he was more definite, like P G Tait, in his opposition to the mechanists. He was studying the creed that had inspired Haldane's anti-mechanistic stance, T H Green's Idealism, for Haldane's physiological concept of reciprocity of the parts of an organism governed by its drive for self preservation (a teleological principle), followed in general outline Green's metaphysics. In opposition to the materialists, who held that knowledge derives from sense impressions of the world written on the blank slate of the mind, Green argued that isolated sense impressions only became 'real' when ordered into a system of relations by the activity of the mind, which cannot be reduced to matter. Green postulated an eternal consciousness (identified with God) which the individual mind becomes aware of as it grows in experience gradually becoming a participant in the eternal consciousness. To him the world was a huge organic unity of interrelated parts governed by an ultimate spiritual principle. It was a monistic creed. [5]

Wilson was considering how to 'best qualify myself for living my part in the life of the huge organism – the world', and concluded that it was by doing just what he was doing – reading, reflecting and experiencing the world. But with the entry of the *Telemachus* into Asian waters, after the long stretch with no landfalls from Aden to Penang, he had fewer quiet hours for reading and reflection. There were more Asian ports of call than on his first voyage, and more passengers: 800 for the return journey from Hong Kong to Singapore causing a water shortage, and among the Europeans proceeding 'home' there was the novelty of several babies. Though he had less privacy he continued his studies in poetry and philosophy, concentrating on Green and Kant. For relief he sketched and described with evident pleasure the strange, rich and exotic life of the Far East.

After Singapore the *Telemachus* entered again an atmosphere of tension, coinciding with the news of General Gordon's death at Khartoum which thoroughly aroused Wilson's blood:

> We hear they are sending out more troops to Egypt. I wonder what they mean to do & what it will all come to. It is futile to try and simply wash our hands of Egypt, as some people would have us do. That is the policy of weakness.

By the time the *Telemachus* reached Shanghai on 25 February 1885 there had been several hostile incidents between the French and the

45

Chinese and relations between China and Japan were precarious. Wilson's opinion was that in the long run the war would help to open China up to modern Western progress and all the power of the Celestial Empire would be unable to stop that tide. The 'dominion of darkness' would soon be broken up.

Something of great importance was breaking up, but if it included the Chinese 'dominion of darkness' it also included the sunshine of European peace. European conflict in Africa, the Pacific and the farthest reaches of the British Empire where Wilson was now a witness, was a disturbing portent of things to come. But in Shanghai this time he had ample opportunity for sightseeing. He surveyed the city, the countryside and the people, at work, at play and at worship. He described the corrupt systems of administration, commerce and justice and pondered the reasons for the decline of a great civilization to its present decadent condition. One thought was that China had missed the 'blending and welding of race with race which has doubtless been such a potent factor in evolving our present western life'. But he concluded that the main cause was moral failure:

China

> The entire lack of *moral principle* and even of *moral sense* among the Chinese is one of the most deplorable features of the national character. This is the great obstacle to the way alike of rational self-government among them & of the progress of Christian faith ... China lacked what was vouchsafed to the West in the same critical situation – the renovating & ennobling influence of the Gospel of Christ which alone perhaps has saved Europe from a degradation to the level of an effete civilization such as we have in China.

These reflections had less to do with China than with Wilson's own search for moral authority. In revolt against hedonism, individualism and the economic materialism of the Manchester School, the 'new liberals' with whom Wilson was aligned were in search of an ethical philosophy by which to live as individuals and as members of society. T H Green of Oxford met their need more than anyone, but as Wilson contemplated China's decrepit empire it was not Green's *Ethics* that was in the forefront of his mind but Hegel's celebration of Western civilization in his philosophies of history and religion: the representation of history as progress in the consciousness of freedom, and religion as progress towards pure spirituality, reaching its highest form in Protestant Christianity. It is clear from his line of thinking and from various turns of phrase in his letters that Wilson was reading the influential *Hegel* by Edward

Caird, professor of moral philosophy at Glasgow and the young D G Ritchie's 'The Rationality of History', in *Essays in Philosophical Criticism* edited by Richard Haldane and Andrew Seth, both published in 1883. Wilson in other words was absorbing the arguments of Caird's Idealism which, unlike T H Green's, was more firmly rooted in Hegelian principles.[6]

Hegel, for Caird, was a theologian seeking 'to restore the moral and religious basis of human existence which a revolutionary scepticism had destroyed' – a circumstance of early nineteenth-century Germany which had its parallel in late nineteenth-century Britain. And in Hegel's dialectics Caird found a method of reconciliation which emboldened him to argue that there are no antagonisms that cannot be reconciled in a 'higher unity'. The conflict between conventional religion and materialistic science could be reconciled, he argued, in a higher unity 'manifesting itself in an organic process of development'. This idea of an evolving truth, fundamental to Hegel's view of history and religion, became fundamental also with Caird who concluded that a philosophy of life cannot be contained in a static system; it required a time dimension. Caird therefore turned with respect to Darwin and Comte for their contributions to the theory of development. For Wilson, Caird's philosophy had a distinct appeal: to a born naturalist with a Darwinian disposition it made profound sense. [7]

Western Europe's outposts in the Far East in 1885 certainly fell short of the moral ideal in Wilson's eyes. The vice and avarice of the trading communities contradicted Christian aims and precepts; a cathedral service he attended in Hong Kong exhibited mere formalism; a visit to a Roman Catholic mission at Ningpo provoked a polemical broadside against their faith, though he credited the missionaries themselves with 'earnestness, assiduity and self-sacrifice'.

He was in a critical state of mind, integrating Idealist teachings with his old convictions, elaborating and renovating his personal philosophy. Though he later claimed that this second voyage was more enjoyable than the first, dissatisfaction with himself was also building. Nearing Aden on his 24th birthday, 14 April 1885, his thoughts were again on his future. It was about this time, after sighting an Orient line steamer bound for Australia – which perhaps reminded him of his aunt Jessie (his mother's sister) and uncle James (his father's brother) who had settled out there – that he wrote to Anderson Stuart enquiring about teaching opportunities in Sydney. London they would reach on 9 May and then he must make haste to Edinburgh to 'see how things are', allowing only a day or two at Moniaive.

> The suspense of the problem of what next is very annoying [he
> wrote to his parents] ... I must not spend more time in this, in one
> sense, idle life ... Even if I cant get fixed for this summer at any
> work a voyage to China would throw me late for next winter & that
> mustn't happen ... if I can now I must buckle to.

In the summer of 1885 he was still debating the respective claims of
practice and teaching. On the advice of David Hepburn, Turner's
right-hand man at the time, he applied for a demonstratorship for
the winter session. In Hepburn Wilson had a strong supporter.
Having known Wilson from the beginning of his medical course,
Hepburn was impressed by his energy, ability and thoroughness, his
'keen scientific instinct' and 'rare gift of an orderly, well-regulated
mind, whereby his information was always ready and easy of access'.[8]
Turner was kind and encouraging. Wilson also sought medical
opinions as to whether general practice or teaching would be better
for his health. All advised against the knock-about work of general
practice and the experience of a locum tenens at Dunbar for three
weeks in June confirmed that opinion. His decision for teaching was
nevertheless a 'closely balanced business' about which he was 'greatly
exercised' and indeed it was not yet settled, since it depended now
on Turner. Wilson was fully aware of the importance of that
appointment, as he wrote to his parents:

> If I get this I know I could easily get an assistantship (university)
> after that and I think I am doing right. We *must* walk by faith after
> using all the wit & foresight which have been given us. Of course
> you know that science is my special love & perhaps forte too &
> now that I have so far decided I am eager about it. [9]

For Wilson's friends Haldane and Lorrain Smith it was also a
consummation devoutly to be wished. Between them were strong
bonds of common interests, including their belief that 'together we
are able to do something which separate we might not'. They had
forged a lifelong friendship. Lorrain Smith was now training for
medicine, having graduated in Arts the previous year, and if Wilson
got Turner's appointment, he would have Smith as his coadjutor,
which was 'no small inducement'. John Haldane was at University
College, Dundee, where after graduating in medicine in 1885 he
had been appointed a demonstrator to Professor Carnelley. He was
investigating the chemical composition and bacterial content of air
in dwellings, schools and sewers, accounts of which were published
in 1887, the foundation of much of his future work.[10]

Wilson did secure a demonstratorship on Turner's staff for the winter session, 1885–6, demonstrating human osteology to junior students, so the three friends were in close enough range to take up their common interests.[11] Over Christmas Wilson visited Cloan, the Haldane estate at Perthshire, mixing a little business (in minor surgery and instructing ambulance classes) with the considerable pleasure of the hospitality of that affectionate family. Mrs Haldane was growing then into the remarkable personality of her later years. She was devout but not dogmatic in her religious views, and well enough read in theology to hold her own in debate with a number of professional theologians, who visited her for that express purpose. Wilson met Richard for the first time, noting he was 'a very jolly fellow and *very* clever', and his political colleague Asquith, the member for Fife. The Haldanes enjoyed 'walks' in the countryside that were more like route marches, so their company was physically as well as intellectually strenuous.[12]

Surprisingly, at the end of the winter session Wilson embarked on a third voyage to China, this time on the SS *Palinurus* of the Ocean Steamship Company, leaving the Mersey on 17 April 1886, three days after his 25th birthday. Perhaps it was his health but more likely his finances that prompted it. He left soon enough to ensure that the beginning of the following winter session was not trespassed. This voyage took a different route, giving him the opportunity to take a look at Malta, a place he found so attractive that he was loth to leave it. He was impressed by the fine harbour, the heavy fortifications and views of the peaks, here and there crowned with Church, Convent or Monastery. He wandered its bright streets speckled with the forms of sleeping Maltese lying about 'promiscuous in all directions' and noted with a caustic eye the ubiquitous 'blackcoated shovelhatted priests, as well as monks and "holy friars" white brown black and grey'. He was transported to delight by the richness and colour of the Cathedral's interior, the marble staircase at Government House and most of all by the tapestry that covered the walls of its Council Chamber. 'It is splendid. There is some very fine tapestry at Drumlanrig but this beats it hollow'. Malta's medieval character had cast a spell.[13]

Wilson was not concerned with moral philosophy on this voyage. The highlight of his Chinese experiences was an evening at the theatre in Shanghai:

> I never saw such a display of gorgeous costumes in my life. The embroidery was simply magnificent, silk & satin stiff with embroidery of gold & gorgeous colours. The dresses were various

49

but the conventional dress is that of old China before the Tartar invasion ... I wish I could describe the music – but I can't ... the orchestra ... was the prominent element wh. consists of about half a dozen performers. The noise these fellows made with their tom-toms & woo-jius was perfectly appalling. There were some fighting scenes & as the fight became more energetic the music (!) became fast & furious until it was impossible to tell whether one had ears or no.

The Chinese empire got off lightly this time. He was now more optimistic about the advance of Christianity and the civilizing influences of railways and manufactures. He touched on the disturbing news of a Russian threat to China's north and her troubles in the south with the Burmese. An alliance with Britain he believed would be China's best diplomatic move. He was in fact much more interested in British politics, his hero Gladstone having been defeated on the Irish Home Rule Bill at the second reading. He had no doubt that in the long run Gladstone would be proved right. Home Rule was the only solution to the Irish problem.

Wilson's main preoccupation was with his studies, now closing in on the field that was to prove his life's work. On the outward journey in the Mediterranean he had science and philosophy again in his sights, reading

Darwin, Mill & Herbert Spencer & that school of which I stand in no fear nowadays when I can be sure of my standpoint. And from said standpoint the views of these writers are at best very imperfect & partial. In fact their science needs nothing short of rethinking on new lines. But Darwin's *Scientific* insight is marvellous!

This revelation marks the beginning of Wilson's unreserved commitment to Darwinian theory, becoming with the years the sturdiest plank in his personal philosophy. It inspired his most serious purpose, the work through which he reached for self-realization. He sensed a difficulty in reconciling Darwin's evolutionary concept – atheist, amoral and opportunist – with the pantheism and progressivism inherent in Hegelian and Idealist philosophy. Decades were to elapse before most people, including biologists, could look the materialist and aprogressive implications of Darwin's theory straight in the eye. The idea of progress which pervaded Victorian thinking, equating evolution with progress, was not easily dislodged. For Wilson the tension of holding together these two irreconcilable creeds, Darwinism and Idealism, fuelled both his research drive and his dedication to high moral principle.

For the rest of this voyage he pegged away at comparative anatomy, dissecting a squirrel he had in spirit and reading according to a programme he set himself. Thoroughly absorbed in some aspects, he grew irritated at his slow progress, especially since he had fewer interruptions than on his previous trips. Nevertheless he was growing more confident, more at ease in social gatherings, an old hand by now in nautical ways. He was ready for the challenge of an unexpected proposition which cut across his bows on his return to Scotland at the end of July.

On 11 April 1886 in Sydney, New South Wales, Anderson Stuart had written to Wilson:

> Well let me make a proposal to you – that is that you should not lose sight of the place here either as Demonstrator or Professor: the former will certainly be vacant in 1887 at the end of the year or 1888 at the beginning of the year ... I am not bidding you leave your native shores for the Land of the Future: I am not even inviting you: But if you would like to come at any time let me know early as I may be able to put you on a good line.

Sydney was a delightful place wrote Stuart, its University 'a really big affair', and in three years he had made excellent progress with the medical school. There were vulgarians of course, but so were there everywhere.[14]

On 15 August Stuart wrote again, giving a more glowing description of Sydney and a more precise account of the medical school and its prospects. And a definite offer this time, clearly bidding him to leave his native shores for an appointment as demonstrator of anatomy at a salary of 350 pounds per annum beginning March 1887. 'The man who has been in Melbourne for 3 years wants to come but I would rather in the first instance have yourself and in the second place a man from the old country straight and if both fail then I shall have to fall back on him'. This letter reached Wilson just as he was settling down in Edinburgh for the winter session, demonstrating to and examining senior students on the brain and organs of special sense. He did not reply at once: 'I'll see by & bye when the next wh. he promises arrives' he wrote to his father on 6 October 1886. But accept he did, probably because Anderson Stuart gave convincing assurances of excellent career prospects and a healthy climate. On the latter Stuart put Sydney's case cogently:

One hears at home accounts of the *heat* of Sydney: the 3 worst months are simply Neapolitan Summer weather and the remaining 9 are *perfect!* Query which is preferable 3 such hot mos. and the 9 perfect or as at home ie. in Britain, 9 beastly ones 2 middling and *perhaps* one good? I vote for Sydney!!! [15]

Wilson completed half the winter session, holding his last class on 17 December in the midst of a busy week of farewells during which he also managed to read an essay lasting an hour and a quarter to 'The Society'; it honoured him by election to honorary membership because he was to leave Scotland.[16]

Haldane, then studying in Berlin, was critical of Wilson's decision to go to Sydney:

I am very sorry indeed to hear that you are going to leave Scotland. Your leaving will make a great difference to me, & doubtless to your other friends. I don't doubt that you will get on very well at Sydney, & soon make a name for yourself there, but I must say that I hope you will come back before very long. Perhaps it is best for yourself to go, but as to this one can't form an opinion on abstract grounds, without knowing all the considerations that have made you decide to go. I only know that it would take a good deal to make me decide to go to Australia! ... Perhaps Australia may not be such a barren place as one pictures it, but to my mind it is a place full of people who are physically very healthy & vigorous, but whose minds are only occupied over matters that are practical in the narrowest sense. Anyhow I hope you will come back before very long.

Haldane extolled the value of experience in Germany if arranged with discrimination and the opportunities opening up in Britain: 'There seems to me just now to be no end of good work waiting to be done in Physiology, Pathology, & Hygiene'. Wilson had made up his mind. With Turner's blessing and testimonials from nine senior teachers he left Edinburgh before Christmas. Cunningham expressed the opinion some years later that Wilson was 'the soundest anatomist Turner had sent out from Edinburgh'.[17]

After a round of farewells in Moniaive, Dumfries, Gatehouse-of-Fleet and Half Morton, Wilson travelled south for a Channel crossing on a cold snowy day, 6 January 1887, looking as he passed Gretna towards Jeanie's home where they had parted a few days before. His journey took in a brief Continental tour, his first and last until 1905, through France and Italy before joining the SS *Orient* – one of the fastest and most comfortable ships afloat – at

Naples for the voyage to Sydney. The French countryside bored him but the magnificent alpine scenery was refreshing. He went through Turin to Genoa where he saw the last of Europe's snow six inches deep in the streets. Then on through Pisa to Florence, the cleanest place he had ever seen and artistically the most absorbing. On to Rome where he inspected the Vatican, the galleries, the Sistine Chapel and the museums. St Peter's surpassed in splendour any church he had ever seen.[18]

Ascetic Protestantism had not robbed Wilson of keen enjoyment of the beautiful, the strange, the magnificent, the gorgeous and the elaborate. Edinburgh had disciplined his mind, widened his intellectual range, strengthened his aspirations and given him lasting friendships. Voyages to the Far East had restored him body and soul, and given him a perspective on his native land in the untidy *from Naples* patchwork of the British Empire Thus equipped he embarked for *1887* the antipodes from Naples on 16 January 1887 with the *Scots &* expectations of advancement that the Scots had come to associate *Empire* with Empire.

Notes

1. JTW's stock of evening shirts: KR to author.
2. Account of first voyage and all quotes from JTW to parents: n.d. (? late Aug/early Sept) 1884; 5.9.84; 16.9.84; 18.11.84; 26.12.84. WP.
3. Jeanie's qualifications, in collection of her personal documents. WP.
4. Account of second voyage and all quotes from JTW to parents: 26.12.84; 29.12.84; n.d.(? Jan.) 1885; 29.1.85; 4.2.85; 16.2.85; 25.2.85; 11.3.85; 17.4.85. WP.
5. Tait: *DNB*, 472–3. Green's philosophy: Passmore, 57–9; Copleston Vol. 8, 194–5; Richter; Green.
6. Idealism: Passmore, 56–7; Ritchie, Ch. V in Seth and Haldane; Caird.
7. *Ibid.*
8. Hepburn on JTW: application for Challis Chair of Anatomy in 1889.
9. 'If I get this': JTW to parents, 4.6.1885. WP.
10. 'together we are able to' and 'no small inducement': JTW to parents, 4.6.1885. WP.
11. JTW demonstratorship: Turner to TPAS, 20.12.1886. WP.
12. Mrs Haldane: Gosse 'The Matriarch' in *Leaves and Fruit*. 'a very jolly fellow': JTW to his mother, 28.12.1885. WP. Visitors to Cloan: JSH to JTW, n.d. (? late 1885). WP.
13. Account of third voyage and all quotes from JTW to parents: 26.4.86; 1.5.86; 21.5.86; 31.5.86; 11.6.86; 18.6.86. WP.

14. 'Well let me make': TPAS to JTW, 11.4.1886.
15. 'The man who' and 'One hears': TPAS to JTW, 15.8.1886. WP. 'I'll see': JTW to father, 6.10.86. WP.
16. 'The Society': probably the D'fries and Galloway Debating and Literary Assoc.
17. 'I am very' and 'There seems': JSH to JTW, 14.11.86. WP. Turner's blessing: JTW to parents, 17.12.1886. WP. 'The soundest': GES to JTW, 15.6.98. WP.
18. Departure, and Genoa: JTW to JCR, 30.12.1936. WP. SS *Orient*: P L Ballantyne, *The Cool Weather Route: To and From Australia by Passenger Steamer in the 1880s*, Adelaide, 1981. Florence and Rome: JTW to parents, 18.1.1887. WP.

4

Colonial Sydney

16 Jan 1887

When Wilson appeared for dinner on his first evening on the RMS *Orient* he found a place reserved for him beside the ship's doctor who turned out to be a friend and fellow Scot, James Struthers, son of Sir John Struthers the Professor of Anatomy at Aberdeen. James Struthers had been a contender for the Sydney position Wilson was about to occupy, but he bore no grudge on that score. 'It was a very pleasant surprise', wrote Wilson to his parents, 'and he was very pleased too'. At the same table 'Just opposite me on the doctor's right I found Prof. and Mrs. MacCallum going out to Sydney. So we were quite a friendly corner immediately ... The Professor is a kind of man I can get on with very well'. So began a friendship that lasted 55 years, until MacCallum's death in 1942.

MacCallum

Wilson's reasons for going to Australia were health and a job offering pay and prospects sufficient to meet his obligations to his parents who were to follow him to Sydney, and to enable him to marry. Probably he appreciated, unlike John Haldane, that Australia offered unique opportunities for the investigative scientist. A chair in anatomy would meet his material ambitions:

> Struthers seems to think that I am in a good way going out as I am and that the appointment will result well. He says something about their splitting Stuart's chair in 1888 and I am rather anxious as this is a bit sooner than I expected or wished for. But all will be well I have no doubt in any case.[1]

Professor Mungo MacCallum had a grander motivation, a dedication to the imperial idea. The son of a Glasgow merchant, Mungo William MacCallum was educated at Glasgow High School and the Universities of Glasgow (where he took the Luke Fellowship

55

for literature, philosophy and classics), Leipzig and Berlin. In 1879 he was appointed to the University College of Wales and in 1884 published his first book, *Studies in Low German and High German Literature*, the first fruits of a talent which was to establish him as a distinguished scholar. In 1887 he was 33 years old, married with two children, confident in his work. Seven years older than Wilson, 'a little man of towering personality', MacCallum had already made a good start on his career. It was with great hesitation that he had applied for the new Chair of Modern Literature in the University of Sydney, and with misgivings that he accepted it. Two factors prompted the venture. The first was J A Froude's *Oceania* published in 1886, which revealed to him 'the brilliant promise of the Australian Colonies'. The second was the dispatch in 1885 of a NSW contingent to join the British forces in the Sudan campaign. MacCallum became convinced 'that coming to this far-off land would not mean anything like exile, that I would still be among our own people, that the transfer would only be from Great to a portion of what Sir Charles Dilke had aptly called "Greater Britain".' It involved no breach of patriotism.[2]

As 'brither Scots' bent on the same enterprise MacCallum and Wilson had much in common. Wilson was delighted to discover they occupied the same platform in philosophy. Empire was not a dominant ideal for Wilson, though very likely his views were similar, if not as formed or definite as MacCallum's. Few Britons then disagreed with the basic concept of empire. As Gladstone wrote in 1878:

> The sentiment of empire may be called innate in every Briton. If there are exceptions, they are like those men born blind or lame among us. It is part of our patrimony: born with our birth, dying only with our death; incorporating itself in the first elements of our knowledge, and interwoven with all our habits of mental action upon public affairs.[3]

Political controversy over the Empire was not about whether Britain should have one or not, but how it should be managed and for what purpose, an important issue in the duel between the two great party leaders, Gladstone and Disraeli. Their point of difference on Empire was clear. Disraeli wanted a powerful, united military empire reinforcing Great Britain's strength as a world power. Gladstone adhered to the settled Liberal Party policy of limited government, informal rule and free trade. By the early 1880s, however, even the anti-expansionist, anti-militaristic Gladstone found himself painting more of the map red, though not as much in the Pacific as Australians would have liked. Against colonial protests he allowed Germany to take over north-east New Guinea in 1884. A quickening change in European politics and in the relations of European powers with the rest of the world brought with it the madness of European expansion, in Africa, the Pacific and the Far East. With complex motives, usually summed up vaguely as 'Commerce, Christianity and Civilization' but with no deliberate policy of aggrandizement, Britain extended her empire. 'We seem, as it were, to have conquered and peopled half the world in a fit of absence of mind', said Sir John Seeley in 1881. Wilson must have applauded the NSW contingent going to the Sudan in 1885. To 'simply wash our hands of Egypt' he had written at the time, would have been 'a policy of weakness'. On board the RMS *Orient* the Sudan campaign was no doubt a topic of conversation with Mungo MacCallum whose other persuader for emigration to Australia, J A Froude, Wilson took the opportunity to read.[4]

The professor, the doctor and Wilson formed 'a sort of trio or triumvirate rather which is located at one end of the table at mealtimes and is otherwise pretty closely associated', wherein Wilson's two dominant interests, science and philosophy, found stimulating hospitality. MacCallum was one of Edward Caird's disciples. With Henry Jones, J H Muirhead, John Watson, J S Mackenzie and William Smart he had sat in the huge classes in moral philosophy in Glasgow where Caird introduced them to Kant and Hegel – heresy to orthodox Presbyterians and traditional Scottish realists – drawing on history, poetry, politics and religion as well as philosophy to reveal a new heaven and a new earth, a world that was through and through intelligible and yet intrinsically spiritual. Wilson's developing friendship with MacCallum, as he told his parents, quelled a persistent anxiety that he would meet only philistines out in Sydney. They arranged to carry on joint studies in philosophy. Mrs MacCallum was German, very nice, simple and unaffected Wilson reported and their two children 'Tibbie' [Isabella] and Mungo – then known simply as 'Boy' – were 'a fascinating pair of fellow-passengers'.[5]

philistines?

Wilson's shipboard routine was promptly established. Rising at 6.30 with a cup of coffee and an intention of reading 'that doesn't usually come off', he breakfasted at 9.00 on porridge which they made 'fairly well', and after a smoke with MacCallum the two men sat down with their books till lunch at 1.00, after which they read again or perhaps played at games till tea at 4.00. They were preparing themselves for their courses in Sydney, MacCallum working away on old French and German, and Wilson 'almost entirely occupied with Anatomy, reading books I had never seen before'. Wilson fell short of his programme but was this time lenient on himself: '... still I have reason to be glad I have got so much done'. He managed also to imbibe some Froude and John Forster's *Life of Dean Swift*. After tea, recreation of various sorts till dinner at six, followed by a walk unless it was too rough, or chess, or whist at which Wilson distinguished himself and won a meerschaum pipe. Meals were good: the new technique of refrigeration delivered fresh milk, meat and vegetables 'just as if we were ashore' and dinner was the highlight of the day:

> The Dr has a wonderful memory & a marvellous fund of good stories with the knack of making them tell and MacCallum is also something of an adept in the same line ... at our end of the table there is prevalent in an aggravated form the vicious habit of punning. Some are as bad as any Papa could make but it may cheer him when I say that in John Forster's opinion (Life of Swift) there are puns which from the nature and extent of their *atrocity* can only be perpetrated by the best intellects and are merely the condescensions of such minds.[6]

Australian news was eagerly sought. A reported outbreak of smallpox in Sydney, reinforced by the advice of Struthers, 'a dab at that disease', decided Wilson to be vaccinated. The first Australian landfall was Adelaide where he admired and was refreshed in the February heat by the botanic gardens and the fruit, especially grapes. Adelaide had good reason to be proud of itself but it was not to Wilson's taste: 'There are many very good buildings but the climate is such that they never mellow with age & always look too brand new'. And it was too hot, burnt up and barren looking. 'MacCallum & I were not sorry that we were *not* to be in Adelaide, on the whole'. Sydney he had been told would be 'an improvement just on all the less inviting features of Adelaide'. He visited the University in Melbourne and found that his first meeting with his father's younger brother, an employee in Melbourne railways, would be in Sydney.[7]

The RMS *Orient* steamed through Sydney heads on the morning of 22 February 1887,

> when of course we 'new chums' were all on the alert to see the famous Sydney harbour. Even out here 'Sydney harbour' is rather proverbial. Certainly it is a lovely place tho' we were not able to see the full beauty of the place by reason of the fog or haze.

famous Sydney harbor

Wilson was greeted by his uncle James accompanied by Anderson Stuart's laboratory assistant John Shewan (Stuart himself being in New Zealand) who had been Professor Rutherford's class attendant when Wilson was a student. The University, where that same day he met H E Barff the registrar, Professor Warren of engineering, W A Haswell lecturer in zoology, and Scott, professor of classics, made a good first impression on Wilson. Built on a hill amidst extensive grounds, it reminded him of Glasgow University except that Sydney's buildings were finer. The medical school was 'a really handsome structure', built in the same perpendicular Gothic style as the older main building, but not yet finished. Roof construction was just beginning. It would provide 'splendid accommodation in every way' when completed, which was expected by the end of the winter term.[8]

He was impressed too by the Prince Alfred Hospital which, in conformity with Scottish tradition, was closely associated with the University – located in fact on university grounds. Built on the same lines as the new Edinburgh Infirmary and opened in 1882, it surpassed in its equipment and accommodation anything Wilson had seen. It had over 200 beds. Sydney's only other hospital, the Sydney Infirmary in the centre of the city, was by comparison primitive. At Prince Alfred, Wilson met the two men who had preceded him in his university post: James Graham, the medical superintendent, 'an exceptionally nice fellow' Wilson thought, despite his conservative political beliefs and poor opinion of Mr Gladstone; and Alexander MacCormick, honorary assistant surgeon at the hospital – 'a sharp man ... and the only good surgeon here but that doesn't mean a very great deal, for the other surgeons are not up to much' – and a demonstrator in physiology (mainly histology) and materia medica at the University.[9]

At Graham's invitation Wilson accepted temporary lodgings at the hospital and the honorary position of resident medical officer till a permanent one was elected, so beginning a long and active association with the hospital which then had a slender resident staff. Wilson was to act several times as a stop-gap resident and at least once as a stop-gap medical superintendent. He was also to be the hospital's first pathologist, part-time of course, from 1888 to 1890, and honorary secretary from 1897 to 1901. It was in this hospital setting in the early months of 1887 that a young fourth-year medical student, Arthur Mills, caught his first glimpse of the man who was to exercise a strong influence on his life. Wilson was then 26 years old, tall, spare and fresh-faced, with a tidy fair moustache.

He had the mannerisms, or 'distinctive tics', which were to become familiar to generations of students: 'The shrugging of the shoulder, the rubbing of the shin of one leg against the calf of the other, the active, almost springing gait, the deep stentorian voice' which, when allied with 'the penetrating glare of his eyes', could jerk a drowsy student to instant attention or instil 'mortal terror into the "gentleman in the last seat but one".' Those disciplinary instruments were not then well developed, though Mills noticed that when Wilson spoke, he spoke with authority. This was 'Jummy',* as he was always called by staff and students alike, except in his presence.[10]

Temporarily settled and working on the then outskirts of the city, Wilson got to know Sydney by shifts and sallies, a gradual revelation like the harbour on the first morning. Nature gave Sydney a similar endowment to Edinburgh. There were cliffs and high prospects from which to view her grand harbour and neighbouring hills. Civilization if more recent clung in similar fashion to the natural lie of the land. The streets were narrow and steep, winding along the ridges like Edinburgh's old town, and there were some fine old public buildings, private mansions and terraced houses. In the centre of the city shops jostled with houses and, as in Edinburgh, wealth lived cheek by jowl with poverty. In 1887 both cities housed around a quarter of a million people who lived by much the same principles and faced much the same problems. They travelled in similar trains, trams and horse-drawn vehicles or they walked as Wilson was accustomed to do. But Sydney could only occasionally look grey. Her climate and the colour of her sandstone buildings were warmer. Her weather was more predictable. In the 1880s Sydney's most treacherous feature was her sanitation, rendering her no more healthy than Edinburgh or London. From 1888 the water supply began to improve, and then by degrees the sewerage and drainage.

Sydney's philistines and vulgarians were obvious enough. 'Politics are rather a one-horse affair out here and politicians are not very admirable in general. [The New South Wales Premier Henry] Parkes, for example, is not by any means a man of high principle or ideas', Wilson observed. Still, he approved of Parkes' free trade policies. His first experience of Australian presbyterianism in the Glebe suburb did not pass muster: 'an awfully poor exhibition [in] the preaching dept.' In the evening, probably for reasons of protocol, he attended St James Church of England with Dr Graham and Professor Anderson Stuart. Afterwards these three, with Professor Scott, Professor MacCallum and one or two others, were entertained at supper by the minister, Mr Jackson.[11]

60

Anderson Stuart had just returned from a visit to New Zealand. It was four years since his arrival in Sydney, newly married and with high hopes as Sydney's first Professor of Anatomy and Physiology. He never forgot his first sight of the partly built four-roomed cottage in a back paddock intended for the medical school and the biology department. He was shown it by Mr Butler the Latin lecturer and Professor Charles Badham the renowned classical scholar who remarked 'that the "stinks" were all to go out at the back'. Anderson Stuart now knew, if he had not realized it before, that the University of Sydney had a classical bias, in the tradition of hallowed Oxford, which, in association with shortage of funds, had for 30 years inhibited the development of science and prohibited several schemes for professional departments, including a medical school.[12]

On the medical school two factors had induced the University authorities to relent. The first was the establishment of the Prince Alfred Hospital. The Act of Parliament of 1873 founding the hospital provided that it be built on university grounds, that the medical staff be appointed by a conjoint board with equal representation from the Senate of the University and the board of directors of the hospital, and that it be open for clinical instruction to medical students. The second was the unexpected and munificent Challis bequest of 1880 which ensured that the university would, on the death of the widow, be comfortably funded. In 1882 the Senate decided to establish a medical school, Anderson Stuart was appointed to head it and Prince Alfred Hospital opened to receive patients and medical students.[13]

The Chancellor of the University, Sir William Manning, representing a substantial body of opinion, held to the classical idea of a university. The teaching of the Arts, he said in his Commemoration Address in 1886 was

> of the very essence of University education, and the chief source of 'culture' and preparation for the world's higher work; whilst Medicine and like professional branches, are simply offshoots of more limited aims, taken under the University's care.[14]

This must have sounded strange to an Edinburgh man whose *alma mater* had for centuries accommodated medicine, law and divinity as respectable academic pursuits, and had in recent years spent considerable funds to outfit its medical school with up-to-date buildings and equipment. But Manning's words were not at all strange to Archibald Liversidge, the London- and Cambridge-trained Professor of Chemistry who, since his appointment in 1872 as Reader in Geology and Assistant in the Laboratory, had campaigned on a broad front for the proper recognition of science. 'After Homeric battles with the forces of Arts' he persuaded the Senate to establish in 1879 a faculty of science of which he was the first Dean. In the same year he proposed the formation of an Australasian Association for the Advancement of Science, which came into being in 1888. He was joined in 1886 by 25-year-old physics professor Richard Threlfall who founded a modern physics department. A Cambridge graduate and former assistant to J J Thomson at the Cavendish Laboratory, Threlfall had while still a student designed and built the first automatic microtome. In 1891 came the geologist T W Edgeworth David, an Oxford classics graduate before he launched himself into geology at the Royal School of Mines, South Kensington. A quiet charming man and gifted orator, David combined erudition with a dedication to science, and he was not above practicalities either, having for eight years done geological survey work for the New South Wales government before accepting the university post. In 1892 he wrote:

Edgeworth David

> In a new country like this, geological thought, like other branches
> of thought, should be new and strong; and though having its source
> in the riper knowledge of men in older countries, it should be free
> to flow in channels which it wears for itself.

Ten years later, when they delivered addresses for the University's jubilee celebrations in 1902, Stuart and David still felt it appropriate to insist that the claims of medicine and science to university status were valid.[15]

By 1902 Anderson Stuart was basking in the sunlight of success, and took the opportunity to remind his audience that, 'When the battle has been fought *and won*, we can afford to look back with equanimity upon our struggles; but while struggling, as I well remember, we were anything but equanimous on either side'. Stuart fought hard and not always in an orthodox fashion. In March 1883 shortly after he took over his two rooms in the cottage in the back paddock – and began teaching four students there before they had windows or a roof – Stuart contrived the speedy exit of the department of biology by making the place smell as disagreeable as possible. That gave him four rooms, to which were added a lecture room, an injection room and a dissecting room. But Stuart had more grandiose ambitions. By 1884 he had turned his attention to

Med in 1883

lobbying the government. In 1885 he persuaded the University Senate to request funds to complete the medical buildings and the Government complied, on the understanding that the money was to be used for extensions to the seven-roomed cottage. With the Colonial Architect, however, Stuart prepared plans for a new and imposing Gothic structure to stand up-front beside the Main Building and the Great Hall whose style it copied and spent the money entirely on the foundations knowing, as he said himself, 'the foundations without any superstructure were an anomaly'. And Stuart made sure that when corrected by more government funds the 'anomaly' remained exclusively medical. Gradually the building rose, and was officially opened on 4 February 1889.[16]

The Medical School became a very handsome stone building in which the few staff and fewer students of the early years enjoyed a wondrous sense of space. It was mocked as "Stuart's Folly" but within 20 years it was overcrowded. Most of the interior finish was plain, serviceable and economical, though fitted with the latest fixtures and equipment for medical teaching. But the corridors were sumptuous: paved in black and white marble of distinctive pattern and crowned by segmented plaster vaults and moulded cornices. As the years went by the exterior was embellished by sandstone gargoyles and escutcheons and, over the front entrance beneath a statue of Asklepios, a curious bird with imposing beak;** the interior received donations from an appreciative medical community of stained-glass windows and a collection of busts of the great physicians and surgeons of history to line the corridors; later still came paintings of local luminaries of medical teaching. By means of this building Anderson Stuart tied the Sydney medical school to its European heritage, and created a cathedral to the glory of the medical profession in Australia. In 1902 Stuart emphasized its importance:

> To this magnificent building as it stands we undoubtedly owe much of the success of the Medical School as an institution. Student and graduate and teacher alike feel proud to belong to it, and its influence in creating an *esprit de corps* and good traditions cannot be overestimated.[17]

It is no wonder that Anderson Stuart and the Chancellor were soon at loggerheads. Sir William Manning was fond of referring to the medical school as distinct from the 'University-proper', and would have liked to sever the finances of one from the other, for while the medical building rose to alter the skyline, the Arts School stagnated

[handwritten margin note:] Stewart (med) vs Manning (arts, th Chancellor)

for want of funds. Manning was forced to accept that circumstance because, as he expressed it in his address in 1886, in medicine 'no starving is possible consistently with the issue of diplomas guaranteeing fitness for the profession', whereas starvation in arts was possible, though regrettable, because Arts men 'can at least do no mischief to life and health, in virtue of a degree in Arts, as would result from degrees in Medicine to men who have been imperfectly taught'. It was unfortunate, he added, 'that medical men alone are assumed to be (and to a large extent must be) the best judges of [the medical school's] requirements and even of its government'.[18]

Manning had a point. Till the advent of the medical school, the University had received a miserable £ 5,000 a year from the government since its beginning 30 years previously and daily he now observed that 'an immense block is in course of erection at a probable cost of £80,000!' for the medical school. These facts he confided in May 1886 to Dr A C Brownless, Vice Chancellor of Melbourne University, whom he privately consulted about how Melbourne governed and financed its medical school. In July he managed to have a resolution adopted by the Senate for consideration of what were the 'full requirements' of providing a medical school equal to any in the world, and how it might be made self-supporting. By December he was in deep chagrin: 'The [Medical] Faculty have just sent in a report demanding a very large additional expenditure – up to £8,000 a year in fact – to include 5 Professors at £900 a year (which is what one Professor now has, with half fees in his school) and a number of lecturers as already existing but with increased salaries', he informed Brownless. Moreover he felt slighted: 'The Report says nothing about fees or of any scheme for self support – nor on the subject of hygiene which was mentd in my resolution'. Brownless replied with sympathy and invidious comparisons: Melbourne University had just spent £10,000 on extensions to its medical building, and students' fees covered all but £1,000 per annum of its school's running costs. The medical cuckoo in Manning's nest proved as clever as he was insatiable and got nearly everything he wanted: except five professors.[19]

Anderson Stuart's appetite was never to be appeased. The Medical School was a vision to which he devoted his great gifts as an organizer, administrator and politician. He was ruthless and overbearing, seeming to invite opposition 'as something to be crushed'. Yet he had 'some flair for diplomacy when there was no other alternative' for his plans were crowned with extraordinary success. For the University, particularly the Medical School, he managed to loosen the purse strings of a succession of governments. A favourite ploy was to interest the wife of a cabinet minister in his schemes. And he had friends at court, notably H N MacLaurin, Arthur Renwick and later James Graham.[20]

The weather was usually stormy around Anderson Stuart, even domestically in the early years. His marriage had proved a calamity from which he was trying to free himself by legal means when his wife died suddenly, early in 1886, probably from an accidental overdose of a sleeping draught. Stuart had by then made enemies in Sydney, some of whom did not scruple to say he had murdered her. Inured to ill-favour, Stuart threw himself with greater intensity into his plans for the school. This dream and a thick epidermis of conceit came to his rescue. On 15 August 1886 he had written this account of himself and his affairs to Wilson:

As to myself my story has been, briefly told, 'worry and work'. Worry from domestic matters over which it is best to draw the veil: worry from the thousand and many troubles that beset him who is called upon while still young and inexperienced to pilot a difficult enterprise into the harbour of success against the currents of prejudice interest and – pure cussedness. But there is an end to all things – and the end of *this* thing is brilliant success.

At Christmas I shall have my courses of junior and senior anatomy *written* up, my physiology lectures *written,* all my stock of diagrams painted, a complete catalogue made of all things in my department, a splendid collection of instruments in the house, 225 beds in the hospital opened, the management of that institution on a sound basis, the first graduate through his exams, the first session of our (Royal) Medical Society over – but beyond all the roof on our splendid new school, stone built, to accommodate 500 and enlargeable to accommodate at least 1200. It will place us far in the van in the Southern Hemisphere, will worthily stand comparison with the mother school. I have done it all myself and having paid great attention to the accommodation for practical work in all the departments you may with some confidence look for Light from the Southern Land...

Physically I have enjoyed perfect health, corporeally I am 12 stone net, facially still bare, capillarily just a shade grey, socially very happy. I am pleased to say that my late troubles have left no trace of detriment to my social position tho' till the proper account of it all was known I had many hard things said of me. But all that too has passed away and now that I am beginning to issue from my seclusion I find everyone very kind very nice and seemingly anxious to show in a quiet way that I still retain their confidence and esteem. Nationally I am an Australian out and out. I mean to live and die in Sydney which is a perfect paradise in my eyes. It has been good to me: it is a beautiful city, and its surroundings are charming: it is a *great* and *growing* city and its climate suits me to a T. So that when Australia has proved felix to me it is only meet that I should entertain, at least in the meantime the most kindly feelings towards it and by identifying myself with everybody that tends to its welfare, repay in part the debt I owe it.[21]

Anderson Stuart had composed this letter carefully, for it was intended to recruit Wilson to his enterprise. It gives a grandiloquent though not essentially inaccurate account of the development of the medical school and of Stuart's command. Evidently he had 'enlargeable' ideas for it even beyond the building which so upset Chancellor Manning and which did materialize years later. Characteristically his account of the Prince Alfred Hospital leaves out the contributions of others, notably Sir Alfred Roberts who was its builder and its dictator until he died in 1898. No detail of hospital management and development, medical and nursing practice or teaching escaped Roberts' eye. Anderson Stuart, the dictator at the medical school, could not rival Roberts on hospital grounds. Yet it is a fact that Stuart, as early as 1883 had the power to appoint the medical staff of the hospital. In August 1886 he explained to Wilson:

> the Board that makes the Hospital Appointments is one half Hospital Board, one half University Senate: *I* am ex officio member of Hospital Board and am on the House Committee so that the University influence is strong everywhere and is growing. This influence always goes for the university man, and it is a recognised principle that the appointments in the School and in the Hospital are to be held by the same person if possible: I have got that put on record by each body acting separately and by both acting together: it is the recognition of a principle I have fought for ever since I landed.[22]

Stuart left little to chance. Before leaving Edinburgh he had recruited from Rutherford's staff a technical assistant, John Shewan, who early in 1883 arrived in the same ship with Alexander

[margin note, handwritten] 1886 Stewart on Aust:

MacCormick, whom Stuart had recruited by cable. Shewan was to do skilled work over many years, preparing models, diagrams and the technical items for Stuart's lectures. MacCormick, an Edinburgh classmate, started as a demonstrator in anatomy and physiology and by 1885 was launched on his surgical career, lecturing part-time at the University. Equipped by his Edinburgh training and a dedication to Listerian principles he quickly made his mark and never stopped advancing in surgery. With energy, courage and the skill of an artist he became in Wilson's mature opinion 'one of the great surgeons of the world and the high standard of Australian surgery ... owed more to him than to any one man'. Another classmate, Robert Scot Skirving, appointed medical superintendent at Prince Alfred Hospital in 1883 later combined part-time teaching with a successful practice in medicine and surgery. With swashbuckling verbal panache he was a colourful teacher, but not interested in research. Yet another, James Graham, succeeded Scot Skirving at Prince Alfred in 1886 and lectured part-time in midwifery for many years but did not justify Stuart's expectations as a teacher. Politics suited Graham better and as a politician he served Stuart well.[23]

The preponderance of Edinburgh men was remarkable. A scandal some said. But there were men of other backgrounds, including four clinical teachers appointed before Anderson Stuart's arrival, of whom the most distinguished was W Camac Wilkinson, lecturer in pathology. Australian born and London trained, he was the only staff member with the FRCP and he became a distinguished pathologist. In 1888, on the recommendation of Michael Foster of Cambridge, an exotic constituent was added with the appointment as physiology demonstrator of the strange, brilliant and cultivated Almroth Wright. Dublin trained, he became famous as an immunologist, immortalized by his friend Bernard Shaw as Sir Colenso Ridgeon in *The Doctor's Dilemma*. Sydney did not suit him and he returned to England in 1891; in 1892 he was appointed Professor of Pathology at the Army Medical School at Netley. Wright was the same age as Wilson and they became lifelong friends with common interests in philosophy and literature as well as medical science. Wright's successor, also recommended by Foster, was Charles James Martin, London- and Leipzig-trained. Younger than Wilson by five years, they became close friends. A fruitful collaboration resulted, satisfying for both and important for Australian science.[24]

In 1887 Sydney University was a small close-knit community in

which all students began with studies in Arts. J T Wilson's presence
was noticed by *Hermes* the undergraduate magazine on 24 March:
'He comes with the style of a Scholar and Anatomist ... we perceive
in him a tower of strength in the Anatomical Department and
general student life of the school'. The intimacy of the community
was in marked contrast with Edinburgh's academic life, not simply
due to its smaller size but also some traditions of English origin.
Sydney from its early years had residential colleges and the more
personal teaching method of Oxford and Cambridge, the tutorial,
had a significant place. If its classical bias offended Stuart's pride, his
lonely soul responded gladly to this English sense of community, as
he had confided to Wilson in April 1886:

> Upon my word I am almost ashamed to say I like the English
> University man better than the Scottish chiefly because of their love
> for Alma Mater, their esprit de corps; there is a sort of fraternality
> which is wholly wanting with us.[25]

In April 1885 he had founded the Medical Society on the Edinburgh
model, for it was one institution which did foster esprit de corps
harmonizing with English traditions. One wonders, however, what
he thought of Wilson's first paper to the Society on 27 April 1888 on
'Some problems of Life and Mind' which, *Hermes* reported,

> although somewhat lengthy, and perhaps difficult to understand in
> parts, was listened to with intense interest, and provoked a
> somewhat animated discussion. The mechanical theory of
> conscious intelligence was contrasted with the purpose of action,
> and the latter was upheld, the former being rejected on the ground
> that it gave an unsatisfactory explanation ... it showed that the
> compiler has given it a great amount of thought and study.

A shaky report, but it attests to Wilson's alignment at this time with
Haldane's rejection of the materialist arguments of William
Rutherford on the workings of the mind.[26]

In the medical school Wilson's duties, demonstrating anatomy
and embryology, were light – there were only 46 students in 1887 –
and so he applied himself to practical needs by starting the Museum
of Normal and Morbid Anatomy, on the ground floor of the new
building. Within two years it held over 700 specimens, earning the
congratulations of the Senate. Wilson never ceased to be fascinated
by laboratory and demonstration techniques, the mounting and
preservation of specimens, photography and photomicrography. So
it was with no sense of penalty that he put in long hours at the

of 1888 to live in a cottage in Stanmore, then a popular suburb with academics, he lived in a boarding house in Macquarie Street, and nearby lived MacCormick. Wilson occasionally assisted MacCormick in emergency operations and went sailing with him. MacCormick looked like a genial farmer, with fingers as fat as sausages, but he was as finely tuned to the art of sailing as he was to that of surgery. Yachts were his only extravagance. Blessed with a strong constitution and a phlegmatic temperament, he was never bothered by heavy seas as many of his guests were, including Almroth Wright and Wilson. Another recreation of the early years was whist with four young cronies at Prince Alfred Hospital. One of them, Cecil Purser a student resident, liked to remember how Wilson 'the mentor of the four, would often stay his hand and remark with emphasis, "This is not whist"', when interest strayed to gossip. Staff and students mixed easily then, for they were few and their age difference small. The 1888 centenary afforded special diversions.[28]

More serious hours were spent studying philosophy with Mungo MacCallum at his new home in Dulwich Hill, where Wilson was a frequent weekend guest. A surviving list of 'Books read' from these years suggests that the pair of them pored over T H Green's *Prolegomena to Ethics*, Edward Caird's *Philosophy of Religion* and *Social Philosophy of Comte*, J S Mill's *Political Economy* and *Autobiography*, R B Haldane's *Adam Smith*, James Seth's 'Inaugural Lecture on Philosophy as the Science of Sciences', Andrew Seth's *Scottish Philosophers and Hegelianism and Personality*, F D Maurice's *The Religions of the World*, Bosanquet's translation of Hegel's *Aesthetics*, Wallace's *Introduction to Hegel's Logic* and various articles in *Mind*. The list also reveals Wilson's wide general reading, with 127 titles ranging over heavy and light literature, old and new. In science he read Darwin's *Life and Letters*, Paget's lecture on cancer in *The Lancet*, W K Parker's *Mammalian Descent*, Foster and Balfour's *Embryology*, Haeckel's *History of Creation Vol I*, Humphry's *Observations in Myology*, T H Huxley's *American Addresses*, Boyd Dawkins' *Early Man in Britain*.[29]

Hermes was right: Wilson really was a scholar. All but a professional student of philosophy, his habitual practice was to read anything worthwhile at least twice. He became known as a formidable man in argument, for he arrived at a point of view only after submitting it to lengthy evaluation. This quality and his real interest in 'broad culture' probably did more to disarm the 'classical' opposition to the medical school than Stuart's bureaucratic politics, clever and successful though he certainly was. Nothing so clearly illustrates the difference between these two men as their attitudes to Chancellor Manning. Stuart treated the old man with ill-concealed contempt. Wilson paid tribute where it was due. Though Manning believed that Arts held the 'very essence' of a university he actively promoted the development of professional schools; it was the extravagance of Stuart's claims for medicine that outraged him. As Chancellor, from 1878, Manning won increased government grants and freed the Challis bequest from English estate duties to provide in the 1880s for schools of law, medicine, science and engineering and he achieved in 1881 the admission of women 'on an equal footing with men', for which reason the women students' union was named Manning House. He also acquired the organ for the Great Hall and proposed a school of music. On his 80th birthday, 20 June 1891, 40 members of the University Musical Society serenaded Sir William, its President, from his garden. Wilson, as Vice-President, proposed the toast and, in the journalese of the day, 'dilated upon the everlasting good which Sir William had done in the interests of The University'.[30]

For his first Australian holiday Wilson took to the bush. In May or September 1887 he visited Theo Barker, his Australian classmate in Edinburgh who had a country practice at Wellington, New South Wales. Wilson learned to ride a horse and accompanied Barker on his rounds. The area reminded him of his native Glencairn and all his life he kept a clear memory of a particular kurrajong tree on a hill overlooking the town. They played whist with the local bank manager and visited the Reverend Fielding whose daughter Una was to become one of Wilson's more distinguished students. Of special interest was an excursion to the Wellington breccia caves, the site of fossil remains of extinct marsupials, discovered in 1831 by the explorer Thomas Mitchell who sent specimens to Sir Richard Owen at the British Museum. Owen's monumental work on these fossils was published in 1877. About the time of his visit Wilson was working on a paper on nerve/muscle relationships in man, including comparative observations from dissections of Australian marsupials. Perhaps he acquired them on this visit. At all events Theo Barker took enough interest in Wilson's work to supply him a few years later with a live platypus.[31]

This most peculiar animal played a role in the federation of Australian science in 1888. In August 1884 when the answer to the long puzzle of platypus reproduction was announced in a telegram to the Biological Section of the British Association for the

Advancement of Science meeting at Montreal, it had a dramatic impact. Proposals to hold a future meeting in Australia foundered but Archibald Liversidge who sent the telegram from Sydney used this international interest to publicize his ambition to form an Australasian Association, its first congress to be during the centennial celebrations planned for Sydney in 1888. And this, with the help of a few others including the distinguished government astronomer H C Russell, he achieved. The first Congress of the Australasian Association for the Advancement of Science, attracting 857 representatives from all the colonies, met at Sydney University on 27 August 1888 for a week of ceremonies, lectures, conversaziones and excursions, H C Russell presiding. Dr E C Stirling of Adelaide announced the discovery of another peculiar Australian animal, the marsupial mole (*Notoryctes typhlops*), which created almost as much interest as the platypus.[32]

When Anderson Stuart wrote to Wilson in August 1886 inviting him to come to Australia, one bait he trailed across the page was the mention of an abundance of research material. MacCormick had exploited this opportunity and in 1885 was awarded the MD with gold medal of Edinburgh University for a thesis on the musculature of the Australian native cat (*Dasyurus viverrinus*). So too had W A Haswell, friend and contemporary of Richard Haldane. With MA and BSc degrees from Edinburgh Haswell was a prize-winning student influenced by Sir Wyville Thomson and T H Huxley in whose wake he followed. He began his Australian research in 1878 in a hut at Watson's Bay, examining material collected by the 'Chevert' expedition to New Guinea; then in 1881 he joined HMS 'Alert' on a marine survey of the Great Barrrier Reef, and with great energy studied the marine fauna of Port Jackson and the adjacent coast. In the 1890s, in collaboration with Professor T J Parker of Otago in New Zealand, he wrote *A Text Book of Zoology*, a standard work which ran through four editions and was translated into Russian.[33]

Wilson's published research began with a study of the innervation of the axillary arch, a small muscle found occasionally in the armpit of humans. Interest centred on the difficulty of establishing its homology,*** the comparative anatomist's main tool for tracing descent. William Turner had earlier suggested it to be a relic of the *panniculus carnosus*, a muscle that moves the skin of loose-skinned mammals. By the 1880s there were three other views, the main one holding that the axillary arch is associated with the musculature of the shoulder girdle. In 1881 Cunningham commended a theory, first advanced by Gegenbaur of the Heidelberg school of anatomy, that nerve-supply is the surest guide to establishing the homology of muscle. This provoked a search for muscle anomalies, especially in the anatomy rooms of Edinburgh University and Trinity College Dublin where Cunningham presided after 1883. So when in 1887, in the Medical School dissecting room, Wilson came across a subject with an axillary muscle in both armpits, he investigated their nerve supply. He found one axillary arch was supplied from a nerve concerned with the innervation of the skin of the upper arm, while the other was supplied from a nerve concerned with the innervation of the inner and back skin of the upper arm. Taking into account the findings of others and his own dissections of a cat, a possum, a kangaroo-rat and a wallaby, he concluded that the evidence supported Turner's view. This paper was published in January 1888 in the *Journal of Anatomy and Physiology*.[34]

The following year Ambrose Birmingham of the National University of Ireland published a more comprehensive study of the subject and concluded that the axillary arch is normally innervated by a nerve which runs at a deeper level and supplies the muscle of the ribcage; this conclusion seemed to exclude Turner's view and conflicted with Wilson's interpretation of the innervation of his two specimens of the axillary arch, one of which Birmingham dismissed as 'an abnormality'. This spurred Wilson to explore the question further. The autopsy room of the Prince Alfred Hospital furnished him with seven more instances of the axillary arch, in five of which he traced the nerve of supply and examined other nerves more or less related to it. In 1890 he reported that three of his five specimens supported Birmingham's thesis but the other two were further examples of 'abnormal' cases. So while accepting Birmingham's main conclusions he challenged the term 'abnormal'. His research had shown they were not by any means rare; they were more like variations.[35]

Other kinds of variations in nerve-muscle relationships came to Wilson's attention in the dissecting room in 1888. One study was concerned with the variation in the nerve supply to the *quadratus femoris*, a member of a group of small muscles concerned in the stabilization of the hip joint. Another was concerned with the first lumbrical muscle of the hand, in which two specimens showed almost identical variations. These two further contributions to the debate led him to conclude that, contrary to accepted theory, nerve and muscle were not uniformly correlated and that 'the essential

73

morphological character of such variations is in all probability a transference of nerve-fibres from one path to another'.[36]

These four short tersely-written papers, the first research results of a lifelong interest in muscle innervation and homologies, show the qualities that made Wilson an important scientist: thorough grasp of the issues under investigation, meticulous observation and keen critical appraisal of the findings. Edinburgh's bias to comparative anatomy is evident and his first paper in 1888 on the axillary arch reveals Turner's influence, but his second on that subject in 1890 established an independent position. His findings in all four papers had sufficient clinical as well as morphological importance to be included in the next revision of Quain's *Anatomy*. 'Turner has a great opinion of you', wrote Jim Smith.[37]

Wilson's abiding interest in neurology probably began in Edinburgh with his demonstrations to senior students on the brain and organs of special sense. His first papers on muscle innervation marked the beginning of the lecture course which so impressed his students, even those most critical of his dry descriptive delivery. He scoured European and American journals for current developments in neurological research to expand and update them and for illustrative material which Louis converted into slides for the epidiascope; his own research furnished him with more information and slides. He assembled a huge arsenal of material to illustrate his neurology lectures to students and to audiences like the Linnean Society and the Royal Society of NSW. From 1897 he supplied material to C J Martin, by then acting professor of physiology at Melbourne University, to help him build a neurology course. These were the beginnings of a distinguished pattern of neuroscience in Australia.[38]

Funds from the Challis bequest began to flow into the University coffers in 1889, and with them were established chairs in Anatomy, Law, Philosophy and History, for which applications were invited from the Australian colonies and the United Kingdom. Wilson completed his application on 31 October 1889. He briefly recorded his qualifications and experience, mentioned his work on the Museum, appended a list of his publications, testimonials from William Turner and Anderson Stuart, also one independently got up by all 70 of his students past and present, testifying to his excellence as a teacher. He addressed himself to the main threat: the short-list prepared by the Selection Committee in Britain. He wrote that he had accepted the post as demonstrator of anatomy in 1887 knowing that a chair was soon to be created and believing that faithful service

early neurology lectures

in this subordinate position would constitute an additional qualification. Sir William Turner in 1886 had mentioned this aspect of his case in recommending acceptance of his present position. By that decision he had given up 'a very fortunate position on the staff of a renowned school of Anatomy' which also meant he was not eligible for consideration by the British Selection Committee. Had he remained in Britain he said he would surely have been on that Committee's short-list.[39]

Anderson Stuart's testimonial strongly supported Wilson's application. He testified to Wilson's excellence in teaching, research and museum work, mentioned the good relations Wilson enjoyed with his colleagues and emphasized his 'high principle and strength of character': Wilson was eminently fitted for the chair and deserved it. He concluded with a telling point:

> I do not say we might not get as good a man, but I do most unhesitatingly say that the chances are all against our getting another man whom we know to be as good. The Senate can otherwise only select one of the European candidates, none of whom it can see or know. The Home Committee can say no more than that these three were the best that have applied and it is precluded from drawing any comparison between them and Dr Wilson. Thus ultimately the Senate has to choose between a man whose efficiency is proved by three years of experience, and men of whose fitness it can only judge by testimonials; and the very best testimonials cannot speak of many personal qualities which go far to make a good teacher ... I would regard the severance of his connection with the University a great loss to the whole institution not only to the medical school.[40]

The three-months' wait for the Senate's decision were anxious ones for Wilson and his parents, being the culmination of three years' labour for a prize on which hung all their fortunes. He had good reason to entertain high hopes but, highly strung by nature and encumbered more than most young men by family responsibilities, his confidence must at times have wavered. It was rumoured that D J Cunningham had applied. Probably Wilson knew that to be false but he also knew that Johnson Symington was a contender and a serious challenge: another product of Turner's school, Symington was ten years older than Wilson with an established reputation and a senior position at Minto House in Edinburgh. As Haswell observed later, 'though all the probabilities seemed in [Wilson's] favour, there was still the possibility that something might miscarry'.[41] The fateful day of the Senate Meeting was 3 February 1890. Three days later Wilson wrote this account of that day to his fiancee Jeanie Smith at Half Morton:

> I can hardly bring myself to think what I did previous to the Senate meeting. The same morning I saw the Chancellor who seemed somewhat favourably disposed. When the Senate met I couldnt help feeling pretty confident as to the result. I had to go to the farewell dinner to Scott the same evg. and so I took down my dress suit in a bag to MacCormicks & I had posted a boy at the door of the Senate meeting place who was to get a note from Stuart with the result and bring it to me. Then I went and had a shave after which I went back to MacCormicks & took possession of his room (he was out) and started 'A Society Clown' by Guy Grossmith. This was after four about five o'clock. I considered with myself what would happen if I failed and I think somehow I could have faced it. Before half past five the boy came with a couple of lines pencilled by Stuart and in opening the paper my hand trembled. All the day before I had been stoically calm. The note contained the information Law Mr Pitt Cobbett Elected Anatomy J T Wilson Elected Philosophy Francis Anderson Elected History postponed. I then sent the boy out to Stanmore with a note to my father & mother and went down to the GPO & telegraphed to Mrs MacCallum at Blackheath according to a promise and cabled to you ... Then I went back to MacCormicks & finished my story book. Then I dressed & went down to Scott's dinner where I received my first congratulations from all the Professors & Lecturers present to the number of about fifteen. Anderson was of course there too. We had a very jolly dinner. MacCallum occupied the foot of the table & Anderson and I were on his left & right. Gurney as Dean of the Faculty of Arts was in the Chair. I neednt describe the dinner. The healths of the new professors were drunk & first I, and then Anderson responded.[42]

The three British candidates were an Englishman, an Irishman and a Scotsman. Dr Anderson of London withdrew his candidature. Dr St John Brooks of Dublin was recommended by an Irishman and in the Senate was proposed by an Irishman, Sir Patrick Jennings, but received only two votes. The Scot, Johnson Symington, the real threat to Wilson, was not even proposed. As Wilson explained to Jeanie: 'This does not mean that his claims were thought lightly of but that everyone of his possible supporters had already weighed his claims against mine & decided that on the whole my claims were greater'. Better a Scot you know than one you don't was perhaps a piece of wisdom the Senate had picked up over the preceding seven years. Wilson's appointment was 'universally approved' in Sydney. *Hermes* expressed the general feeling on 3 April 1890 when it registered pleasure that 'Those two trusty and well-beloved erswhile lecturers – Mr F Anderson and Mr J T Wilson – have been appointed to Challis Professorships in their respective subjects'.[43]

Mr and Mrs Thomas Wilson in Stanmore were overjoyed when the news arrived by messenger late on the afternoon of 3 February. A close friend Alexander McKinley who was staying with them at the time recorded the moment: 'Your mother's face was burning with joy. And your father's heart was welling into his eyes as they told me the good news. "Laus Deo" your mother repeated'. Soon afterwards both parents were busy with preparations to receive a daughter-in-law. It involved the fitting out of another cottage, for which Wilson again committed himself to debt, this time to his uncle Henry Glover.[44]

Jeanie's reaction was lively: 'My dearest Professor', she addressed her letter of 5 February. 'The joyful tidings of your appointment came on Monday evening after six o'clock. I can't say we were surprised but it is a wonderful relief. Still I have to stop and assure myself that it is really true'. Jeanie and her sister Maggie were occupied in the drawing room with visitors when the cablegram arrived: 'I heard the machine stop', Jeanie continued, '& so did my heart. Maggie went out & then when she asked me to go I knew it was the dear message'.[45]

Jeanie and Maggie were just then overburdened with anxiety about their father who, now ill and weary of life, faced retirement under the distressing renewal of sectarian friction in the parish, which of all things promised to install an Englishman in the Free Church and Manse of Half Morton. The Free Church all over Scotland was on the decline. As the brothers were away building their careers, and Annie courageously doing the same, Jeanie and Maggie bore the brunt of the domestic crisis. The news from Sydney gave clear definition to Jeanie's future and the domestic arrangements of the Smith family. They decided to move to Edinburgh. But first holidays were badly needed. Maggie would take their father to Bridge of Allan to restore his health and spirits, but that waited on improved weather. Jeanie decided to visit brother Jim in Oxford.

Classic Oxford was a welcome change from the gloom of Half Morton. Jeanie stayed a month at Jim's lodgings at 37 Walton Street. She found him well but too busy with physiology, philosophy and John Haldane to spare her much time, even for their planned study of German. But Jeanie quickly got to know Mrs Wilson, the young bride of a local medical practitioner and together they explored the ancient town. They sampled public lectures at the Sheldonian Theatre, heard a service at Magdalen Chapel, looked in on Jim at work in a physiology laboratory, heard the Union debate 'that in the opinion of this House the tone of thought in Oxford is not conducive to originality or greatness', and watched the university sports and the college boat races. The best part was Jeanie's feast of music: she attended as many of John Farmer's Sunday evening concerts and Monday 'hall singings' as she could, as well as Keble College concerts on Thursday evenings. On Sundays when Jim was free they explored the countryside, for Oxford was still a small town. 'It was a profitable way of spending church time' commented Jeanie who for a daughter of the manse carried her religion lightly. One particular Sunday, appropriately in the teeth of an east wind, they walked to Cumnor and saw where Cumnor Hall once stood, and the grave of Tony Foster whose tablet proclaimed him a saint and not the villain portrayed in Scott's *Kenilworth*.

Oxford's academic community was hospitable but Jeanie maintained a Scottish wariness. She was bracing herself for her new life as the wife of a university professor which, after more than three years of weekly letters, was presenting more distinct outlines. Unreality was dissolving: 'I can now take all your proposals in earnest' she had written from Half Morton on 5 February. From Oxford on 27 February she wrote 'I don't mind anyone knowing now when the end can be seen', for the news of their engagement was out on both sides of the world, associated as it was with Wilson's appointment to the Sydney chair.

In some quarters it added warmth to her reception, for instance with Dr and Mrs J Arthur Thomson. A frank warm-hearted man and another Turner product, Arthur Thomson was then a lecturer in anatomy in Oxford. He had been on the 'home' selection committee for the Sydney chair and told Jeanie of the bad feeling that bedevilled its proceedings and those of the Anatomical Society meeting in London which on the proposal of Turner and Hepburn elected Wilson as its first overseas member. In one quarter Jeanie had a cool reception, from the Fairbrothers, which she attributed to his not getting the Sydney chair of Philosophy: 'I suppose if Fairbrother had run the risk you ran in going out as you did he would have had a better chance'.[46]

Jeanie was learning that beneath the surface of monastic Oxford there flowed hazardous worldly currents. As in all universities material ambition muddied the pure streams of intellectual, moral and spiritual aspiration. With some apprehension she noticed another component of academic life, the self-conscious efforts of wives to further their husbands' careers. Mrs Sanderson turned the gas off and on for her husband's lantern lectures, and looked 'immensely satisfied to be able to assist her dear husband'; Mrs Gotch was 'studying physiology zealously to help her husband'; Mrs Thomson 'has an ambition to be a help to her husband. She says so herself but she is too fragile to do heavy work'. Like Mrs Garran who 'entertains undergraduates every day from 5 to 6 & has a smoking party every Sunday evening', Mrs Thomson put her efforts into hospitality. For her part Jeanie welcomed her brother Jim's friends and colleagues to lunch and dinner and made a point 'as in duty bound' to call on Mrs Sanderson and Mrs Thomson. The social highlight of her stay was dinner at the Burdon Sandersons. 'We survived it' she reported on 12 March.

> There were some others there. Miss Haldane her brother Mrs Birkbeck Hill & Miss Hill. And three students beside our honoured selves. I was taken in by His Silent Mightiness John Scott Haldane. I made a brave attempt to converse with him but I simply gave it up when he did not respond.[47]

Haldane was making Oxford his base under the patronage of his eminent uncle Professor Burdon Sanderson and wanted both of his Edinburgh friends with him. Jim Smith was drawn to comply. Previously he had been inclined to try Sydney. Now he joined forces with Haldane to persuade Wilson to visit Oxford. Plans may even have been floated for an Edinburgh wedding but at all events through Jeanie they recommended Oxford to Wilson:

> Jim regrets very much that you can't see your way to strip yr. summer session and come here to study – he thinks it of immense benefit. He is also not so sure whether he will go to Sydney even if he were to get the offer – he thinks it would be so much better if he could manage to stay at Oxford & it seems possible, but I can say nothing definite – only I have assured you before about certainty & I may as well tell you of doubt.

Jim Smith did stay on in Oxford to collaborate with Haldane and, as Jeanie knew in advance, Wilson declined. To 'strip the summer session' was quite unreal, if only for the reason that Wilson's senior colleague in Sydney had precisely the same idea.[48]

In Oxford another young man was then weighing the pros and cons of accepting the chair in Modern History in Sydney. Against the advantage of 'a tidy berth' as Jim Smith referred to Wilson's chair, George Arnold Wood considered the disadvantages. He would be half the world away from his family and Oxford and the historical sources that held his interest. Professor Scott, on leave from Sydney, had a mission to persuade Wood to accept the Sydney chair and Wood's Australian friend at Oxford G W Thatcher advised him:

> If you want to study old European historical records, don't go. But
> if you want to study history in the making and become yourself a
> maker of men – go!

By a few days Jeanie missed meeting Professor Scott. 'As it is I must wait for the pleasure a little longer' she wrote on 20 March: till 1891, when she would meet Arnold Wood also, in Sydney.[49]

Jeanie was refreshed by Oxford and felt equal to 'the flitting and then the trousseau' when she returned to Half Morton. She had acquired, she remarked wryly, a 'cosmopolitan mind' and felt none too patient with dreary parish affairs: 'They are all so serious & oppressed by their afflictions and especially by their religion' she reported after a meeting of church office bearers. 'Mr Johnston asked me if I had been at the Eng. Ch. Service. Luckily I had but I did not describe the service particularly – only a choral service on a week day'. A church on the defensive and an epidemic of influenza in the parish would have been depressing enough, but in addition Jeanie found her father again very ill. He was in fact in a final decline and died soon after the Smiths moved to 33 Leamington Terrace, Edinburgh. So Jeanie and Maggie, in the sadness of mourning and impending separation, put together Jeanie's trousseau. On 27 June she paid on deposit half the fare for her passage to Australia on the P&O ship *Carthage*, and on 24 July 1890 she left London for Sydney. 'Of course I shall like Australia' she had written on 5 February, 'people make places'. But it was a comfort that in a few years they could return: 'It is delightful to think of your getting a year off after a few years – we must be very economical so as to go when we will'.[50]

Wilson greeted Jeanie in Adelaide at 6.30am on 4 September, and they were married later that day at the Chalmers Presbyterian Church on North Terrace. By happy coincidence the ceremony was conducted by the Reverend Dr Paton who hailed from Dalton, the parish of Jeanie's mother's people in Dumfriesshire. In Sydney they went to live in a cottage they called 'Glencairn' in Stanmore Road, within neighbourly distance of Mr and Mrs Wilson. At the beginning of term a detachment of the Musical Society serenaded the newlyweds.[51]

Jeanie had thought about her new life and was prepared to tackle

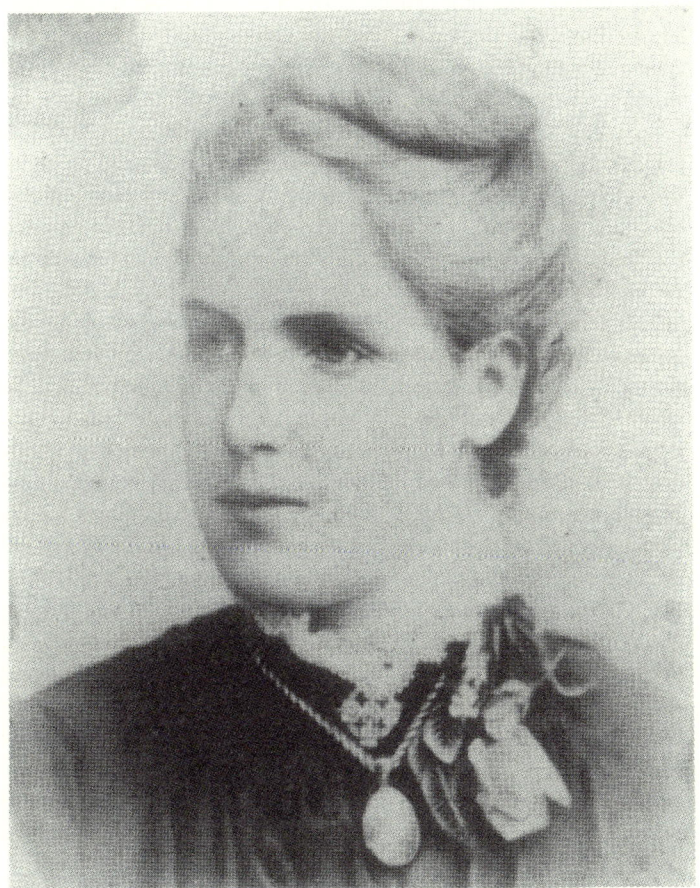

Jane Elizabeth Wilson (née Smith), c.1890   Wilson Papers, SUA

it with energy and resource. The Burwood Presbyterian Church offered a familiar outlet for her but a more lively one was the University Musical Society of which Wilson was currently Vice-President; it had a lot of female associate members and gave young men like Christopher Brennan opportunities to meet young ladies with serious as well as light-hearted interests. Brennan was then 'a rollicking carefree' classics student and the editor of *Hermes*, showing already the brilliance and waywardness of his life as a poet and scholar. The Students' Union welcomed women to its debates and Jeanie did her philanthropic bit for the University Women's Society.[52]

The final term of 1890 was very busy for Wilson as Acting Dean.

With the first phase of the medical school completed Anderson Stuart left for Europe in September and the Fates conspired to gratify his appetite for limelight. In November Robert Koch startled the medical world by announcing he had discovered in tuberculin a cure for tuberculosis and the NSW Government cabled Anderson Stuart to enquire about Koch's method and, if practicable, to secure a supply of the vaccine. The Governments of South Australia and New Zealand extended this brief. Stuart interviewed Koch in Berlin and reported that his discovery was 'great ... not so much for what it actually accomplishes, as for what it promises for the future'. While in Europe he met other great scientists including Louis Pasteur to whom he was introduced by Pasteur's nephew, M Loir, who had been investigating Australia's rabbit problem, which Stuart also discussed with Koch. So when he returned to Sydney in March 1891 Anderson Stuart had a lot of people waiting to hear what he had to say. This trip was highly successful and he repeated the exercise the following year, probably aiming this time at the distinction of Fellowship of the Royal Society for his research on the eye and the larynx, published in the *Lancet* and the *Philosophical Transactions of the Royal Society* in 1891 and 1892. His visit was noticed by *The Times*, he addressed the British Association and the Royal College of Physicians and was entertained by the presidents of both medical colleges. He saw Pasteur again and made further enquiries about Koch's tuberculosis treatment which confirmed his first opinion: 'The indications ... in my first report have been fully borne out, and although the Koch treatment is in practice, I think I might say it is all an utter failure so far'. These efforts opened a new avenue for Anderson Stuart's ambitions. In June 1891 he was appointed to the NSW Board of Health.[53]

Wilson was immersed in his duties at the Medical School and in his private world. Jeanie was expecting their first child. On Monday 13 July 1891 a daughter was born, and in the anatomy class that day the news was greeted with cheering. Then tragedy struck. Three days later, on Thursday 16 July, Jeanie died, according to her death certificate of 'cystic tumour of ovary'. She haemorrhaged. The facts were recorded briefly in the *Sydney Morning Herald* and the *Australasian Medical Gazette*. From Wilson's pen one brief message survives from this moment, written to this hapless daughter 27 years later:

Do you know that you are now just about the age that your mother reached. She was born on 9th April, 1864. She was so pleased with her little baby girl for the very brief period before she sank.[54]

Perhaps, as the eyes of one man might reflect the pain of his friend, we see Wilson's anguish in the lines Jeanie's brother Jim wrote to him from Freiburg in Germany:

> My dear Jim, I simply do not know what to say to you. I think that long after we might talk of Jeanie. I do not know what we would say. Yet we must do it some day. I often wonder if the baby remains to us to be another Jeanie. I do hope she will just be her mother again.

And so, in many ways, she was. She was given her mother's names, and that of her mother's sister and family, Jane Elizabeth Margaret Lorrain. And like her mother she was always called Jeanie. Like her mother too she grew to be beautiful, musical and spirited.[55]

Haldane heard the news from Jim Smith and wrote immediately:

> I am indeed very very sorry for you – what else to write I don't know. It is just the saddest thing that can come upon a man. Of course I had got to know your wife while she was with her brother in Oxford. She belonged to the best & strongest of what Scotland can produce, & few of the people I have met impressed me as much as she did. She seemed so strong both in her beliefs and disbeliefs and in the keenness of her feelings about the big things of life ... I wonder what you think now of some of the things we used to discuss. I think they trouble me less than they used to. I can see enough just to make me content to leave them & my life in God's hands, & work at what there does seem a prospect of settling. Perhaps it is something the same with you. And if it is it will take away the hopelessness of your sorrow.

It was a good thing that Wilson had his parents in Sydney at this time Haldane thought; nevertheless he pressed the claims of Oxford as a refuge.[56]

Almroth Wright, holidaying in Ireland, wrote with a better grasp of the realities of Wilson's predicament, for he had left Sydney only six months before:

> We were dreadfully shocked and I have had you in my mind ever since. I wish I had been near enough to come to you ... I am looking out over the bay that stretches away to underneath the hills from the window at which I sit and yet a good deal of me is in Sydney with you. The term will be beginning again when this reaches you and I shall be working in the London fogs. One has simply to grope one's way through them and yet our work is very like only you have yours to do in solitude again.[57]

'Bright beautiful Jeanie' was gone, but life went on. Anxiety over his infant daughter prevailed for a year. His parents again made their home with him and during the summer the bereaved family went to Blackheath. But Jeanie's life was endangered there by 'infantile diarrhoea' and what was later called 'dietary deficiency in vitamins'. Mrs Martin probably saved her life by recommending a wet nurse, advice to which Mrs MacCallum was 'most well meaningly averse'. As well as a devoted father and two devoted grandparents, little Jeanie had in these women two self-appointed guardian angels. Wilson took up the violin and photography and went about his university duties, taking the leadership of the faculty for the third term while Anderson Stuart was in Europe, and groped his way through grief and anxiety. Excerpts from the Scriptures became embedded in his being: 'Whoso followeth Christ shall not walk in darkness but shall have the light of Life'; and 'The eternal god is thy refuge, and underneath are the everlasting arms'.[58]

Notes

1. JTW to parents, 18.1.1887. [Also for first paragraph.]
2. 'a little man': Crawford, 114. 'the brilliant' and 'that coming': MWM, quoted in *The Union Recorder*, 8.10.1942, 192.
3. 'The sentiment of': Harrison, 349.
4. Empire, economy, non-intervention: Eldridge, 118–19, 153. Pacific interests: Meaney, 18. 'We seem, as it were': Eldridge. 'simply wash our': JTW to parents, 16.2.1885 and 17.2.1887.
5. 'a sort of trio': JTW to parents, 17.2.1887. 'a fascinating pair': JTW in *Southerly*, No. 2, 1944, 8. Caird: Mackenzie, 510–12; Muirhead 1942, 30–5.
6. JTW to parents, 18.2.1887.
7. 'a dab at': JTW to parents, 18.2.1887. 'there are many' and 'an improvement': JTW to parents, 17.2.1887. 'MacCallum and I': JTW to parents, 3.3.1887.
8. 'when of course' and university people: JTW to parents, 3.3.1887. The medical school & PAH buildings: JTW to JLS (fragment n.d. ? March 1887).
9. 'an exceptionally nice' and 'a sharp man': JTW to JLS (fragment n.d. ? March 1887).
   * 'Jummy' was probably the Australian rendition of the Scot's accented 'Jimmy'.
10. Appointment to PAH: JTW to JES, Feb. 1890. Pathologist and Hon. Sec. positions: Alfred Roberts to JTW, 9.4.1892.; JTW to Dr Schlink, 29.1.1945, in Maddox, 179; Epps, 88. 'mortal terror': *Senior*

Year Book 1922, 8. 'The shrugging': AEM, Valedictory Speech 'Professor Wilson', in *SUMJ*, Oct. 1920, 5, 6.

11. 'Politics are a rather': JTW to parents, 3.3.1887. 'an awfully': JTW to JES (fragment n.d.? March 1887).

12. TPAS, 1903, 77.

13. Senate – Hospital link: Blackburn, 1948, 114–16.

14. 'of the very': Manning, Chancellor's Address 1886. SUA.

15. 'After Homeric' etc.: Liversidge was a driving force in the Royal Society of NSW, an original member of the Board of Technical Education, and the Industrial Technological and Sanitary Museum, a trustee of the Australian Museum, the founder of AAAS and the Sydney section of Society of Chemical Industry. D P Mellor on Liversidge, *ADB*. Threlfall: Mulvaney & Calaby, 138. 'In a new country': TWED, quoted in M E David, 24.

16. 'When the battle': TPAS, 1903, 77. 'the foundations': quoted in Epps, 51, 58. *Centenary Book* 174–5.
    ** A riddle set by Anderson Stuart, probably referring to his own beak-like nose.

17. Medical Bldg: *Centenary Book,* Ch. 10 (riddle, f.n. 485). 'To this magnificent': TPAS, 1903, 81.

18. 'no starving' etc: Manning, 1886 address.

19. Univ. funding and 'an immense block': Manning to Brownless, 3.5.1886, Melb. Univ. Archives, M142, 7–8. 'The [Medical] Faculty' and 'The Report': Manning to Brownless, 6.12.1886, 9. Brownless to Manning, 11.5.1886, Melb. Univ. Arch.

20. 'as something' and 'some flair': Blackburn, 122, 132. Careers, MacLaurin & Renwick: *Centenary Book.*

21. TPAS' wife's death and 'thick epidermis': *SSM,* 137–8. 'As to myself': TPAS to JTW, 15.8.1886.

22. TPAS' powers of appointment: *SSM.* 'enlargeable' and 'the Board': TPAS to JTW, 15.8.1886.

23. Shewan's work: Epps, 53. Selection of MacCormick: TPAS to JTW, 11.4.1886. MacCormick as surgeon: Sir Douglas Miller, 191 and *SSM.* 'one of the great': JTW to Carslaw, 22.7.1943. Graham: TPAS to JTW, 11.4.1886; and *Centenary Book.* James Graham: alderman on Sydney City Council from 1888, Lord Mayor 1901, an MLA 1894–1901, 1907–10.

24. Edinburgh men: Catherine Mackerras, interview with author 1971. Individual staff: *Centenary Book.* Almroth Wright: Colebrook in *RSO* (1948), and corresp. Wright and JTW. CJM: corresp. with JTW.

25. 'He comes with': *Hermes,* 24.3.1887, 8. 'Upon my word': TPAS to JTW, 11.4.1886.

26. Foundation of Medical Society: *ibid.* 'although somewhat lengthy': *Hermes,* 23.5.1888. Wilson relied heavily on, and quoted extensively from, Haldane's exposition in a published essay, probably 'Life and Mechanism' in *Mind,* 27–47. See JTW, 1899, 9.

27. Student numbers 1887: TPAS, Common Place Book. Anatomy Museum (now the Burkitt Library): TPAS in testimonial supporting JTW's application for Challis Chair, 20.11.1889. WP and Brodsky, 114. 'small common-looking' and 'splendid man': JTW to J, 22.7.1936; Brodsky, 109. Museum Curators: *Centenary Book.*

28. Wilson's residence: Family photograph. Sailing: MacCormick to JTW, 26.12.1941. 'the mentor of': Cecil Purser to JTW, 11.10.1941.

29. Studies with MWM: JTW, 'Memories of MacCallum' in *Southerly,* No. 2, 1944, 9. 'Books read': list in Wilson Papers.

30. TPAS' treatment of Manning: Catherine Mackerras to J. (n.d.).Manning's work: Rutledge, *ADB* 1851–90. 'dilated upon': *SMH,* 21 or 23 June 1891.

31. Sir Richard Owen and Wellington Caves: JTW to KR, 7.9.1941; Moyal 1986, 62. Live platypus: JTW and CJM, 1893d, 190–200.

32. Platypus and Australian science: MacLeod (ed.), 28–35, 40–2. Marsupial mole: *ibid.* 41; Troughton, 57.

33. MacCormick's thesis: Miller. Haswell: *PLS* 1928, 485–98. *** Homology: attributes of two organisms are homologous when they are derived from an equivalent characteristic of a common ancestor.

34. Cunningham's 1881 paper, Int. Medical Congress, London. Published 1882.

35. Birmingham's paper: *J of A* 1889, 206–17. JTW, 1890b. 52, 60. Cunningham 1891.

36. JTW, 1890a, 26.

37. 'Turner has': JLS to JTW, 19.3.1889.

38. Illustrative material: S A Smith, 7. 'Recent investigations': Royal Society of NSW, *Journal,* Vol. 27, 489. Neurology material to CJM: CJM to JTW, 16.8.97.

39. Testimonial for JTW was initiated by Dr H V C Hinder. 'a very fortunate': JTW to Senate of U of S, 31.10.1889.

40. TPAS, Testimonial, 20.11.1889 attached to JTW application to Senate.

41. 'though all the': WAH to JTW, 6.4.1890.

42. 'I can hardly': JTW to JES, 6.2.1890.

43. 'This does not mean' and 'universally approved': JTW to JES, 11.2.1890. 'Those two trusty': *Hermes* , 3.4.1890, 2.

44. 'Your mother's face': A McKinley to JTW, 1.6.1920. Debt to Henry Glover: F 7.2a. in WP.

45. JES to JTW, 5.2.1890, 27.2.1890, 6.3.1890, 12.3.1890 and 20.3.1890. [Also for next three paras].
46. Arthur Thomson was opposed to JLS going to Oxford to work on pathology, which JSH was trying to achieve. Thomson apparently had different ideas for development of pathology there. JLS did not find Thomson 'frank and warm-hearted', but conceited: JLS to JTW, 4.8.1891. 'I suppose if': JES to JTW, 27.2.1890. Samuel Alexander also thought of applying for the philosophy chair but did not, assuming (correctly) that the local man would be appointed: JES to JTW, 20.3.1890.
47. 'immensely satisfied' and 'studying physiology': JES to JTW, 27.2.1890. 'has an ambition': JES to JTW, 6.3.1890. 'entertains undergraduates' and 'as in duty bound': JES to JTW, 12.3.1890. 'There were some': JES to JTW, 12.3.1890.
48. 'Jim regrets': JES to JTW, 20.2.1890. TPAS' summer trip: *Hermes*, 20.10.1890.
49. Arnold Wood's decision and 'If you want': Crawford, 108–10.
50. 'the flitting', 'They are all' and 'Mr Johnston': JES to JTW, 20.3.1890. Fare deposit and departure date: ticket from P & O. 'Of course I', and 'It is delightful': JES to JTW, 5.2.1890.
51. Jeanie's arrival in Adelaide: *The Times*, 5.9.1890. Marriage details supplied to author by *ADB* Office, Canberra. Dr Paton: JTW to J, 4.9.1935. *Hermes*, 20.10.1890, 2.
52. University Musical Society, and 'a rollicking carefree': Axel Clark, 30. Jeanie was a Vice President of the University Women's Society in 1891: *Hermes*, 19.8.1891.
53. TPAS' trip: U of S Calendar for 1891, 367–8. *AMG*, Sept. 1890, 331. 'great ... not so much' and 'The indications': quoted Epps, 69. Roy MacLeod drew the author's attention to a letter from Liversidge in Sydney to Thistelton Dyer, Director of Kew Gardens, 26.9.1891, discussing Stuart's ambition and prospects of an FRS.
54. Cheering by anatomy class: J, 'The Story of the Shaping of one tutorial lecturer in psychology', Dept of Adult Education, Univ. of Sydney, 1924–1970 (unpub. notes). 'Do you know': JTW to J, 12.7.1918.
55. 'My dear Jim': JLS to JTW, 4.8.1891.
56. 'I am indeed': JSH to JTW, 20.7.1891.
57. 'We were dreadfully': Wright to JTW, 10.9.1891.
58. 'Bright beautiful Jeanie': JLS to JTW, 4.8.1891. 'infantile diarrhoea', 'dietary deficiency' and 'most well meaningly': JTW to J, 18.10.1933. JTW's new hobbies: J, early draft, biographical sketch of JTW. 'Whoso followeth': Deuteronomy, 33:27.

5

The Fraternity of Duckmaloi

Early in 1892 Wilson opened a new window on the world. He began
to look closely at Australia's marsupials and monotremes which from
the earliest years of white settlement had attracted international
scientific interest. Australia's fauna confounded established
taxonomic principles. The platypus for example, first described in
1799 by Dr George Shaw from a skin at the British Museum, was
thought to be a taxidermist's creation until anatomical research was
done on further specimens in 1802 by Everard Home. Shaw's generic
name of *Platypus* had to be changed to *Ornithorynchus* but the term
platypus stuck. Although J F Meckel discovered its mammary gland
in 1824 and its production of milk was demonstrated in 1832 by L
Maule, controversy still surrounded *Ornithorynchus*: should it be
classified as a mammal and how did it reproduce? Sir John Jamison
wrote from Sydney in 1817 that it was oviparous but European
zoologists continued to argue about this until 1884 when the
Cambridge embryologist W H Caldwell reported on eggs unearthed
from the banks of the Burnett River in Queensland. In a dramatic
telegram relayed by Liversidge in Sydney he announced to the British
Association meeting in Montreal on 29 August: '*Monotreme
oviparous, ovum meroblastic*' which, being interpreted, means that
monotremes lay eggs with large yolks which do not divide into cells
but are absorbed as food by the developing young, as with birds. Yet
like mammals they suckle their young. So where did it fit in the
evolutionary scheme of things? In 1848 Verreaux had observed that
the internal structure of *Ornithorynchus* 'resembles that of certain
reptiles, and appears to form a link between the Mammals and
Lizards'. Now, nearly 40 years on, Professor Parker in *Mammalian
Descent* was still at a loss on where to place the monotremes.[1]

88

Until the 1880s naturalists in Australia had been collectors showing little interest in theories of descent, even though they might stand or fall on the evidence of Australian fauna. Sir Richard Owen's commanding stature as Britain's leading comparative anatomist and palaeontologist had held Australian naturalists in thrall for 50 years. From the 1830s they had sent him large consignments of specimens for his classification and speculation on the Creator's inscrutable design. By 1840 when in his mid-thirties Owen had become an authority on marsupials and monotremes, which of all the exotic forms that came under his notice interested him most. Owen was a creationist who, while admitting that animals have 'an innate tendency to deviate from the parental type', liked to think they deviated according to a divine plan. Evolution occurred, but only within the boundaries of ideal types. He clarified the concept of homology (as distinct from analogy),* the comparative anatomist's main tool for tracing descent, but rejected Darwin's theory that the mechanism of evolution was natural selection. For Owen the pouch of the marsupial was 'irrefragable evidence of Creative foresight'.[2]

[handwritten margin note: Sir Richard Owen, a creationist]

[handwritten margin note: homology]

[handwritten margin note: pouch = creation]

Owen's authority gradually eroded from about 1870 at home and abroad. It was vanquished in Australia in the 1890s by a new generation of professionally trained scientists for whom Darwinian theory was the organizing principle. Their first spokesman in NSW, William Haswell, in his Presidential Address to the Biology Section of the Australasian Association for the Advancement of Science in 1891 said:

> this illuminating influence, which has lent tenfold interest to the work of every investigator of animated nature, had also shown to him ... that, while not leaving his particular corner of the field, he is doing work that is of interest to a comparatively wide circle of thinking men.[3]

Haswell, MacCormick and Wilson in Sydney, Stirling in Adelaide and Baldwin Spencer and his assistant Arthur Dendy in Melbourne were the pioneers of this new era in Australian biology. Steeped in modern evolutionary concepts, skilled in histology and microscopy, they mounted sustained Australian-based investigations into Australian fauna. They were looking to fill in the gaps in the genealogical tree of

---

* Analogy: denotes different organs of functional similarity among different animals (e.g. fins of fish and wings of birds) whereas homology – a term coined by Owen – refers to the same organs in different animals under every variety of form and function.

89

Darwin's inspiration, or the 'missing links' in the evolutionary sequence of T H Huxley's hierarchies. Australia's peculiar animals which had never fitted comfortably in Owen's morphological system might help them solve some of the puzzles of evolution.

Wilson's research started with an investigation of the strange little silky-furred burrowing animal without external ears or eyes, the marsupial mole (*Notoryctes typhlops*), whose discovery in South Australia in 1888 had created a sensation among mammologists around the world akin to that attending the discovery of the platypus. With specimens and other material contributed by Dr Stirling, Baldwin Spencer, the Australian Museum in Sydney, and Jim Smith (then at Cambridge with a research studentship), Wilson started on the myology of the marsupial mole. It was a long and frustrating job, due to the lack of comparative data, and was not published until 1894. Running to 60 pages of text and 15 plates this paper reveals Wilson at his most relentless. He added to his research on the specimens an exhaustive comparative review of British, European and Australian sources so as to discuss more thoroughly the numerous anomalous features which gave rise to doubts about the mole's systematic position and affinities. As well as *Marsupialia* he gave attention to the *Monotremata, Edentata, Insectivora, Rodentia* and *Carnivora*. His prime interest was not so much this animal's muscles as their nerve supply, which was to be the subject of a second study. This did not eventuate, but it indicates Wilson's continued preoccupation with nerve/muscle relationships, the subject of his first four papers published in 1888/9. Comparative neurology was his dominant research focus.[4]

In 1892 Wilson was juggling several projects. For the Intercolonial Medical Congress held in Sydney in September 1892 he wrote two papers; one on the closure of the central canal of the spinal cord in the foetal lamb which showed he was fully up to date with embryology studies in Britain, Europe and America; the other on a series of varieties in human anatomy. He also wrote a short abstract on the craniology of the Australian Aborigines appended to an account of Aborigines by a certain Dr Fraser for the Chicago Exhibition. As well he was collaborating with a former student W J Stewart McKay in research on the homologies of the borders and surfaces of the scapula in monotremes. McKay went on to do an extensive investigation of the shoulder girdle of the monotremes. What focused their interest in this area was the fact that the platypus grew an inter-clavicle bone in its shoulder girdle, a feature of reptiles not found in mammals. In 1893 Wilson and McKay presented a joint paper to the Linnean Society which supported the view that the shoulder blades of both species of monotremes, though superficially different, were in fact homologous as revealed by comparative study of their muscle attachments.[5]

Wilson's work on the marsupial mole attracted comment from the platform of the Royal Society of NSW: 'It is a gratifying indication of our scientific progress', observed H C Russell the government astronomer in his Presidential address in 1892, 'that such work should now be carried out in Australia, and in our Medical school, instead of being, as a matter of course, entrusted to English or foreign scientific observers' who included Sir Richard Owen of the British Museum, William Turner of Edinburgh, Johnson Symington of Belfast, E B Poulton of Oxford and Henry Flower of London. Europeans who had studied preserved Antipodean material included K E von Baer, J F Meckel, H M D de Blainville, J F Blumenbach, Geoffroy St-Hilaire, Emil Selenka and Charlotte Westling. Then there was the Cambridge embryologist W H Caldwell who in 1884 perpetrated wanton slaughter of marsupials and monotremes along the Burnett River in Queensland on a generously-financed expedition which was also to collect lungfish (*Ceratodus*). Lungfish, which could breathe air in fouled water, were thought by the evolutionists of the day to be a 'missing link' between fish and amphibians in the evolutionary ladder as propounded by T H Huxley; similarly the monotremes, because of their reproduction system and other features, were believed to link reptiles and mammals. Caldwell returned to Cambridge with over 1300 *echidna* specimens alone, comprising 'a fairly complete series of stages', for studies he soon abandoned for a career in paper manufacture.[6]

While Russell was addressing the Royal Society in Sydney on 5 May 1892 an extraordinary event, again on Queensland's Burnett River, illustrated the rising authority of Australian scientists in the international arena. After travelling over a thousand miles to the Burnett to collect lungfish specimens, Baldwin Spencer, Melbourne's biology professor, learnt that a German zoologist Richard Semon, after a three-month journey, had preceded him by a fortnight on precisely the same mission. Feelings of personal rivalry were compounded by the sense of national honour at stake: some of Baldwin Spencer's Melbourne colleagues construed the episode as an international incident. When the two scientists met, however, their misgivings were dispelled. Science spoke an international language after all. They exchanged information useful to their respective researches, dissected a lungfish together, and parted friends. The encounter marked a new phase in Australian science: scientists might pride themselves on their international outlook but Australia-based scientists, nearly a decade before the Australian colonies became a nation, were raising a national banner.[7]

In Sydney a group of these new researchers congregated around Wilson at the University. The first was Charles James Martin who had arrived in Sydney in early 1891 to succeed Almroth Wright as demonstrator in physiology. Martin, newly married, took a cottage in Stanmore Road just 300 yards away from the Wilsons and the two families became intimate friends. Martin was a gangling sensitive soul but a tough-minded scientist and a confirmed mechanist. He was a Londoner, born in 1866 into a large family, 'a Nonconformist middle class one characteristic of the period, with lots of children, a fading flavour of piety and a small revenue'. At 15 he discovered science and embarked on part-time medical training at Birkbeck and King's Colleges and St Thomas's Hospital. Evening classes, second-hand books and apparatus of his own devising were his means of enlightenment. By 1886 he had a BSc with honours and a gold medal, by 1888 the MRCS and LSA and by 1890 the London MB degree. His teaching and research work included six months in Leipzig with Carl Ludwig, his hero and exemplar in physiology. Martin accepted the position in Sydney for frank material reasons: it was better than anything offering in Britain at the time. But Australia suited him well: he liked the people, the climate, the freedom from constraint and the camaraderie of young scientists channelling new grooves; and there was J T Wilson, just five years his senior, who stood in similar relationship to him as his favourite brother. Wilson the anatomist and Martin the physiologist fitted like hand and glove: they supplied the leadership and inspiration to a small but distinguished group of researchers into Australia's native fauna, self-styled a few years later 'The Fraternity of Duckmaloi', commemorating a favourite hunting ground for platypus.[8]

In the middle of 1892 C J Martin joined forces with Wilson on two papers on the platypus. It was probably Wilson's Edinburgh classmate, Dr Theo Barker of Wellington NSW, who sparked their interest by sending Wilson a live specimen. In their first paper Wilson and Martin focused their attention on the so-called 'duckbill' or snout of the platypus, which had puzzled previous investigators. They found it was not 'leathery', 'pergamenous', 'coriaceous', or 'horny' as described by some eminent comparative anatomists in Britain and Europe, who only had access to preserved specimens. Misconceptions had therefore arisen about its homology. Careful examination of the plate of cartilage forming a major part of the base of the snout enabled them to establish its morphological status, previously obscure, as 'a true cartilagenous homologue to the prenasal of the pig'. The name *Ornithorynchus anatinus,* meaning 'duck-billed' platypus, was singularly inappropriate.[9]

Curiosity about 'the markedly sensitive nature' of the snout (remarked on by Everard Home, who in 1802 showed great insight in comparing it to a human hand), led them in their second paper to investigate the nervous system of that organ histologically, to examine the destinations in the snout of its enormous fifth pair of nerves. They examined the peculiar rod-like tactile structures, the primary sense organ of the snout found in 1884 by Professor E B Poulton of Oxford whose work they confirmed in substantially greater detail. This second paper was a pioneer neurological study in peripheral sensibilities and a technically impressive piece of work. The mechano-receptor functions they postulated from their material, using simple optical microscopes, were later confirmed by electro-physiological studies and still later by electron microscopic findings. Further work just then was prevented by lack of specimens but they had made a start on what was to become for Wilson an enduring interest in the platypus.[10]

The Wilsons moved again in 1892 to a larger house, called 'Linden', at 77 Cavendish Street, Stanmore, and towards the end of that year they took in a young boarder, J P Hill, who in time was to become Wilson's most important collaborator. James Peter Hill was born in 1873 at Kennoway, Fifeshire, the younger son of a farmer and cattle breeder, and educated at the Royal High School in Edinburgh. After a year's study of botany and zoology at Edinburgh University, where he was particularly influenced by Dr John Beard, lecturer in comparative embryology and vertebrate morphology, Hill went to London in 1890 to study under G B Howes FRS, the associate and successor of T H Huxley at the Royal College of Science, South Kensington. When Haswell wrote to Howes in 1892 seeking a demonstrator in botany and zoology, Howes recommended Hill who set sail for Australia on 19 August, aged 19 and with no degree. He found Sydney a lively place for scientific work and within three years published some six papers on marine biology under Haswell.[11]

Wilson's private world settled down to a steady throb. His mother, now assisted by a maid, managed the household as thoroughly as ever but on one occasion caused chaos in Wilson's

93

study where she sought to bring order. It went into family lore as 'the deluge'. His father retained his vigour and took a lively interest in colonial as well as 'home' politics, church affairs, astronomy and bowls. The infant Jeanie saw him as kindly and unobtrusive, 'always there' in case of need. Her memories of these years included being taught her letters by her grandmother; also a dog, a monkey, a wallaby and a mulberry tree, all landing her in trouble now and then; and there were her father's friends: Mr Barff 'with a hairy beard like a genial bear', Professor Wood 'with a beaming smile', Dr Purser, Dr MacLaurin, Dr Mills, Dr Hinder and his little girl 'who strangely had no mother either', the Davids whose children were 'more awesome than their parents', the Anderson Stuarts who lived 'a day's journey away in Double Bay'. There were tennis parties at weekends at 'Linden' and there was the time her father and J P Hill learned to ride a bicycle by careering around the court, falling off at the corners. The long vacations meant Blackheath in the Blue Mountains and relaxed companionship with Hill, the MacCallums, the Martins and the Dockers, all of whom were good at climbing and exploring. There her father learnt to play golf. Behind all these memories was the tenderness of her busy father, who got as much fun as she did from her toys and whom she always wanted to please, though one memorable effort brought disaster: observing him tearing pages out of journals for her 'delectation' she concluded this was a fine thing and did the same to a row of books before she was put wise. This child's view of Wilson and Hill at work was of the pair of them bent over microscopes in the study-laboratory joined 'in a blue haze of pipesmoke', a picture she would always associate with platypus.[12]

Every last Wednesday of the month her father and Hill went off with Dr Martin to meetings of the Linnean Society, at the Linnean Hall in Ithaca Road, Elizabeth Bay. The Society had been founded in 1874 by Sir William MacLeay who endowed it with handsome accommodation, salaries for its permanent officers, research funds and the nucleus of a library. Though its membership was never large the Linnean Society was important, being for many years the only major society in Australia devoted exclusively to the natural sciences. A significant change took place in the early nineties when J J Fletcher, an authority on the *Amphibia,* became director of the Society and editor of its *Proceedings.* By then many original members were fading away, their places being taken by vigorous younger men like Liversidge, Haswell, Edgeworth David, Wilson, Martin and Hill from the University, and scientists from the

94

Australian Museum like R Etheridge Jnr the palaeontologist, J H Maiden the botanist, C Hedley the conchologist, E R Waite and J T Ogilby the zoologists and W J Rainbow the entomologist. Liversidge, Haswell, Edgeworth David and Wilson became trustees *Trustees* of the Australian Museum during the nineties, and each served as president of the Linnean Society for the customary two years. They contributed to the Royal Society of NSW and worked hard for the fledgling Australasian Association for the Advancement of Science. It was a concerted effort to stimulate, lift and gain recognition for science.[13]

J J Fletcher called Wilson, Martin and Hill 'the three musketeers'. Their enterprise provided Sydney's Medical School with one avenue for post-graduate research. The first recruit was W J Stewart McKay, who was followed by Grafton Elliot Smith, C G Wilson, H V C Hinder, Cecil Purser, Frank Tidswell, J F Flashman and A E Mills in the 1890s. Some were motivated by high scientific purpose and others just by the fun of it, like Cecil Purser who 50 years later reminded Wilson of one episode:

> Do you recollect the 'possum excursion on the banks of the flooded South Creek with the flood waters up around the willows, the willow trees harbouring many 'possums and how excited C.J.Martin was extracting the young 'possums from the pouch when the old retriever dog swam in and brought the 'possums to land, and I was often called to come along with the double barreled breech loading shot gun, to bring the 'possums down when the rifle bullets missed their quarry?

Wilson relaxed in this company and grew a beard. The days were physically and mentally strenuous, the evenings comradely around the camp fire. But nights under canvas were freezing in August and September, the prime time for hunting pregnant platypus, colder than anything in Wilson's Scottish experience.[14]

It was not an exclusive club. Friends, relations, local collectors and scientists were all welcome provided they pulled their weight and paid their share of expenses, of which they kept a careful record, for these were lean years: a severe economic depression caused the government to reduce its funding of the university progressively from 1892 to 1900 and this resulted in retrenchments, salary cuts and the *research during* abolition of grants for scientific apparatus. Field trips were often the *depression* result of information or hospitality supplied by country people. An informal network of naturalists and collectors sent specimens: Dr T L Bancroft of Eidevold and P Kenny from Gayndah in Queensland,

95

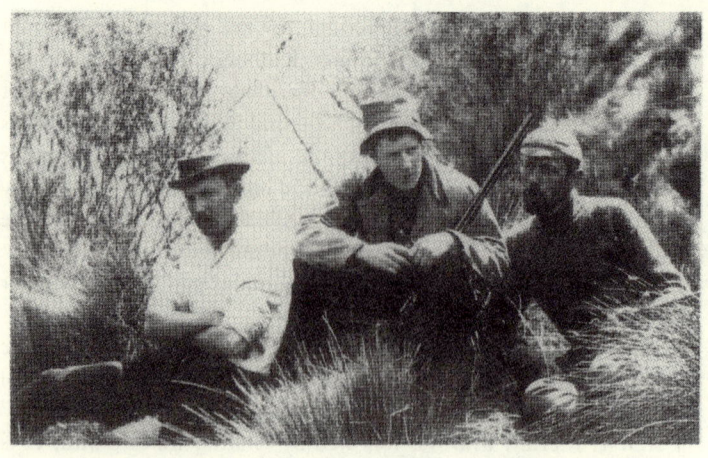

Hunting Platypus, Duckmaloi River, Sept. 1895: Grafton Elliot Smith,
J P Hill, J T Wilson.

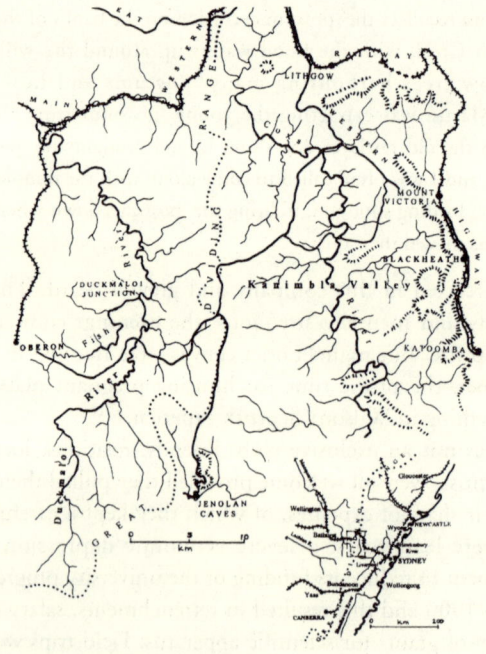

The Fraternity's Principal Collecting Areas, the Blue Mountains of New South Wales.

the blood vessels, and a blood coagulating enzyme which caused intravascular clotting. This work clarified prevailing confusion about the physiological action of snake venoms, and had important clinical relevance in Australia where snakebite was a nightmare. The NSW branch of the BMA provided a grant of 50 pounds to defray expenses for this work. Martin went on some years later to develop antidotes which brought him into collision with Albert Calmette of Paris, Eduard Buchner of Berlin and others: vitalists who held that neutralization of bacterial toxins with anti-toxins, and snake venoms with antivenenes, could not occur *in vitro* but only *in corpore*. Martin demonstrated in a test tube that there was no profound mystery about the process; it was simple chemistry.[17]

In 1894 Martin, in collaboration with Frank Tidswell (who succeeded him as demonstrator in physiology early in 1897) presented a paper to the Linnean Society on the spur on the hind limb of the male platypus which transmits a poisonous secretion from the duct of the femoral gland, a weapon that they concluded was used against other males during the pairing season.[18]

Grafton Elliot Smith, a graduate of 1892, joined the enterprise in 1894 when, after a year as house surgeon at Prince Alfred Hospital, Wilson chose him as a demonstrator. He had not yet decided on a career in research rather than surgery, though he was sure of the field: it was neurology.

> I had been a subscriber to the journal *Brain* from my first year and had become deeply interested in the new work on the thalamus and the sensory paths and decided to do experimental work in the afferent nervous system in the cat. But Dr. Martin pointed out in emphatic terms how stupid this was – that in every physiological laboratory in the world people with every help could work at the spino-thalamic tract in the cat, whereas in Australia there were marsupials and monotremes which most people would give anything to have for examination.... Hence I decided to work on marsupials.[19]

Elliot Smith had been a distinguished student and a prosector; as a demonstrator Wilson found him a 'helpful, enthusiastic and effective teacher' while in research 'his interest and his initiative ... developed with astonishing rapidity'. Wilson set him to work on the myology of the bandicoot *Perameles* to enlarge the comparative data for his own work on the myology of the marsupial mole. But it was not long before Elliot Smith's precocious fascination for the brain asserted itself. Wilson guided Elliot Smith's first steps in research –

98

introducing him for instance to the work of Edinger, Kölliker, Gustaf Retzius and others, the leading European authorities in neurology – but soon realized that this young man was 'emphatically an independent worker'. Elliot Smith examined the brains of marsupials and monotremes and with iconoclastic originality came up with the germ of the brilliant conception which was later to revolutionize knowledge of brain morphology, more especially that part concerned with the sense of smell (*rhinencephalon*). He discovered that the marsupial brain lacks the *corpus collosum*, the thick band of commissural fibres connecting the cerebral hemispheres. His first paper on brain structure published in the *Proceedings of the Linnean Society of NSW* in 1894 was later hailed as a classic by the world's foremost comparative neurologist, Ludwig Edinger of Frankfurt. The following year a thesis making an important contribution to the anatomy and histology of the brain of the non-placental mammals won him the MD (by examination) of the University of Sydney and a gold medal. Before he left for England on a travelling scholarship in April 1896 he turned out about a dozen vigorous papers advancing the view that in the study of the cerebral commissures (strands of nerve fibres uniting like structures in the two sides of the brain) lay the road to understanding the morphology of the vertebrate brain. It was work of genius.[20]

Wilson's recollection of his association with this young man who was ten years his junior was, from the outset, 'of the happiest'. But Elliot Smith's memory held more ambivalent feelings: he harboured resentment toward Wilson for his boring osteology lectures which 'rapidly killed all interest in the subject'; he resisted Wilson's efforts to make him extend his proficiency in technique; and initially he rejected Wilson's recommendation that he pursue anatomical research in Britain. This second son of a schoolmaster had problems with authority and at times he challenged authority to the point of perversity. Nevertheless Wilson and Elliot Smith were great friends for life.[21]

In Elliot Smith conspicuous ability and originality were joined to a fertile pen and boundless ambition. Even before he left Australia he had established a reputation abroad. As well as testimonials and letters of introduction to eminent scientists in Britain, Wilson, Martin, Robert Broom and Baldwin Spencer armed him with an abundance of valuable marsupial material including two rare marsupial moles (*Notoryctes*), one of the exceedingly rare pig-footed bandicoots (*Choeropus*) and a whole series of the narrow-footed marsupial mouse (*Sminthopsis*) for which, at the time, he was extremely grateful. In the northern hemisphere he quickly made his mark and became an agent and roving ambassador for the antipodean fraternity. He was welcomed by the anatomists Alexander Macalister and W L H Duckworth, both working at anthropology, but he found that the Cambridge anatomy department was not well equipped for neurology. It did not even have a microtome until Elliot Smith harassed Macalister into buying one out of his own pocket. More congenial were the physiologists H K Anderson, J N Langley and W H Gaskell who had neurological interests. He established his work station in the physiological laboratory. Also in Cambridge to sharpen Elliot Smith's competitive instincts was the physicist Ernest Rutherford who had travelled with him in the same ship to England.[22]

Wilson's attention in 1894 was claimed by the enigmatic structure in the skull of the platypus known as the dumb-bell shaped bone or '*os paradoxum*' which, as the name suggests, had given rise to much controversy. It is a nose bone of imposing, almost reptilian, proportions and in relative terms nearly the largest among mammals. Wilson reviewed the literature – the most important contributors being William Turner, Johnson Symington and G B Howes – gave an account of its anatomical relations in the skull and homologized it with the anterior nose bone (vomer) of other mammals, taking its origin from a pair of fused pre-vomers as G B Howes postulated rather than, as Turner and Symington held, from the bones of the palate. Its significance in mammalian development Wilson concluded could 'only be decided by actual embryological investigation, for which, unfortunately, the material has hitherto not been available'.[23]

into embryology Wilson was getting deeper into embryology but opportunities for studying the embryos of the platypus were rare, for its nesting burrows were both difficult to find and difficult of access, and not enough was known of the animal's diet and habits to keep it alive in captivity. Indeed so great was the difficulty of obtaining the right specimens that Wilson looked for 'more abundant light' from the mass of monotreme material collected by W H Caldwell in 1883/4 and Richard Semon of Jena in 1891–3, in their expensive expeditions to Australia. Neither shed any light. So when Wilson found a foetal specimen in the Australian Museum he made a careful description of its external features. It revealed nothing new but it did arm him with evidence to refute continuing references to the snout of the platypus as a horny duckbill. With the exception of the very limited area of the caruncle (shell breaker) Wilson found the epidermis of the platypus foetal snout – and for that matter the snouts of two young *echidna* he also examined – no more 'horny' than that of a mammary foetus of a marsupial. The term 'duckbill' persisted nevertheless and it continued to irritate Wilson, even as late as 1928 when he reviewed Harry Burrell's book on the platypus.[24]

Next came a second paper with Martin on the rod-like tactile structures in the platypus snout to answer certain criticisms by Poulton. They elaborated and largely confirmed their previous findings with special reference to the nerve supply of those organs, and went on to give an account of their observations of the remarkable sweat glands, also previously described by Poulton, whose interpretation they accepted: that the epidermal down-growth, through which the terminal part of the sweat-duct reaches the surface, represents a modified hair follicle. They went further, postulating that its rich nerve supply and the projection of the cells of its core on the surface showed it is an active sensory structure.[25]

On 1 October 1894 at Wellington NSW four female platypus were shot. Three had just laid their eggs but the fourth had two in her left uterus ready to be laid. One of these launched J P Hill on his life-long investigations into the embryology and reproduction of monotremes and marsupials. On 28 November Hill and Martin delivered to a meeting of the Linnean Society in Sydney a joint paper giving the first precise description of the structure of a platypus embryo (at the 17-somite stage of development) and its foetal membranes, advancing many new facts and interpretations which have stood the test of time. Two of their revelations were particularly interesting. The first was the greatly increased size of the egg at this stage of development – nearly ready to be laid – since it left the ovary, due to the yolk's absorption of uterine secretions. The embryo itself they found was markedly retarded in development, a mechanical effect, Wilson suggested, of the nutrient fluid of the yolk pressing the embryo against the egg's resistant shell. This characteristic was distinctly different from oviparous reptiles and birds. The second remarkable discovery concerned the foetal membranes or vesicle containing the embryo and yolk: the platypus vesicle suggested 'a striking connecting link between the conditions obtaining in the *Sauropsida* [reptiles] and in the Placental Mammals'. Hill and Martin had uncovered a clue to understanding that the basic pattern of foetal membrane development is phylogenetically instructive.[26]

It was about this time, late in 1894 or early in 1895, that Hill began to collaborate with Wilson in a study of the dentition of the

101

marsupial bandicoot, *Perameles*, entering a lively controversy in England and Europe about mammalian dentition. This subject had rested traditionally in the territory of palaeontologists and comparative morphologists as a means of determining the position of various mammals in the genealogical tree, but during the early 1890s embryologists, attacking the problem from a new point of view produced new information and hypotheses about the affinities of mammalian sub-classes. Stimulated by this debate and in particular the divided opinion about whether the one functional set of marsupial teeth is homologous to the first or second set of teeth in higher mammals (the *diphyodonts,* meaning successions of teeth), Wilson and Hill investigated for themselves the early development and succession of teeth in the bandicoot, chosen because it represented a fairly generalized marsupial type. They had abundant material, sufficient to reveal 14 different stages in the development of bandicoot young. The result was a detailed paper of 161 pages, published in 1897 in the prestigious English *Quarterly Journal of Microscopical Science*, edited by E Ray Lankester FRS, the Linacre Professor of Comparative Anatomy at Oxford. They concluded that it is the first teeth, not the permanent teeth (as Sir Henry Flower of London had argued in 1867), that are almost completely suppressed as the direct result of the permanent attachment of the young to their mother's teat in the pouch, the suckling condition peculiar to the marsupials. This meant that, in respect of their tooth equipment, marsupials could be seen in their view as 'degenerate' rather than 'primitive' mammals. The dentition of the bandicoot – supported by Hill's early findings on its placentation – led them to the view that the marsupial order as a whole was 'at least an offshoot from a diphyodont stock common to both Metatheria [marsupials] and Eutheria [mammals]'. The same reasoning led them to suggest that the monotremes must also represent an offshoot of a common 'Promammalian' ancestor (Hypotherian). Eleven years later they found evidence of vestigial milk teeth in each jaw of two mammary foetuses of platypus, which supported the theory that at some remote period the monotremes did conform to a true mammalian pattern. In Cambridge Grafton Elliot Smith read the proofs and dispatched reprints to interested authorities, 18 of them, in England and Europe.[27]

This work with Hill was interrupted by shorter pieces. For the Intercolonial Medical Congress of Australasia held in Dunedin in February 1896 Wilson contributed two short papers on human anatomy. In the first he returned to the subject of variation in the innervation of the thoracic musculature of man, to support D J Cunningham and his British colleagues in an argument with Professor Bardeleben of Jena. The second paper was an inquiry into the discrepancies of various studies on cranial measurements. He rejected the notion of racial correlation in the arrangement of cranial bones, supporting the view of Hyrtl that 'The lines on the human skull answer exactly to those of the skulls of anthropoid apes'.[28]

Hill meanwhile had made a very important discovery concerning the short-nosed bandicoot, *Perameles obesulus*. In a preliminary note to the Linnean Society in November 1895, just one year after he and Martin had read their paper on the platypus embryo, Hill announced his discovery of an allantoic placental connection between maternal and foetal tissues in the bandicoot uterus extending to the serous membrane, thus allowing ready transfusion between the two blood streams and performing both nutritive and respiratory functions. It was, therefore, concluded Hill, 'a true allantoic placenta of the discoidal type'. This meant that the marsupials as a whole could no longer be classified aplacental as contemporary scientific opinion would have it.[29]

The question was topical. G B Howes, writing in *Nature* in 1896, proclaimed Hill's discovery both welcome and important. Richard Semon in 1894 had described and illustrated a similar condition in the koala, *Phascolarctas*, and both of these studies would help to clarify conceptions of the interrelationships of marsupials and mammals, then being debated largely in terms of tooth generation. That the bandicoot allantois was discoidal, continued Howes, lent support to the view which for some years had been steadily gaining ground, that such a placenta was the most primitive type, as the Cambridge embryologist F M Balfour had hypothesized in 1881. In Sydney Wilson publicly congratulated Hill on 'a discovery of the highest biological import', while Edgeworth David pronounced it comparable with Röntgen's X-rays, 'perhaps one of the most important, if not the most important scientific discovery as yet made in Australia'. From the platform of the Royal Society of NSW he appealed to 'any person residing in the country desirous of helping Mr Hill in his interesting and important investigations' to send him specimens of opossums, native cats, bandicoots, or any other kind of marsupial.[30]

Foetal specimens of marsupials were scarce. When Hill embarked on a detailed developmental study of the placentation of the bandicoot he had only enough material to describe six stages, of which two were post-partum – not much of a reward for two years collecting by the Sydney fraternity and others who had answered Edgeworth David's call. But it did enable him to amplify and confirm the brief statement of his preliminary note, and to give in detail a connected account of the process of placentation in the bandicoot. He was now able to state that an allantoic placenta, in all respects similar to that of the southern short-nosed bandicoot, *Perameles obesula*, also occurs in the closely related long-nosed bandicoot *Perameles nasuta*. The phylogenetic significance of this invasive discoidal chorio-allantoic placenta in bandicoots gave rise to a great controversy (still unresolved) as to whether this process of placentation evolved convergently in bandicoots and placental mammals (*Eutherians*), or whether it represents a primitive marsupial (*Metatherian*) condition. Hill and Wilson had addressed this question in their dentition paper, to which Hill in his conclusion returned.

> Has the allantoic placenta of *Perameles* been independently evolved within the limits of the Marsupial order or is it directly and genetically related to that of Eutheria through the common ancestry of the Meta- and Eu- theria from an earlier diphyodont protoplacental stock? In a previous paper in this Journal, on the tooth development of *Perameles,* by Professor J T Wilson and myself [1897], we incidentally touched upon this question, and expressed our preference for the latter of these two views; and I may here at once say that a much fuller knowledge of the details of the placentation process in *Perameles* has in no whit served to weaken our previously expressed opinion.[31]

The alternative, that the allantoic placenta had twice been acquired independently within the mammalian class, they now considered highly improbable. Their interpretation, that the marsupials and the mammals were divergent branches of a common ancestral stock (most marsupials having discarded the placentation process) called into question the hierarchical 'scale of nature' outlook of the times. In evolutionary terms the marsupials and the 'higher' mammals had with equal success met the challenge of environmental adjustment.[32]

Hill dispatched this paper to Ray Lankester of Oxford in April 1897, for publication in the *Quarterly Journal of Microscopical Science*. He had come a long way in less than five years. Under Haswell he had written six papers on marine life, accurate and useful descriptions but of no great consequence compared with the three papers he produced in the 18 months following the transfer of his research focus to Australia's terrestrial vertebrates, the first in collaboration with Martin, the second in collaboration with Wilson, the third on his own. They were of enduring importance, the last two inducing a fundamental change in the understanding of mammals. At 24 he was an embryologist of note. Yet he still had no degree. In 1897 the University granted him leave without pay for two terms to enable him to complete the requirements for a BSc at Edinburgh. During his absence his place was filled by Gregg Wilson, a biology demonstrator from Edinburgh. In other words a temporary exchange of demonstrators was arranged and Hill must have paid his own fares since the Senate was able to report, piously, that the arrangement was at no cost to the University.[33]

In August 1897 Hill departed for Edinburgh with a sheaf of introductions from various people, and some commissions from Wilson for books and apparatus. His reputation had preceded him. In London he found an invitation from the Dutch embryologist A A W Hubrecht to attend in mid-September a meeting of the *Verein für Naturforschen* featuring placentation in its discussions at Brunswick in Germany; it was to be attended by men of considerable stature: Wilhelm His, Emil Selenka and Richard Semon. But commitments in Edinburgh precluded his acceptance. From Oxford came the gratifying praise, and greetings, of Ray Lankester who was engrossed in Hill's placentation paper. By mid-September it was in type.[34]

Though a Scot born and bred Hill did not rejoice in his homecoming. The family home on a farm at Kennoway in Fife was cheerless, his mother having died during his five years in Sydney, and it was so cold that he found himself cowering indoors for much of the time. Edinburgh University he found, was a 'stagnation place' where folk took things easy. 'To find the Dean you wait a week and then get two mins'. The zoology laboratory was not up to Sydney standards and John Beard was away for a lengthy period. He wished himself back among the marsupials in New South Wales as was Gregg Wilson he imagined. 'From what people tell me here Gregg Wilson has gone out with the intention of clearing the continent. Be aisy with him,' he wrote to J T Wilson, who had strong opinions about extravagant foreign collectors.[35]

Hill had a strenuous time juggling chemistry, botany and geology which kept him away from the zoology laboratory where he was itching to investigate a new-born possum *Trichosures* and a new-born native cat *Dasyurus* and experiment with the wonderful effects of Mann's Methyl Blue-Eosin stain. Beard had 'some lovely stuff especially in the way of Elasmobranch and other fish embryos', and

[handwritten margin note: Hill returning to Scot: Edin. Not up to Sydney]

105

in the museum he noticed there was a lot of Australian material including some of Robert Broom's collection of Aboriginal skulls. One morning in Frazer's bookshop he bumped into Professor Anderson Stuart and his wife, fresh from the Toronto meeting of the British Association. Back from the same meeting was Grafton Elliot Smith where he had made a considerable impact with a paper on the cerebral commissures. Smith was 'getting fat, quite fat,' Hill reported, 'so the climate seems to suit him.' News reached him in January that T J Parker had died in Dunedin and that Wilson and Haswell were putting his name forward for that zoology chair, an initiative that was not successful. It was testimony of the esteem of his peers, however, and a sign that Sydney might not long be blessed with his services.[36]

Hill graduated BSc (Edin.) with special distinction in March 1898. In the following year Edinburgh awarded him the Gunning Victoria Jubilee prize for research in zoology and a George Heriot Research Fellowship of 100 pounds, renewed in 1900. In addition the Government Grants Committee of the Royal Society of London awarded him funds for four years to study marsupial and monotreme development. He arrived back in Sydney in late May 1898 with his degree, a medal, a microscope (probably a binocular, stereoscopic Braus-Drüner), a bike and some of Beard's embryos.[37]

Between 1899 and 1901 Hill was to publish four more important papers, further expanding knowledge of placentation, parturition and embryological development in bandicoots and other marsupials. One arresting find, which fascinated Hill for many years because it also characterized South American marsupials, was the strange phenomenon that the bandicoot is born by rupturing the connective tissue between the median vagina and the perineum. During these years he took to breeding the eastern native cat or quoll (*Dasyurus viverrinus*) in captivity, accumulating a great collection of eggs and precise breeding records, in preparation for further work.[38]

At the end of the decade C J Martin and J T Wilson took the opportunity of scientific platforms to survey the field of biological thought. In Sydney on 7 January 1898 Martin, as President of the Biology Section, addressed the Australasian Association for the Advancement of Science on the history of relations between morphology and physiology over the last 50 years. It was a vigorous appeal for these two great divisions of biology to repair the split that opened between them in mid-century when physiologists, after the brilliant discoveries of German and French scientists, became preoccupied with making physiology an exact science like physics and

chemistry; and anatomists became absorbed, after the publication of
Darwin's *Origin of Species,* in constructing a huge genealogical tree of
life on earth. The understanding of the cell, the frontier at which
biological inquiry had arrived would need the joint efforts of the
students of form and the students of function. Delivered a year after
he left Sydney for Melbourne, this address celebrates his association
with Wilson and the Fraternity of Duckmaloi, in which biology's two
major divisions were in fact united.[39]

On 30 March 1898, as President of the Linnean Society of
NSW, Wilson addressed the question of how far mechanical theories
are capable of explaining the phenomena of living activity, a
question that had preoccupied him since his student days in
Edinburgh. His own research, his reading of European and
American research and his work with Martin had persuaded him of
the value of applying the methods of physics and chemistry to
biological problems. Work on these lines had delivered abundant
proof that the essential questions in physiology had been tracked
from the outworks of the cell complex to the citadel of the living
cell itself. The cell still held its secrets but there was no reason to
believe that the same principles of investigation would not yield
results. Mechanism had to be pre-supposed if the scientist's work
was to be made intelligible: 'some definite chain of physical events
there *must* be'. What the mechanisms are is the business of the
scientists to discover.[40]

At the root of the Darwinian doctrine of natural selection there
lay, Wilson stressed, 'the mechanical principle of external necessity in
a determining environment'. The *micella* theory (that protoplasm is
composed of crystalline granules) proposed by the Swiss botanist Karl
Nägeli was a hypothesis derived from mechanical principles which
could open up fruitful fields of discovery. The recent work of August
Weismann of Freiburg, proposing the theory of the continuity of
'germ-plasma' to explain the process of heredity 'by the transmission
from one generation to another of a substance with a definite
chemical and, above all, molecular constitution', he acclaimed as 'a
strictly logical continuation of the effort [by Darwin] to account for
the phenomena of life on the lines of physical causation'. Wilson saw
that Weismann's concept supplied a material basis for the mechanism
of inheritance in the ultra-microscopical structure of the chromatin of
the germ cell. Though the concept could not then be tested or verified
because of technical limitations, he asserted that science would make
those investigations, perhaps by 'other than optical means'. 'Who can
tell' he asked, 'what structural facts may not be borne witness to by

107

future instruments of research?'[41]

But, continued Wilson, science had its limits. It was only one aspect of reality. To the question 'how?' of natural phenomena he saw no limits to the efforts of science. As to their 'why?' – their object, purpose or final cause – that was a matter on which science 'must be forever dumb'. He believed that Darwin's great apostle T H Huxley had fallen into confusion in his statement in 1893, *Evolution and Ethics,* when he posed the 'apparent paradox' of man's ethical nature being at war with 'the cosmic process' of evolution. In the words of Professor Burdon Sanderson, Wilson urged 'Let us willingly and with our hearts do homage to "divine philosophy", but let that homage be rendered outside the limits of our science.' Their competing claims to explain the reality of life had ultimately to be brought before the tribunal of philosophical criticism.[42]

When Wilson wrote this address he probably believed that most reputable scientists held similar views. He certainly believed the vitalism-versus-mechanism argument was threadbare. He was laying to rest the puzzle of teleology in biology that the Haldanes had raised in their essay of 1883. Although he knew that Haldane and Lorrain Smith still entertained vitalist tendencies he probably did not realize their strength when, as usual, he sent Haldane a copy of his address. The sharp retort it provoked gave Wilson the measure of that difference. In a letter of 3 January 1899 Haldane wrote in his usual affectionate style but it contained these uncompromising passages:

> The more I work at physiology the more sure do I become that physico-chemical working hypotheses cannot be made the basis of scientific biology, & I'm rather surprised that you should think otherwise, considering the general philosophical position of the last part of your address. Why on earth do you lay any stress on the theories of Weissman &c? Surely they have no value except as a sort of beacon and warning, or perhaps as a means of making people realise what the questions of heredity, development and nutrition really mean?
>
> You lay great stress on the theory of Natural Selection as a causal explanation of evolution but I am sure this theory won't stand. It certainly doesn't seem to me to explain any of the characteristic features of organisms. You seem also to argue that the use of accurate physical & chemical methods in physiology implies an acknowledgement that physico-chemical methods of explanation are the only possible ones. I think you might as well argue that the application of mathematics in physical & chemical work implies

that physics & chemistry are nothing but mathematics. It seems to me that it is in the application of rigorously accurate physical & chemical methods that the salvation of biology from mechanical conceptions really lies. Everywhere the old mechanical ideas have gone to the wall in physiology when accurate investigation has been substituted for loose hypotheses.[43]

With this letter Haldane enclosed his article 'Vitalism' published in the prestigious journal *Nineteenth Century* in September 1898, setting forth his outlook on biological inquiry. His philosophical position was still as it was in 1883. He had adduced more physiological evidence from recent research on respiration which he believed refuted mechanical theory. Always, he insisted, there is the conundrum of Life itself, 'one of those ultimate facts in experience we may try to explain but cannot get rid of'. He sought for biology fundamentally different conceptions from those of physics and chemistry, but beyond the fact that they must be vitalistic, purposive or teleological Wilson could not fathom what those conceptions might be.[44]

Haldane was by now a distinguished physiologist, having in 1897 been elected a Fellow of the Royal Society of London. Criticism from him carried weight so in Wilson's second presidential address, delivered on 29 March 1899, he took the question further. He accommodated Haldane's argument as far as he could. He admitted that, in the progress of physiology, physico-chemical theories had broken down many times; but they had succeeded many times too. He agreed that residual phenomena remained unexplained. That was inevitable: 'the mystery ever recedes as we pursue it further into the recesses of organisation'. But the mechanical theory had given splendid proof of its capabilities, and Haldane himself accepted that 'by the further application of these principles we shall continue to extend our knowledge'. Haldane used mechanical methods as much as anyone.[45]

What then was the difference between them? It seemed to be that, as soon as a new discovery was made by mechanical methods, Haldane claimed it was non-vital: 'If we look ... at the phenomena which are capable of being stated or explained in physico-chemical terms, we see at once that there is nothing in them characteristic of life.' Wilson viewed such distinctions as meaningless: 'Surely any and every process carried on as a part of the life of an organism is characteristic of life.' And defeatist. On this point Wilson contrasted the attitudes of Haldane and Martin over a respiratory phenomenon on which both were qualified to speak: 'that the tension [more accurately, pressure] of oxygen in arterial blood is frequently higher than it is in the air of the lung alveoli'. Haldane saw this as a 'defiance of physico-chemical law, i.e. that the physical laws of diffusion of gases do not hold in this case', and therewith dismissed altogether the validity of applying mechanical principles and methods to this question. Martin on the other hand, while acknowledging the anomalous behaviour of respiratory oxygen, adhered to mechanical principles. The question for Martin was always:

> if this be not a case of the operation of known mechanism, what is the actual and genuine mechanism underlying it; if the originally supposed mechanism is not the true cause of the operation, what is the real and actual antecedent cause?

This, said Wilson emphatically, was 'the only genuinely scientific question, the only kind of question answerable by means of experimental scientific procedure'.[46]

Haldane appealed to the development of modern anatomy as a way out of the physiologists' difficulties. His views of modern anatomy, in Wilson's opinion, were misconceived. In adhering to the 'immanent type or plan' view of morphology Haldane voiced the faith of Sir Richard Owen, which certainly was not the view of contemporary morphologists. For Wilson 'the true guiding hypothesis of modern morphology' was 'the natural-historical interpretation of homology' which should not be abandoned 'simply because we cannot effect a definitive analysis of its more important factors'. Certainly the phenomenon of regeneration presented perplexing problems but American and German workers were making inroads on them. Certainly anatomists were in urgent need of a tenable theory of heredity. Weismann and Nägeli were pushing towards that. In the meantime, said Wilson, the absence of a tenable theory,

> does not ... deprive me of the solid conviction that the morphological relationship between, say, the presence of a marsupial pouch and an inflected mandibular angle, is to be interpreted simply as a common family character, transmitted by descent, and deriving its whole meaning from the fact of this transmission; and not as an instance of any recondite conformity to an immanent ideal 'type'.[47]

Wilson denied that progress in anatomy assisted vitalist arguments. Quite otherwise: 'For in reality, morphology, just as much as physiology, has been advancing by the aid of hypotheses which are conceived as every bit as mechanical as those which have achieved no small measure of success in physiological science.' That there was another viewpoint of life above mechanism Wilson freely admitted, and reiterated from his previous address. Haldane had, he believed, committed the error of allowing the teleological explanation of life to intrude into the scientific one.[48]

For Haldane biology was a functional system whose unknowable dynamo was an integral factor; for Wilson biology was an organic process of development whose unknowable first cause was not the concern of the biologist. That there is a spiritual aspect to reality Wilson not only acknowledged but gave precedence, and he bore witness to it forcefully and persistently in this and other arenas:

> The full significance of Nature is not to be apprehended by the externalising operation of purely scientific interpretation, be the scope of its investigations never so extended. Not even a complete 'astronomical knowledge' of the molecular dance of elementary physical particles could absolve us from the necessity of finding the ultimate explanation of all phenomena in terms of that single spiritual principle which alone makes knowledge possible and for which alone even material bodies either live or move or have any being at all.

This was Wilson's final attitude to the problem. Haldane and Wilson remained friends all their lives but this argument marked a definite change in their relationship.[49]

By the end of 1897 the cadre of Wilson's research fraternity had dispersed. Martin had for a year been lecturing in Melbourne and Hill had left in August for Edinburgh. Abroad again in 1897 was Professor Anderson Stuart, accompanied by his beautiful young wife of three years standing. With her he at last found domestic stability and four sons were born to them. On this trip Stuart visited the scenes of his youth including old academic haunts and, while investigating the teaching of dentistry, reminded British and European scientists and medical men of his life and work. Edinburgh University awarded him an honorary LLD. He visited the United States and Canada, attending in August the Toronto meeting of the British Association for the Advancement of Science where Grafton Elliot Smith read a paper on the vertebrate brain, establishing him as an international authority in anatomy and neurology. Elliot Smith's star was in the ascendant and Anderson Stuart enjoyed the glory it reflected on Sydney's Medical School.[50]

111

For Wilson 1897 had been another heavy year. It began in the shadow of his father's death from cancer on 29 December 1896. During May and June Wilson himself was unwell and in September Jeanie became seriously ill. With Anderson Stuart away for the last two terms he once more carried practical responsibility for the faculty – though he was not this time Acting Dean – in addition to his normal teaching duties. But a marvellous alleviation of his tribulations was at hand.[51]

During the first term of 1898 there began a new and tender relationship for Wilson. Miss Mabel Salomons, younger daughter of the eminent and controversial Sydney barrister and politician Sir Julian Salomons, entered his life. She had studied art in London – the Salomons were great travellers – and continued her studies at Julian Ashton's School in Sydney which lacked instruction in artistic anatomy. Seeking to remedy this deficiency, and backed by the resourceful principal of the Women's College Miss Louisa MacDonald, Miss Salomons applied to attend lectures in anatomy at the medical school. Professor Wilson did not welcome this unusual mid-term application but was persuaded by Miss MacDonald's appeal to his duty to give instruction in his subject. It was designated a Class in Artistic Anatomy, and when asked a few months later how it was proceeding Wilson replied 'I married it!'[52]

Events had moved swiftly despite many difficulties which came from both families. Sir Julian did not smile on the proposal: his attractive 24-year-old daughter was 13 years younger than her suitor, a widower with a young daughter. For her part Mrs Thomas Wilson did not welcome so drastic a family change – the Salomons were much grander folk – and neither did Jeanie. In this delicate situation Wilson displayed some ineptitude: for their first meeting he arranged that seven-year-old Jeanie be taken by her stepmother-to-be to the dentist. Jeanie screamed and clung to a lamp post and poor Mabel knew not what to do, being quite inexperienced with children. 'Poor both of them!' commented a sister- and daughter-in-law years later.[53]

James Thomas Wilson and Mabel Mildred Millicent Salomons were married in a quiet ceremony at Woollahra Presbyterian Church on 14 September 1898, the bride's father and H E Barff acting as witnesses. Although Jewish by birth Mabel had been instructed in Protestantism and quickly adjusted to Presbyterian practice. She was in fact very adjustable all round and soon schooled herself to instant motherhood and household management. Intelligent and practical, she had about her a liveliness and unconcern for convention that were for Wilson a source of infinite joy. It was a very happy marriage, blessed by three daughters and three sons. 'They all adored him', said one family friend, 'and *he* adored *her*'. [54]

Wilson's second marriage surprized the University. Young, light-hearted and very different in background and interests from Wilson's close friends, Mabel must have seemed an unlikely partner. 'How are the mighty fallen' commented *Hermes* with undergraduate impertinence, for which it was induced to apologize in the next issue. The news hit Martin like a thunderclap. Labouring under a sense of loss since leaving Sydney early in 1897, he now had to contend with jealousy. After a visit from the newlyweds in June 1899, he wrote in contrite terms to Wilson

> Tell Mabel I was not as nice to her as I ought to have been but I was beastly jealous. I remember distinctly the same feeling when my favourite brother was married. In time I became reconciled, so I ask her please to bear with me and I will love her so very much.

Hill moved out of the Wilson household to join A E Mills in his bachelor quarters in Strathfield.[55]

The century ended in a clamour of jingoism around the Empire. Queen Victoria's Diamond Jubilee celebrations of 1897 acclaimed the splendour of an Empire which for some had the sanctity of a religion. But Britain could no longer match her imperial will, whatever motivated it, with imperial might. The Boer War demonstrated that. The hysteria evoked by the relief of Mafeking in August 1900 exposed a new sense of vulnerability in the British people as they faced a world now cataloguing their guilt and calculating their weakness. The *Pax Brittanica* was breaking up. Under challenge from America and Germany in industrial and technological power, with few friends and no allies, Britain looked to her Empire for support.

Wilson had always supported the idea of Empire and as a citizen accepted its obligations. He had studied the military arts, drilled, paraded, camped and manoeuvred with a host of other Sydney militiamen. In April 1898 he had received his commission as First Lieutenant in the Scottish Rifles, Fifth Infantry Regiment NSW, commanded by Lt Col G R Campbell, and by the outbreak of the Boer War he was a Captain.[56] He would have gone to that war but for one circumstance: his young wife was expecting their first child. At that juncture private responsibilities took priority over the obligations of a citizen.

Notes

1. Background on platypus: Burrell, 7, 28, 29, 32, 45. 'resembles that of': Verreaux, quoted Burrell, 6. Parker at a loss: quoted Burrell, 8.

2. Owen's authority in Australia was challenged from 1870 by a Darwinian, Gerard Krefft, of the Aust Museum: Moyal 1986. 'an innate tendency': Owen 1868, quoted in W C Williams, DSB, Vol. 10, 262. 'irrefragable evidence': quoted Moyal, 1975, 47.

3. 'this illuminating': WAH 1891, 174.

4. The marsupial mole: Troughton, 57. JTW, 1894a.

5. JTW, 1893a, 1893b. Craniology abstract: Warren, in Anniversary Address, *JRS of NSW*, Vol. 27, 1893, 13. JTW 1894b (with McKay). Focus on clavicle: Gould 1991, 272.

6. 'It is a gratifying': Russell, 35. European biologists and Australia: Caldwell, 480–3; Moyal 1975. 'a fairly complete': Caldwell, 465–6. Caldwell's later career: Mulvaney and Calaby, 144.

7. Encounter of Semon, Baldwin Spencer: Mulvaney & Calaby, 105–6.

8. Martin's residence: JTW to J, 18.10.1933. 'a Non-conformist': CJM quoted in Chick, *RSO* 1956, 173. Fraternity of Duckmaloi: Dawson, 118; Wilson family.

9. JTW, 1893c (with CJM). 'a true cartilagenous': 185.

10. JTW, 1893d (with CJM). Later confirmation: M J Blunt to author, 8.7.1982.

11. JPH: Watson, *RSO* 1955.

12. All from J's early draft of Biographical Sketch of JTW.

13. Linnean Society: Walkom. Names referred to: *PLS* and Strahan.

14. The three musketeers: Fletcher. 'Do you recollect': Cecil Purser to JTW, 11.10.1942.

15. Names of people & places: catalogue of JPH Collection, Hubrecht Laboratory.
The meaning of the name Duckmaloi is not known. It was used for this stretch of the Fish River by local settlers from Ireland and by the 1890s had supplanted the official name.

16. Robert Broom and 'unknown man': Watson in *RSO* 1952, 38, 9. Organ of Jacobson: Hyman, 450. Johnson Symington: obituary notice *J of A*, 1924, 275.

17. CJM and snake venom: TWE David, 1896, 31–2; Chick, 187 & *Centenary Book*, 241 (on constituent poisons). *Science Progress* Sept. 1894, No. 7, Vol. II, 1–9. Grant from the BMA: *JRS of NSW*, 1893, Vol. 27, 15. CJM's own view: Chick, 189.

18. CJM and Tidswell, 1894.

19. 'I had been': GES quoted in Dawson, 118.

20. JTW in Dawson, 123–9. 'his interest', 'emphatically': *ibid.*, 125. Introductions: JTW to Woollard, 26.7.1937. Edinger's view: Oppenheimer, 63. GES research work: Woollard 1937–8, 280–94.

21. 'of the happiest': JTW in Dawson, 125. 'rapidly killed': GES 1918, 8. No particular encouragement: Abbie, 107.

22. Armed with specimens: GES to JTW n.d. (?April 1896); GES to Broom, 18.8.1896, Abbie m/film Ms56/1, BL. Dawson, 19. Cambridge people: GES to JTW, 18.11.1896, 5.2.99. GES and microtome: Abbie, 109.

23. JTW 1894d: 'only be decided', 141.

24. JTW, 1895b, 683.

25. JTW, 1895a (with CJM). JPH, *RSO* 1949, 647.

26. CJM and JPH, 1894. 'a striking': CJM and JPH, 1895, 68. Significance of discoveries: Watson, *RSO* on Hill, 106; Luckett, 444.

27. JTW, 1897c (with JPH). 'at least an': *ibid.*, 577. Later paper: JTW, 1907a (with JPH).

28. JTW, 1897a. 'The lines on': quoted JTW, 1897b, 366.

29. 'a true allantoic': JPH, 1895, 581.

30. Howes, *Nature*, 23.1.1896, 270–1. 'a discovery': JTW in *PLS* 1898, 819. 'perhaps one' and 'any person': TWED, *JRS of NSW*, 1896, 29–30.

31. Hill's work on placentation: Watson, *RSO* on Hill 1955, 102; Luckett, 475. 'Has the allantoic': JPH in *QJMS*, 1898, 432–3.

32. . Discussion: *ibid.*, 433–6.

33. No cost to university: *Calendar* 1898.

34. Letters JPH to JTW.

35. 'a stagnation' and 'From what people': JPH to JTW, 12.10.1897.

36. 'some lovely stuff' and Broom's skulls: JPH to JTW, 10.3.1898. 'getting fat': 23.1.1898. GES paper on cerebral commissures: GES to JTW, 5.10.97.

37. Letters JPH to JTW.

38. Hill, 1899–1901: Watson, *RSO,* 106–8.

39. CJM 1898, 408–9, 412–13.

40. 'some definite': JTW, 1898, 834.

41. 'the mechanical', 'a strictly': JTW, 1898, 845, 828. ('by the transmission'): Weismann, *Essays upon Heredity* 1889 [2nd edn Oxford 1892, 167.] quoted in Mayr, 699. Explanation of micella theory: Nordenskiold, 554. JTW on Weismann: JTW, 1898, 827–35. 'other than': etc., JTW, 1898, 836. Weismann's theory brilliantly foreshadowed the disclosure of the DNA genetic code through the techniques of crystallography and molecular biology: Judson, Foreword; JMGW to Author.

42. 'must be': JTW, 1898, 836. 'Let us willingly': JTW, 1898, 831.

43. Threadbare argument: JTW, *PLS* 1899, 6. Vitalist tendencies: JSH to JTW, 29.11.1896. 'The more I work': JSH to JTW, 3.1.1898.

44. 'one of those': JRH & JSH, 1883.

45. JTW 1899: 'the mystery', 10; 'by the further', quoting JSH, 12.

46. JTW 1899: 'If we look', quoting JSH, 13; 'Surely any', 13; 'that the tension', 15; 'if this be not', quoting CJM, 16; 'the only genuinely', 16. Haldane quotes from 'Vitalism', 407, *Nineteenth Century*, Vol. XLIV, July–Dec. 1898. The behaviour of respiratory oxygen was later explained in physico-chemical terms, thus vindicating Martin's comment.[JMGW to author, 23.11.1981.]

47. 'immanent type': JSH quoted in JTW 1899, 23. 'the true guiding', 'simply because' and 'does not': JTW 1899, 27–8. [Owen believed the marsupial pouch was evidence of 'creative foresight'.]

48. 'For in reality': JTW 1899, 28.

49. Haldane's important achievement was to draw biologists' attention to the need for a more holistic approach: Garland Allen, 74. 'The full significance': JTW 1899, quoted in his *RSO* by Hill, 648.

50. GES: Keith 1950, 201–2.

51. Death of Thomas Wilson: CJM to JTW, 26.5.97 & 1.6.97. Jeanie's illness: G S Miles to JTW, 12.9.97.

52. Miss MacDonald to JTW (n.d.? 1898). 'I married': J, Biographical Sketch of JTW, 11.

53. 'poor both of them': AW to author, 1979. Mabel Wilson: LH notes.

54. 'They all adored': Mary Edgeworth David, to author, 1979.

55. 'How are the': *Hermes*, 1898. 'Tell Mabel': CJM to JTW, 14.6.99.

56. Documents relating to JTW's military career.

6

Foundations

The turn of the century was a time for rejoicings and reappraisals. Federation of the Australian colonies after ten years of political contention was given a week of celebrations in Sydney, starting at midnight on 31 December 1900. The city, decked with flags and bunting, was packed with visitors to witness the inauguration of the new Commonwealth of Australia. Crowds gathered at vantage points on the morning of 1 January for the great procession which left the Domain at 10.30 for a five-mile wind through the city to the official ceremony in Centennial Park. The Wilson family was seated in a stand in College Street outside the Australian Museum. All sections of Australian society were represented in the cavalcade but the centre of attention was the new Governor-General, Lord Hopetoun, in full court dress riding in an open carriage and accompanied by a thousand colourful British Imperial troops as well as khaki-clad Australian contingents.[1] If Federation was a national achievement, this was an Imperial occasion, and most Australians believed it fitting that 7,000 miles away on the veldts of South Africa their soldiers were fighting in the cause of Empire.

The Boer War was a very popular war. Feted and farewelled at their ports of embarkation more than 16,000 Australian troops sailed off to South Africa to win reputations for themselves, their country and the Empire. Sydney's medical profession answered the call with exuberance sending the only medical corps from the Australian colonies, a well-equipped and impressively mobile corps of about 240 personnel. The ambulance idea – horse or mule-drawn spring carts carrying medical equipment – was an Australian innovation which drew special praise from Lord Roberts. Many university men joined the adventure, among them Robert Scot

117

Skirving and Alexander MacCormick who paid their own fares, took their own expensive instruments and a small X-ray apparatus donated by the prominent Sydney merchant, Sam Hordern. But they were not well received by the military and after six months, in June 1900, Scot Skirving left South Africa for England to write a critique of the NSW Medical Corps in the field, and MacCormick, after toying with the idea of a tiger hunt as an alternative, followed in September. As for the X-ray apparatus, it fell off the cliff-like bank of the Orange River during a stampede of mules.[2]

At the University Wilson and Edgeworth David sponsored the formation of a University Volunteer Rifle Corps. Wilson chaired its inaugural meeting in Michaelmas term 1900. It began as an approved student body under the command of R C Simpson, a demonstrator in physics, and was supported by a small grant from the Senate to cover expenses. Its first formal parade was for the Duke of York's visit to the University in May 1901. The Scottish Rifles assisted the fledgling corps in many ways and the two groups developed a friendly rapport on the rifle range and at camps around Sydney during Easter, September and January. National Park was the usual rallying ground.[3]

Hermes gave the war light-hearted cover till August 1900 when it announced the death of Lieutenant Keith Mackellar, eldest son of the influential Dr C K Mackellar, member of the Legislative Council and the Board of Health. A memorial for all university men killed in the war was proposed. Disillusion grew as the long misery of the commando phase took its toll, and reached its climax in an ugly public controversy.

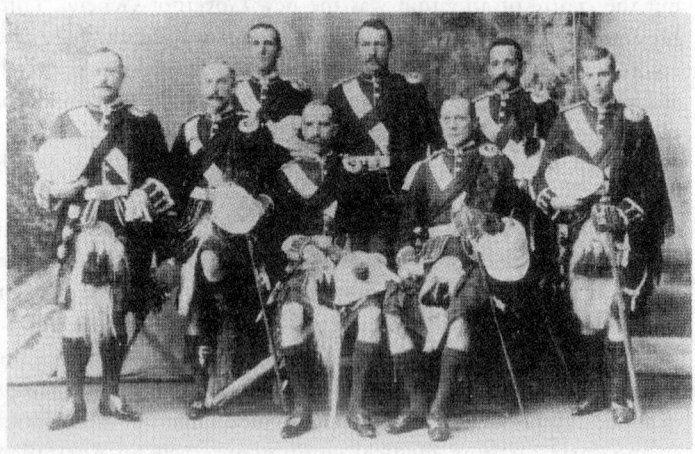

Officers of the NSW Scottish Rifles, c.1900. Seated: Lt.-Col. Campbell, Capt Wilson.
(Photo, courtesy Major T F Wade Ferrell and the Australian National Library)

At the beginning of the war the quiet historian Arnold Wood, just back from a year in England where opposition was fervent and widespread, wrote to the *Daily Telegraph* protesting against support for the war on the basis of 'our country right or wrong'. His letter gave rise to shrill accusations of base motives from the general public; more penetrating was the able reply from his senior colleague Mungo MacCallum, Dean of the Faculty of Arts, who held that while views of what was right might differ, all dispute should cease in the interests of national unity once war was declared. Wood kept silence for two years, until December 1901 when he wrote again to the *Daily Telegraph* criticizing Kitchener's severe counter measures to Boer commando tactics – farm destruction and concentration camps which produced an appalling mortality among South African women and children – and appealing for 'English patriotism to protest against a policy that is bringing everlasting infamy upon the English name'. Again MacCallum joined battle, arguing that Kitchener's tactics were necessary to finish the war quickly against an unscrupulous enemy. The editor closed the debate in January 1902 and Wood then gave expression to his views in speeches to the Anti-War League, of which he reluctantly became President on 30 January. The following week he sent an article on Australian opinion of the war to the *Manchester Guardian*, a brief and distorted report of which was telegraphed to the Australian press. It led to a witch-hunt: 'Professor Wood must go' was the cry. The University Senate to its shame censured Wood for 'highly reprehensible' utterances, 'unworthy of a Professor of History', and might have gone to the length of dismissing him if MacCallum, Edgeworth David and Edmund Barton (who as Prime Minister of the day had declared himself for 'the Empire right or wrong') in the Senate had not supported Wood's right to express his opinion.[4]

The argument between Wood and MacCallum was bitter but rational. For Wood the humanitarian issue weighed heaviest, for MacCallum the imperial cause. On Empire Wilson and MacCallum were of one mind though Wilson must have regretted that MacCallum in his intemperance supplied intellectual ammunition to Wood's denigrators in a public brawl, gave the Senate the opportunity to demean itself and subjected Wood to a severe mauling. MacCallum, he knew, was only too prone to violence in debate, though he knew too that 'he can, when he will, preserve a very judicial mind'. Had MacCallum been in England and not at the Australian outpost of Empire he might well, like Wood, have criticized the war in the same moral terms as his revered teacher

119

Edward Caird did, along with many of his Idealist friends in Britain like John Muirhead and Henry Jones. Yet it was Caird's teachings too which gave the cause of Empire an ideological rationale and a spiritual force.[5] In 1902 MacCallum's thoughts were dominated by a perception of crisis in its condition. As the Boer War and the fracas over Wood fizzled out MacCallum voiced his concern for the well-being of the Empire:

> We certainly do not wish that spirit to flag. We are filled with apprehension at any symptom of its doing so. The grasp of the British Empire and its constituent States and its constituent members, on the industrial and mercantile world needs to be tightened rather than relaxed, and one of the problems of the time is to infuse new intelligence and efficacy into the methods of its enterprise.[6]

One of these methods was through science and technology.

In Britain the Boer War was felt as a national failure, reinforcing fears about the deterioration of the race. It focused a spotlight on the inadequacies of British science and technology in comparison with Germany where science had been harnessed to industry through a carefully articulated national education system. Germany had won industrial supremacy not only in iron and steel production but also in the chemical and electrical industries, sectors in which Britain until recently had been a world leader. Criticism of Britain's neglect of scientific and technical education went back 40 years, and efforts to correct the deficiency went back 20 years: too little too late said the critics. The Boer War, together with faith in education as the engine of progress, supplied the spur to change quickly. The political catchcry became 'national efficiency', first proclaimed by the Liberal Imperialist Lord Rosebery but endorsed across the political spectrum, uniting unionists like Joseph Chamberlain, liberals like Richard Haldane and socialists like the Webbs.[7]

There was one conviction that all shared: that the universities would be the main means of fostering the talent to maintain and increase the might of Great Britain and her Empire. Richard Haldane's prescription was Hegelian. In 1902 he recommended a system of independent regional universities throughout Britain following the German model and crowned by a postgraduate research college for London University 'where students from every part of the empire could come to carry their scientific training further than is possible in the less specialized colonial and other Universities and colleges'. It resulted in 1907 in the foundation of the Imperial College of Science and Technology, South Kensington. Haldane envisaged it as 'a new link in Imperial Federation of probably the only type, apart from that of sentiment, that is possible'.[8]

The same idea prompted the Canadian-born Tory member for Gravesend, Sir Gilbert Parker, to organize an Allied Colonial Universities Conference in July 1903, to which all the universities of the Empire (except the Indian ones) sent representatives. Chaired by James Bryce and addressed by Prime Minister Balfour, the conference extolled research as an educational instrument and sought to induce more hospitality for postgraduate colonial students at British Universities to stem the tide flowing to French and German Universities (the only endowment for this purpose being at Cambridge) and to declare the need for more scholarships along the lines of the 1851 Exhibitioners. A precedent for future conferences was thus established.[9]

Sydney's scientific leaders picked up British concern for the backward condition of British science in comparison with German and American science, to focus attention on the unsatisfactory state of Australian science, though the Australian case was not strictly comparable. Science was popular enough in Australia, as the success of the great exhibitions in Sydney and Melbourne in the 1870s and 1880s had shown, but it was not taken seriously. It had entertainment value as a hobby for amateurs and eccentrics, but was not a vocation. Before 1900 there would have been only about a hundred 'cultivators of science' in the whole of Australia. Sydney's civic leaders, complained the engineer and botanist Henry Deane, had not even officially welcomed the many distinguished scientists who had attended the Australasian Association for the Advancement of Science (AAAS) meeting in 1898. He recommended a campaign to get science into the schools to stimulate at grass-roots level a proper appreciation of the methods and value of science. Endorsing this idea, Liversidge berated the University for removing science from the Matriculation Examination in 1887 while he was abroad, a decision that had checked the development of science teaching generally and in some schools killed it completely. He enjoined scientists who were parents to take the campaign personally into the schools their children attended. Liversidge also tried to found a 'National Australian Academy' to grace the new federated nation and an Australasian *Nature,* but both projects met a disappointing response.[10]

At the University science had made steady progress but scientific research still had no recognized place. It was done by weary teachers in their spare time and at no small expense to themselves. Yet they had chalked up a creditable record: by 1902 Liversidge, Threlfall, Edgeworth David, Haswell and Martin had been elected to Fellowships of the Royal Society of London, while Wilson, Hill and Elliot Smith had achieved recognition in Australasia, Britain and even Europe for their research on Australian native fauna. 'The science schools of the University, are in every instance fine monuments of the earnestness of purpose of the professors in charge, to whose untiring efforts their equipment is largely due,' said the statistician, astronomer and lecturer in engineering at the university, G H Knibbs, addressing the Royal Society of NSW in 1899. 'But for their proper utilization they are not sufficiently endowed; in fact, it is not putting the case too strongly to say that their energies are sadly crippled by that very fact.'[11]

In 1902 the University of Sydney celebrated its Jubilee with a week of festivities beginning on 30 September. It was a hot week and colourful. Flags from all nations decorated the grey walls of the Great Hall and pathways between the various departments were festooned and canopied. At night they were ablaze with electric light. There were receptions, garden parties, dinners, a smoke concert, a ball, a conversazione, a regatta and a cruise around Sydney Harbour to entertain distinguished guests representing universities around the world as well as local dignitaries. Academic gowns of many colours were paraded and there was a boom in tall hats and panamas. The museums and laboratories displayed their wares, on sale were H E Barff's commemorative history of the University, the Student Union's volume of selected presidential addresses (including Wilson's for 1901–2) and the special Jubilee number of *Hermes*. A portrait of the Chancellor, Sir Normand MacLaurin, was unveiled by the Governor, Sir Harry Rawson, and the deans of arts, medicine and science delivered addresses. *Hermes* reported a triumphant week.[12]

Anderson Stuart's address on the growth of the Medical School – the most impressive feature of the university's history in the last 20 years – revelled in the refutation of his early critics. With one professor, a demonstrator, four clinical lecturers and four students in 1883, by 1902 it boasted three professors, three demonstrators, 11 lecturers and 202 students. Rivalling the Arts faculty in student members it was housed in a noble building that made 'Student and graduate and teacher alike feel proud'. The medical and law faculties (and engineering, incorporated at its beginning, in 1883, within the science faculty), had won the argument for '*Brodstudien*', widening the gate for pharmacy, dentistry, veterinary science, education and commerce in the first decade of the new century. Sydney's 'intensely practical community' had responded emphatically to opportunities for vocational training.[13]

MacCallum in loftier terms endorsed Stuart's implicit proposition: that the university ideal – to enlighten the mind, refine the understanding and elevate mankind – could as well be maintained by professional studies as by the liberal arts and the theoretical sciences. The house of culture had many doors. Wilson agreed but he did harbour fears for the security of the traditional university ideal, which in his shorthand was a school for the three Cs: character, culture and craftsmanship. Certainly vocational studies had a legitimate place within the university but not if they degenerated into mere courses in craftsmanship. The guiding impulse of university research, scientific or otherwise, must ever be that of the scholar he insisted, reasserting in updated form Sir Charles Badham and Sir William Manning's side of the argument against Anderson Stuart and the medical school in the 1880s. To promote broad and disinterested intellectual sympathies in both 'the humanities' and 'the bestialities', Wilson recommended the introduction of German as a compulsory preliminary subject for all students: it had the educational value of linguistic discipline and it gave access to the riches of great literature, philosophy and science.[14]

Anderson Stuart was in a celebratory mood. Wilson, concentrating on the future prospects of the Medical School, was more sober about the demands that a proper medical education made on the resources of universities and, directly and indirectly, on the resources of government. His comparative study of medical courses showed it would cost much more to equip and run schools to the standard of the best in America and Germany, the world's leaders in medical research and education. Once a professor and a lecture room had sufficed to teach a subject to any class, however large. Now there must be laboratories, workshops, highly expensive apparatus, abundant perishable material, huge amounts of literature and more teachers. No one teacher could cope with all the requirements of one subject, even to comparatively small classes. If Australian medical schools were to progress beyond their 'present third-rate status' they would require at least a four-fold increase in their endowment just to lift them to the US or German standard, without any thought of future expansion. Medical schools in the United Kingdom, in similar straits, were making strenuous efforts to remedy this 'deplorable inferiority in means and equipment'.

123

Cambridge, despite its princely inheritance, was now asking for 100,000 pounds to repair its deficiencies, while Owens College in Manchester was appealing for 150,000 pounds and the four Scottish Universities estimated their needs at not less than two million pounds. Andrew Carnegie's munificent gift of that amount in 1901 eased the plight of Scotland's universities by providing capital for buildings, laboratories, equipment, chairs, lectureships and scholarships which in turn gave research a much-needed stimulus.[15]

Wilson agreed with what Edgeworth David had to say on the condition of the science faculty. Not as well housed or equipped as medicine – for it had no political 'fixer' of the calibre of Anderson Stuart – there were 117 students enrolled in the science faculty in 1901, all but a handful of them in engineering and most of those doing mining which, observed Edgeworth David, was 'natural and right in a country of such vast mineral wealth'. Science wore a distinctly utilitarian aspect. Classes in physics, chemistry and biology were swelled by engineering, medical, dentistry and pharmacy students. Only 12 students in 1901 were enrolled for the BSc. Pure science, as in Britain, was not lucrative, had few patrons and few openings. Australian politicians were blind to its value and perhaps that was one reason why Richard Threlfall in 1898 returned to England, where lobbying for the basic necessities of research was not such a frustration. Science at Sydney University needed a massive injection of funds. Edgeworth David listed the needs: a chair in botany, a department of agriculture, scientific surveys and expeditions, more laboratories and equipment, better scientific libraries, postgraduate courses, more travelling scholarships to give graduates research experience overseas and, more importantly, research fellowships to regain the services of those scholars so that they might contribute to Sydney's reputation rather than the reputations of overseas universities. These were the needs, but David's hopes for their fulfilment would not have been high. He put his finger on the main hindrance:

> we, in Australia, suffer under a disability from which most of the older countries are exempt – there is practically little or no scientific opinion in the people of Australia.[16]

As Anderson Stuart's interests gradually expanded beyond the medical school – to public health, hospital administration, the creation of a dentistry school and other less-august concerns – Wilson's commitment within it deepened. As student numbers grew so did the administrative burden on Wilson who had only one full-time assistant, Louis Schaeffer. In the shade of Wilson's increasing stature Louis grew into 'the prince of technicians' and a skilled photographer and photomicrographer. With a perfect understanding of Wilson's exacting requirements he presided over the dissecting room, gave 'unwearied assistance' to his research, operated the epidiascope in lectures punctuated with the urgent whisper 'focus, Louis, focus', and at other times remained on the alert for the louder whisper 'Loo-ee' resounding down the corridor. Wilson was also assisted by a string of part-time graduate demonstrators recruited from his best students on appointments of one to two years; in the nineties they were A E Mills, John Morton, Robert Dick, Grafton Elliot Smith, G L Murray, F J T Sawkins and E Ludowici. Like his great exemplar William Turner, Wilson was an efficient and economical administrator, and his department was, on the testimony of J P Hill, 'in its equipment and facilities for teaching and research, far in advance of any comparable department in [Great Britain] at the time.'[17]

Wilson was pre-occupied with the medical curriculum which

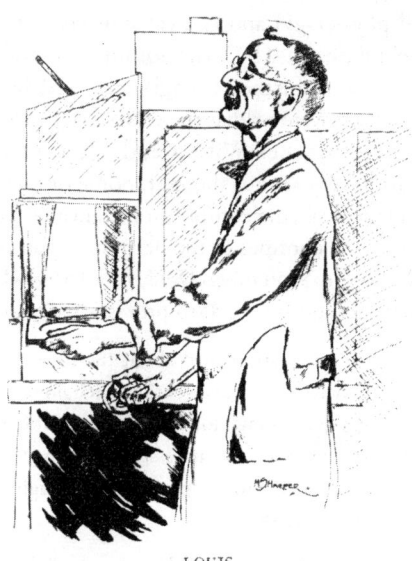

LOUIS.

'Louie' [Louis Schaeffer]
(Sydney University Medical Journal, June 1919)

had become a perennial problem, always threatening to get out of hand as science made ever-accelerating strides, as specialisms proliferated, as the relative importance of subjects changed and as teaching techniques improved. Until 1889 Sydney's medical course was taught in 'somewhat anarchical conditions', with the basic sciences, medical sciences and clinical work alongside one another. Nominally a five-year course – since all medical students had to begin with a year in the arts faculty – it became actually a five-year medical course by a revision in 1889, the first year arts course being made an alternative to passing a medical entrance examination equivalent to the Senior Public Examination at a high standard. Wilson regretted the loss of the first year in Arts for it was one of his strongest convictions that professional studies, or craftsmanship, should be integrated with the general intellectual life of the university and it did not escape his notice in September 1901 that Harvard's medical school enacted the requirement of a four-year arts course as a condition of entry to its four-year medical course. He knew that was a Utopian suggestion for Australian conditions but at least a medical training should have a stronger scientific foundation. The 1889 curriculum established a logical order of progression – basic sciences (physics, chemistry and biology), medical sciences (anatomy and physiology) and clinical subjects – with clean breaks between each phase. In 1892 the foundations in the basic and medical sciences were further strengthened and for the first time barrier examinations were held at the end of each calendar year.[18]

From the mid-nineties Wilson and Martin had been giving medical education very serious thought. Some of their ideas changed the Melbourne medical curriculum, 'an instance of your far-reaching influence outside the confines of the petty state you inhabit!' Martin quipped to Wilson in September 1898, in a letter which disparaged Anderson Stuart's crude approach to professional training:

> Stuart came down here and talked about the necessity of cleaning one's teeth, of having a little conventional religion, and of having successfully negotiated exams, for a prosperous professional career! Also, tips for passing exams, as successfully practised by T.P.A.S. in Edin! The Chief Justice and people like he thought it very fine, because they quite understood.

Martin's representation was apt. This standard lecture of Stuart's entitled 'Medicine as a Career', delivered to countless undergraduates over the years, was indeed a long list of hints and strategies for 'getting on' in the lucrative practice of medicine.[19]

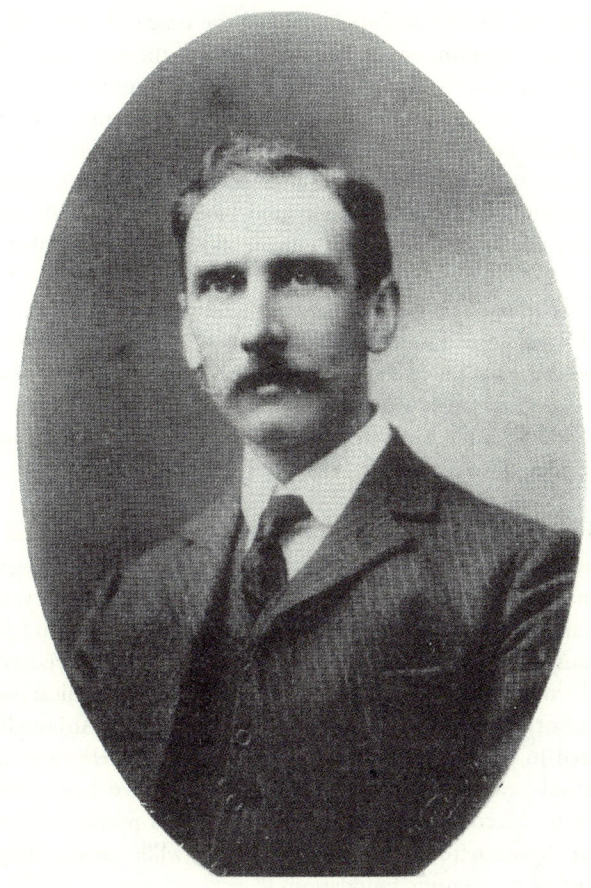

Charles James Martin c.1898   (Wilson Papers, SUA)

At Martin's invitation Wilson gave his views on medical education in an address to the Melbourne Medical Students Society in September 1901. He was convinced that the traditional curriculum had reached the limits of ingenious adjustment. Efforts to secure all-round completeness, equilibrium and the best distribution of time in a logical progression had led to a cast-iron system that blocked the student's initiative, enthusiasm and intellectual growth, so defeating the real aim of education. To add another year to the course would compound the problem; to return to the simpler programme was reactionary. And to cut back the basic sciences would compromise fundamental principles: what, he asked, is the science of Physiology but the practical application to the human organism of the knowledge which these sciences afford? He believed that 'in the generality and the comprehensiveness of biological teaching resides much of its value' for men who were about to be concentrated on its details: physicians should have 'an even more thorough discipline and absorption in [the] radical and fertile truths' of physics chemistry and biology. In marked contrast to Anderson Stuart, Wilson was putting the case for scholarship:

> .... the true student [he concluded] will wisely ignore altogether the achievement of future social and financial success. The key of knowledge lies before him. Let him take it up and use it with what dexterity he may. It will tax all his capacity, and all his energies ... He will probably find that the joys of craftsmanship itself are his exceeding great reward.[20]

So what was to be done with the curriculum? Wilson believed that an entirely new model was needed. The most promising was the system of elective studies being introduced in the final two years of medical courses in the best American schools, Harvard and Johns Hopkins. Harvard's anatomy professor Charles Minot envisaged the introduction of elective subjects to every year of the medical course, compulsory subjects being reduced to a minimum. Although not prepared to go that far Wilson was convinced that electives in the two final years were the educational answer to proliferating specialism. Electives would relieve the student of pressures from the clinical superstructure of the medical course while safeguarding the integrity of its scientific foundations.[21]

After prolonged consideration the new curriculum was adopted in 1902. The answer to an overcrowded course, unbalanced by too many lectures and too little clinical work, was to shift all subjects forward at the expense of the basic sciences in the first year, more particularly biology. That would not have pleased Wilson – it was contrary to his advice – but elsewhere the curriculum bore marks of his counsel. First, the elective principle was introduced for the fifth year: of five minor clinical subjects (diseases of children, diseases of the skin, diseases of the ear, nose and throat, special bacteriology and special therapeutics) the student had to select two. Second, examinations which had increased to an irregularly-timed five, once again marked the end of the three phases of the course (basic science, medical science and clinical work). Third and most important, materia medica, regarded by Wilson as 'an anachronism' was abolished as a separate subject as he had prescribed: pharmacognosy (the knowledge of drugs) went to pharmacy; therapeutics (application of remedies in the treatment of diseases) went to special therapeutics as an elective in the fifth year; and pharmacology 'the scientific basis' went to practical physiology.[22]

The same year saw the foundation of the pathology chair, to which another Edinburgh man, David Arthur Welsh, was appointed. That this, in Wilson's words, 'large and important subject ... with its hardly subordinate domain of bacteriology' had suffered neglect was curious, considering that the elevation of bacteriology to the first rank of medical disciplines had coincided with the foundation of the medical school. (In isolating the tubercle bacillus in 1882 Robert Koch had ushered in an exciting decade of discovery of bacteria causing contagious diseases.) Moreover in 1882 the Senate had made comparatively generous provision for pathology, its importance was appreciated by both Wilson and Anderson Stuart, and on the spot was a well-qualified candidate in W Camac Wilkinson whom the Senate had appointed lecturer in pathology early in 1883, before Anderson Stuart's arrival. Wilkinson's availability may have been the problem: from the start there was ill-feeling between him and Anderson Stuart who would not likely promote the fortunes of a rival, and initially Wilson too had an interest in keeping Wilkinson out, for he did in those early years have hopes that Jim Smith would be the first occupant of Sydney's pathology chair. But he would not have endorsed the Senate's rejection in 1895 of a bequest of 11,400 pounds from Sir William Macleay to found a bacteriology chair or lectureship on the extraordinary grounds that bacteriology was not taught as a separate compulsory course anywhere in the world, that it would further burden the students and that it would add to maintenance costs. In 1896 Camac Wilkinson instituted a postgraduate evening course in bacteriology to meet the needs of busy practitioners. Whatever the reasons for the neglect of pathology and bacteriology, it was only after Wilkinson ceased to be available that the Senate established a pathology chair. The Macleay money went to the Linnean Society to found the Macleay Fellowship, the first research post in bacteriology in Australia, attached to Australia's first microbiological laboratory, an earlier benefaction of Sir William Macleay.[23]

The related field of public health continued to be neglected also by the medical school. It had low status in the curriculum despite Sydney's appalling sanitary condition and high incidence of epidemic disease. Anderson Stuart was better acquainted than most with public health problems: in 1890 he had reported to the Governments of New South Wales, South Australia and New Zealand on Koch's method of treating tuberculosis; as a member of the Board of Health from 1891 and its President from 1893 to 1896 he had had a hand in initiating the Board's bacteriological laboratory in Macquarie St in 1895. At a time when Sydney was suffering an outbreak of bubonic plague, Anderson Stuart met pressures for a Sydney postgraduate Diploma in Public Health with strange reasoning:

> the DPH of Cambridge has been a convenient Qualification for our graduates to obtain while visiting Europe, and in this way 8 out of the 36 graduates who have visited Europe have obtained it. In so far as it has acted as an inducement to graduates to visit Europe, it has been a good thing, because that visit in itself, not before graduation, but after it, is of immense value, precisely as a visit to Australia is of use to the European graduate.[24]

The real reason may once again have been personal. Public health in NSW was professionalized mainly by one man, John Ashburton Thompson. With London and Brussels degrees in medicine and a DPH from Cambridge, Thompson was the only trained epidemiologist in the colony when he joined the Board of Health in 1884 as a temporary medical officer. He became the Board's driving force. When the public service was restructured in 1896 Thompson was appointed the first executive director of the Board, displacing Anderson Stuart from the lucrative offices of President of the Board and Medical Adviser to the Government, which had doubled his income. Stuart's appointment to these positions had been controversial from the beginning (December 1892), and while he accepted his defeat with outward good grace he was convinced that it was the result of a plot by his enemies. He retained membership of the Board until his death in 1920.[25]

New South Wales' first public health Bill was passed in November 1896. Thompson built a small but effective service, publicized the problems and travelled indefatigably to provide first-hand reports on outbreaks of 'sanitary nuisances' and epidemic disease. An essay on leprosy in 1897 won him a world-wide reputation but the pinnacle of his achievement as an epidemiologist was his analysis and management of Sydney's bubonic plague epidemic of 1900 and its recurrences. Wilson was well acquainted with Thompson who from 1892 to 1899 was the Medical School's examiner in public health and attended faculty meetings when public health education was discussed. In August 1902 he became Wilson's brother-in-law when he married Mabel's elder sister Lilian Simpson, a widow with three children. He also became a neighbour.[26]

At the end of 1898 the Wilsons had moved to Woollahra, Sydney's stateliest suburb. Charming, leafy, well-administered and clean – among the first to adopt tar paving – it was the only suburb in all Australia with *haut ton* according to a contemporary Sydney journalist. Woollahra and the adjoining suburbs with beautiful harbour frontages – Darling Point, Point Piper, Rose Bay, Vaucluse – attracted the wealthy, the influential and the successful which by the turn of the century included many of the University's senior men. Little more than three miles from the GPO, Woollahra had an excellent tram service which the Wilsons relied upon, though many of its inhabitants had their own private carriages or the chauffeur-driven cars that came into vogue in the first decade of the new century.[27]

Wilson would have preferred Rose Bay, probably because it was near a golf course, but Sir Julian insisted on Woollahra. Witty, cultivated and benevolent, but also temperamental, pugnacious and acutely vulnerable, Sir Julian was very much the *pater familias* who wanted to keep a close eye on his daughter's welfare. Another consideration was the unusually strong bond between his wife and daughter. So the Wilsons took 'Dela Kaba' in Wallis Street, just around the corner from the Salomons' mansion 'Sherbourne' in Nelson Street. Four years later they moved to a new and larger house called 'Apheta' on the recently subdivided Glenhead estate, next door to 'Sherbourne'.[28]

Mabel's influence on Wilson was soon apparent. He became clean-shaven and remained so for the rest of his life, and he discarded a disreputable mustard-coloured overcoat. His social life expanded beyond academic and scientific circles and Wilsonian hospitality acquired a degree of formality. Of the two, however, it was Mabel who made the more basic adjustments. Accommodating herself to a household in which she was the only newcomer could not have been easy and she had to cope with the inherently difficult relationships with mother-in-law and step-daughter. But Mabel had a positive, sanguine nature. She added Scottish literature to her reading, even Carlyle's mighty *French Revolution*, went camping on the Hawkesbury with Wilson and Hill in the summer of 1898/9 and continued with 'artistic anatomy' at the University to within

131

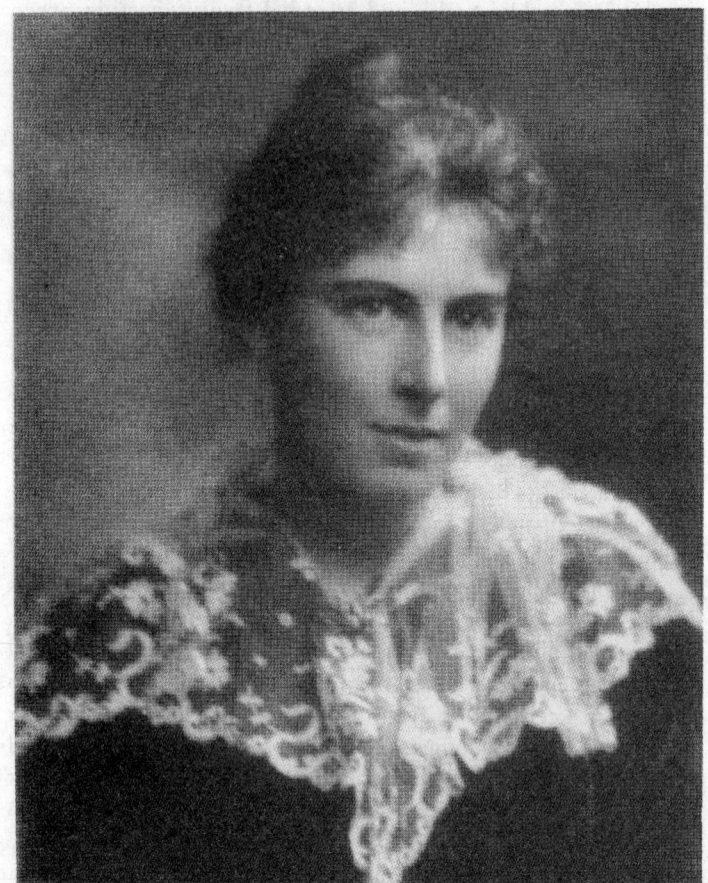

Mabel M M Wilson (née Salomons), c.1890 (Courtesy Wilson family)

weeks of the birth of her first child. Perhaps domestic difficulties accounted for separate holidays in those early years. While Jeanie and her grandmother went to Blackheath, Mabel and Wilson went to Melbourne in June 1899 and to the Huon Valley in Tasmania in January 1901.[29]

The first of the babies who arrived at roughly two-year intervals in the new century lightened the last years of Mrs Wilson senior who died of cancer in October 1902. And if reservations persisted in Jeanie's attitude to Mabel – their relationship never became easy – her reception of new sisters and brothers was wholehearted. First, on 18 March 1900, came Louise Helen Henrietta Mondell, given two names from each parent's family. Lady Salomons' was Louisa and by coincidence so was the unsuspecting matchmaker of the marriage, Miss Louisa MacDonald. Another daughter, born on 26 July 1902 was named simply Dorothea – always called Dorette as the Germans pronounce it – after Mrs MacCallum. A third, Katharine Mabel, was born on 18 June 1904.[30]

A block or two away in Ocean Street lived Mabel's only sister Lilian Simpson. Widowed in 1898, Lilian moved back to Woollahra about the same time as the Wilsons transferred there and probably for the same reason, to be near the Salomons. Her children, Brian, Julian and Norah were around Jeanie's age, but the two families were never really close, for the sisters were quite different in interests and outlook. Eight years older than Mabel, Lilian held 'advanced' opinions and enjoyed the company of celebrities. In August 1902 Lilian married John Ashburton Thompson. Eldest of the large family of a struggling London solicitor who died young, Thompson seemed fated to the role of guardian in his private life, first to his younger brothers and sisters, then from 1894 to two young sons of a brother who died in Adelaide, and then to the Simpson children to whom he must have seemed rather like a grandfather for he was 20 years older than Lilian. Though forceful and somewhat feared at the Board of Health, to the young Wilsons 'Uncle Atty' seemed shy and ill-at-ease. He watched their welfare from a distance. He was the authority who decreed that they had 'cooked' milk instead of the 'raw' which they preferred. With Wilson, however, both Ashburton Thompson and their father-in-law Sir Julian Salomons developed close friendships.[31]

Three other new households were being established at the turn of the century. During the long summer vacation of 1899–1900 Hill returned 'home' to marry Miss Marjorie Steele at the Presbyterian Church, Finchley, London in January, and to honeymoon in Scotland. They returned to settle in a house they called 'Langside', in Livingstone Road, Petersham. At the end of 1902, when they took a holiday in Britain, Hill was a candidate for the newly established Chair of Biology at Victoria College, Wellington, New Zealand. Despite excellent testimonials from Wilson and Haswell of Sydney, Martin and Baldwin Spencer of Melbourne, Professors Beard and Cossar Ewart of Edinburgh, G B Howes of London, A A W Hubrecht of Utrecht and a particularly fulsome one from the usually restrained Ray Lankester of Oxford, Hill did not get that appointment. In 1904 he was awarded a DSc from Edinburgh University and in October of that year, in recognition of his long service as a demonstrator and 'valuable contributions to science', Sydney University created a new position for him as Lecturer in Embryology. His annual salary rose from 323 to 450 pounds. At about this time the funds awarded him by the Royal Society in 1900 to study marsupial and monotreme development would have run out.[32]

When Grafton Elliot Smith attended Hill's wedding in January 1900 he seemed settled in Cambridge. In three struggling years he had accomplished an astonishing feat of research in brain morphology – on the origin of the *corpus callosum*, on the brain of the *Edentata* (a group of mammals with unconvoluted cerebrum that includes the armadillo and aardvark of South America), and on the margin of the cerebral cortex and other features of the mammalian brain. He had also begun work on his celebrated descriptive catalogue of the brain collection in the Museum of the Royal College of Surgeons which gave him an 'unrivalled grasp of the comparative morphology of the brain'. The Anatomical Society in 1900 recorded its appreciation of the stimulus he had given to the study of the central nervous system in Great Britain, till then almost the exclusive property of the physiologists.[33]

St John's College in Cambridge had elected Elliot Smith to a Fellowship in November 1899 and a university appointment seemed likely. His future was settled for six years, he had assured Wilson on 10 November 1899. Eight months later, however, on the recommendation of Professor Alexander Macalister of Cambridge, he accepted the newly created chair in anatomy (carrying an annual salary of 600 pounds, rising to 800) at Cairo's government medical school, and by October 1900 he was installed there with his bride, a Sydney 'colleen', Kathleen Macredie whom he had married in London in September. But Cairo's cost of living was high and he thought wistfully of translation to Melbourne where the establishment of an anatomy chair was mooted. Martin made discreet enquiries. By August 1902, however, when he returned to Sydney for the first time since 1896, accompanied by his wife and baby son, Elliot Smith was content with his lot in Cairo. Egyptology, whose attractions he had been resisting for some time, had claimed another victim. From 1902 Elliot Smith carried a dual professional commission, in anatomy and anthropology.[34]

In Melbourne in March 1900 Martin was moving his wife and 18-month-old daughter Maisie into a new house and shortly afterwards he took charge of a new laboratory at the University. With challenging research in train, notably on thermal adjustment and respiratory exchange in monotremes and marsupials, he savoured the prospect of many more years in Melbourne. An inspiring teacher and now a distinguished physiologist – elected Fellow of the Royal Society in 1901 – he was invited to apply for chairs at King's College London in 1899 to succeed W D Halliburton, and at Queen's College Belfast in 1901. The first he dismissed lightly, the second he considered over several months. Melbourne University, in dismay, expressed its appreciation of his 'stimulating influence' and its regrets that it could not yet confer on him the position and emoluments he deserved. Martin replied that he was more concerned about keeping in touch with scientific work abroad. So the Council of the University gave him five months leave every second year to visit Europe and America. 'This seems to me to be good enough!' Martin advised Wilson in May 1902. 'I am glad to have the beastly thing settled one way or another. It was undermining my constitution.' But it was not settled, and Martin accepted the next proposition, to become Director of the Lister Institute in London and left Melbourne in September 1903. It was a surprise development, conducted by cable, and Martin accepted with reluctance. 'Why are we leaving?' asked his five-year-old daughter Maisie as they were about to board ship. 'Because your mother is homesick,' replied her father. 'It is the only reason.' Martin went to Sydney at the end of July 1903 to have 'a quiet time' with Wilson, and before leaving gave him information on salaries and requirements at Belfast in the hope that Wilson would also consider returning to Britain.[35]

But Wilson's thoughts at that time were dominated by his research with Hill on the embryology of the platypus. He had realized by 1900 that if he were to contribute anything important to the world of science he would have to shed some of his more mundane and time-consuming activities. Early in 1901 he resigned from the Council of the Linnean Society and he cast off the onerous position of honorary secretary to Prince Alfred Hospital which he had carried since the final illness of Sir Alfred Roberts in 1897. Anderson Stuart succeeded him at the hospital on condition that a paid secretary also be appointed. Soon afterwards Stuart became the chairman, in time to organize the laying of the foundation stone of the Victoria and Albert Pavilion by His Royal Highness the Duke of York, on 30 May 1901. With royal eclat Anderson Stuart took up duty as Prince Alfred's second autocrat, while from abroad Elliot Smith applauded Wilson's riddance of 'extraneous work: 'for there are scores of people who might be an efficient Secretary to the hospital, but only one who can write anatomical memoirs'.[36]

Notes

1. Inauguration of Commonwealth & Opening of Parliament: Cuneen, 1–2, 18.
2. Boer War contingents & medical corps: Field, Preface, 35–7, 103, 108–9; *SSM,* Vol. 3, 23, 244.
3. In the student mind Wilson had long been associated with military affairs, *Hermes* observing on 29.10.1898, 'If the long talked of Varsity Volunteer Corps ever comes to anything Professor Wilson will be the man to lead us as he is a lieutenant in the Scottish Rifles with whom he recently spent a fortnight in barracks'. Senate grant: Senate Minutes, 1.7.1901. First parade: Mosher, 217. Rapport with Scottish Rifles: *Hermes,* 6.12.1902, 13.
4. Arnold Wood controversy: Crawford, 153. 'English patriotism': quoted in Crawford, 173. Wood's censure: Crawford 183–223. 'highly reprehensible': Senate Minutes, 10.2.1902. Support for Wood: Meaney, 47.
5. 'he can': JTW to J, 1.5.1935. Caird's view: Muirhead, 112.
6. 'We certainly': MacCallum address, 'University Influence', 1.10.1902, 43.
7. British industry and science: Searle, Ch. 1; *Nature* and Lockyer; Meadows, Ch. X.
8. Haldane: Ashby & Anderson, xiii–xv, 44, 47, 49. Common conviction: Sanderson, 207. 'where students' and 'a new link': R B Haldane, 1902, 36–7.
9. University Conference 1903: *Report of Proceedings* 1912, ix–xi; Univs Conference as precedent: *Nature,* 16.7.03, 250–2.
10. Appeal of science in Australia: Moyal 1986, 101–2. 'cultivators' of science: Nathan Reingold in MacLeod, 6. Sydney's failure: Deane, 44–5. Sydney Univ. exclusion of science: Liversidge, *RS NSW* J, Vol. 35, 1901, 16. Disappointing response: MacLeod, 55.
11. Liversidge: *ADB;* 'The Science' etc. Knibbs, 42. JTW on research: S A Smith 1950, 9.
12. Jubilee celebrations: University of Sydney, 1903.
13. For statistics on growth of Sydney Univ.: Barff, 94–104. Lecturing staff: *Centenary Book,* 106–23. In 1883 lecturers were all part-time: Medicine (Cox); Surgery (Mitford); Midwifery (Chambers); Medical Jurisprudence (Goode). Dixson (Materia Medica) and Wilkinson (Pathology) were then overseas. By 1902 the Medical school in addition had 3 honorary demonstrators and 4 honorary lecturers (Barff, 100). 'Student and': TPAS, 81. 'intensely practical': JTW, Inaugural Lecture, Cambridge, 1921 (unpub).

14. University ideal: MacCallum 39. Wilson's views: JTW 1902c, 90–2, and 1901, 410–14, 431.
15. 'present third rate' and 'deplorable inferiority': JTW 1901, 429, 107 resp. Carnegie Trust: Turner, 372–6.
16. 'natural and': TWED 1902, 111–12. Science students: U of S *Calendar* for 1903, 358. Threlfall: *RSO* Vol. 1, 47; Home 351. 'we in Australia': TWED 1902, 117.
17. 'unwearied assistance': JTW 1907b, 36. 'focus, Louis': *Senior Year Book*, 1920 and interview with Catherine Mackerras. Wilson's demonstrators were recent graduates who began their duties in Lent Term and were paid £200 a year: *Centenary Book*, 280–1. 'in its equipment': JPH 1949, 646.
18. Review of curricula: JTW 1920. 'somewhat anarchical': *ibid.*, 275. Details 1884, 1890: *Centenary Book*, 178–9.
19. Melbourne's curriculum: Russell, 102–3. 'an instance' and 'Stuart came': CJM to JTW, 29.9.1898 and 21.7.1901.
20. 'in the generality': JTW 1901,427. 'an even more': JTW 1902a, 64. '... the true': JTW 1901, 431.
21. On electives: JTW 1901, 425–31.
22. Changes in curricula: Faculty of Medicine Minutes 21.10.1902, 117; Centenary Book, 318. 'an anachronism' and 'the scientific basis': JTW 1901, 418–19.
23. For problems experienced by Welsh: *Centenary Book*, 333; U of S *Calendar* 1902, 364–5. 'large and important': JTW 1901, 421. Background on bacteriology: *Centenary Book*, 340. Camac Wilkinson: *Centenary Book*, 48, 122–4, 331–2. JTW's hopes for JLS: JES to JTW, 20.2.1890. Bacteriology Chair: *Centenary Book* 340; *Hermes* 17.7.1896, 11. Macleay bequest: *Centenary Book*, 340–1; *Proceedings* of Linnean Society, 1895, 137–8 and 1896, 621; Walkom, 38. Micro-biological lab of 1885: Fenner, 3, 6–7.
24. TPAS and Public Health: Epps, Ch. 5. 'the DPH of Cambridge': TPAS 1902, 87.
25. Ashburton Thompson: *ADB*. Sydney Univ. decisions on Diploma of Public Health: Senate Minutes of 4.9.1905, 9.10.1905 and 11.6.1906; Faculty of Medicine Minutes of 9.11.1905.
26. Armstrong, 97–8; 'Obituary J Ashburton Thompson', *J of Royal Sanitary Institute*, Vol. 36, 1915. Public Health Act: Thompson, 130.
27. Woollahra: *The Echo*, 15.5.1890, 3.
28. Sir Julian Salomons: *ADB*. Family communications to author.
29. Family communications to author.
30. Family communications to author.
31. Family communications to author.

32. Hill & 'valuable contributions': U of S *Calendar* 1905, 396. DSc: Branagan, 155. Hill's salary: Syd. Uni. Archivist, Ken Smith, to author 13.4.87. Funds from RS: *RSO* on Hill, 102.
33. Elliot Smith: letters to JTW from Oct. 1896;. 'unrivalled grasp': Bishop, 1974, in Elkin & Macintosh, 53. Barclay Smith, 24.
34. JTW 1936 and 1938.
35. Offers to Martin: CJM to JTW, 19.8.1899. Melbourne Univ. response: Russell, 93. 'This seems to': CJM to JTW, 10.5.1902. 'Why are we' and 'Because your': Maisie Gibbs (née Martin) to LH, 28.8.1980. Martin's visit to Sydney, etc.: CJM to JTW, 7.7.1903, 18.8.1903, 29.8.1903.
36. Wilson's activities: *Centenary Book*, 226, 277; letters, JTW to J; PLS for 1901. Anderson Stuart and the PAH: Epps, 88–91; Maddox, 24. 'extraneous work': GES to JTW 24.2.1901.

7

Embryology and the Platypus

Wilson, like many comparative anatomists of his generation, had become a comparative embryologist. 'Johnson Symington is at present reading up Embryology in order to bring the Quain part up to date.' J P Hill reported from Scotland in January 1903, 'but you needn't fear that the ground will be cut from beneath your [large?] feet.'[1]

Darwin had given embryology a powerful stimulus by recommending it as a means of determining phylogenies, or lines of descent from a common ancestor. British biologists were belated in following his advice and British embryology lost a vital force with the accidental death in 1882 of the brilliant young F M Balfour. His death took the heart out of the embryology research school (which included William Bateson, W F R Weldon, A E Shipley, Walter Heape, Richard Assheton, Adam Sedgwick and W H Caldwell) that had gathered around him in Cambridge. His two-volume textbook, *A Treatise on Comparative Embryology* (1880–1) was his enduring monument. Balfour's friend and contemporary, the Oxford-trained zoologist E Ray Lankester had been an enthusiastic embryologist in the 1870s but by 1891 when he was appointed to the Linacre Chair of Comparative Anatomy at Oxford he had discarded the idea that embryology was a better method than comparative anatomy for determining phylogenies. He made important contributions to embryology without establishing a research school.[2]

In Scotland embryology struck no secure roots though a few individuals made contributions to it. In Edinburgh, William Turner did some valuable comparative work on mammalian placentation and the intra-uterine mammalian brain while the zoologist John Beard, who launched J P Hill on his career, worked on elasmobranch embryos for many years drawing his inspiration from Franz Keibel of Freiburg, a leading comparative embryologist, and from Anton Dohrn (1840–1909), a marine embryologist and founder of the Zoological Station at Naples, the great Mediterranean clearing house of German zoology.[3]

Germany produced most of the great embryologists in the nineteenth century, most of the important embryological ideas and most of the technology to explore and test them. Modern embryology was founded by Karl von Baer of Königsberg (1792–1876) on his 'biogenetic law' of 1828 which held that the embryos of 'higher' and 'lower' animals resemble each other more closely the further back they are tracked in the evolutionary line. This was revised in 1866 by Darwin's ardent German champion Ernst Haeckel of Jena (1834–1919) with his 'principle of recapitulation', meaning that individual organisms pass through successive stages corresponding to the adult forms of their ancestors in the phylogenetic sequence or, as it is usually summarized 'ontogeny recapitulates phylogeny'. He went on to assert that the gastrulation stage of embryonic development – when by invagination the simple cell mass forms dual walls – marks the emergence of vertebrates in the evolutionary process. To a hypothetical, double-walled, cup-like creature, his common ancestor of all vertebrates, Haeckel gave the name Gastraea. Implied in this theory is the idea that there is in living things an intrinsic drive towards perfection and further, that acquired characteristics are heritable. Haeckel's biogenetic law is now almost entirely discredited along with the assumption that human history is subject to a law of progress, which the biogenetic law seemed to guarantee, placing man at the pinnacle of biological achievement. Evolution, it is now recognized, does not proceed by scaling an improvement ladder but by aimless branching as species diversify in response to fortuitous nature. Nevertheless the biogenetic law supplied the foundation on which the imposing edifice of descriptive embryology was built.[4]

Naturalists and comparative anatomists like Wilson and Hill, whose main interest was evolutionary biology, favoured the descriptive approach. Others, more interested in functional biology, were drawn to the mechanistic outlook and methods of experimental physiology. With improvements in histological techniques in the 1860s and 1870s – in microscopy and the fixing, staining, sectioning and mounting of tissues – the way was opened for experimental embryology pioneered by the morphologist Wilhelm His (1831–1904) who sought to explain embryological development on purely mechanical grounds.[5]

Experiments by Wilhelm Roux (1850–1924), founder of the 'developmental mechanics' school in Breslau, and Hans Driesch of Heidelberg (1867–1941), reached contradictory conclusions about embryonic cell differentiation. Roux found the process was governed by internal, or hereditary forces, Driesch that it was determined by regulative responses to conditions external to the cell, or environmental forces. An energetic controversy arose among biologists, resurrecting the ancient issue of preformation (determined in germ) versus epigenesis (formed by gradual elaboration) – as old as Aristotle and still not settled – but converted by modern tools from a mainly speculative debate into a concrete scientific one.[6]

Also in the 1870s and 1880s yet another German embryologist, August Weismann of Freiburg (1834–1914), trained in the traditional descriptive methods of comparative anatomy but with initial epigenetic sympathies, came up with a theory of profound significance that endorsed the concept of preformation. On the solid basis of extensive microscopical observations of the origin and distribution of germ cells in 43 species of hydroids, and drawing on the concepts of phylogenetic and experimental embryology, Weismann in the 1880s propounded his theory of 'the continuity of germ plasm'. He distinguished two kinds of cells: germ cells and somatic cells. To the nucleus of the germ cells alone he ascribed the role of hereditary transmission, concluding that internal factors or material units in its nucleus were the sole determinants of heredity and development (particulate inheritance). Weismann represented the 'germ plasm' as an immortal substance around which each new generation builds a body (or soma) that serves as a carrier of the germ cells from one generation to the next.[7]

If then there is a strict law of heredity, whence variation? As Weismann elaborated his germ-plasm theory he saw heredity, rich with possibilities, as the source of variation with natural selection acting as the mechanism of evolution. Weismann realigned the debate on heredity and variation into a Darwinian perspective so that when the Abbé Gregor Mendel's laws of inheritance were rediscovered in 1900 they were soon recognized by most thinking biologists as filling the gap in Darwin's theory.

Weismann had attempted the sort of rapprochement between anatomy and physiology – relating evolution theory to cell theory – that C J Martin called for in 1898, and Martin duly applauded his effort. He was sceptical, however, of the 'highly speculative' cell

141

constituents Weismann postulated, which could not be verified by observation, micro-technique of the day being unequal to the task; nor did he think Weismann was justified in choosing the cell nucleus as the vehicle of hereditary transmission; and he suspected that the very interesting 'chromatin filaments', the stainable material in the nucleus (now known to consist of DNA) might have been assigned undue importance simply because it stained while the cytoplasm (or protoplasm) did not. Martin was not attracted by the conception of a germ of 'such an infinitely complicated architecture'. Weismann's theory he concluded was 'too complex in detail, too simple in principle'.[8]

Martin's opinion reflected biological opinion generally: reserved. John Haldane was dismissive. 'Weismann's theories have gone to the wall', he wrote to Wilson on 3 January 1899. But Wilson was more receptive. He grasped the paradox that Weismann presented, of 'wholly to eliminate the action of environment in the *production* of variations, while assigning to it the exclusive privilege of perpetuating the lucky ones by its selective influence'. He was inclined to think Weismann too absolute in denying the modifying influence of the environment on the soma and agreed with Martin that the evidence did not validate the theory, hidden as it was in the chromatin of the germ cell. But he did appreciate Weismann's 'mechanical imagination' in producing a strictly logical material explanation of Darwin's doctrine of evolution by natural selection. Complex it was, but complexity, Wilson argued, constituted no valid objection; indeed he foresaw that 'the future advance of biological investigation must consist in unravelling the enormous structural complexity with which we are bound to credit [the nucleus of an ovum]'. The starting point was the recognition of the germ as a material system possessing 'either in its physical structure, or in its chemical composition, or in both together, potential equivalents of those properties in which it resembles the parental organisation'. Wilson upheld Weismann's particulate theory of inheritance although it could not at the time be demonstrated and despite severe criticism which induced Weismann himself to retreat to the defensive position that the hereditary determinants should not be taken to have physical reality and that his theory was merely an attractive guiding concept or working assumption.[9]

Wilson's ready acceptance of Weismann's theory may indicate a prepared mind, or an emotional need, or both. It affirmed his philosophical belief in 'the Eternal Now' and religious belief in 'the

142

Life Everlasting'. Many years later he wrote of it to his daughter Jeanie with all the wonder of a new discovery:

> What a wonderful phenomenon this hereditary transmission is! And how infinitely complex the physical & psychical substratum of it all! Yet we take it as a matter of course – as, of course, it is. Nor can I believe that human personality, as an element of Reality, is merely transitory. Rather do I feel that it is the time-continuum which is – not exactly illusory – but at most only a half truth. 'All that is at all lasts ever past recall', in some sense a permanent value .... One of the articles of my creed is a *non credo*: *I do not believe* in the absolute reality of Time. Surely Kant was right in regarding it as a necessary mode of human perception, albeit constitutive for our apprehension of the universe.[10]

Wilson's two aspects of reality, Science and Spirit, seemed on this question to endorse each other.

Attacked even by orthodox Darwinians, Weismann's theory received a better reception in England than in his own country or America. The question was controversial for decades, and not unequivocally settled until the 1940s. Wilson declared his belief in particulate inheritance in a paper on variation in mammalian dentition published in 1905. In that paper he also registered his decided opposition to the fanciful epigenetic or 'dynamic' view of inheritance postulated by the maverick morphologist William Bateson of Cambridge (1861–1926), the geneticist who had recently validated Mendel's ratios on inheritance characteristics. Bateson believed that 'the new body is made again from the beginning, just as if the wax model had gone back into the melting-pot before the new model was begun'. Wilson's objection was emphatic:

> It is obviously untrue to fact to suggest, by means of such a metaphor as that of the melted wax, that with each germinal generation there is a return to morphological indifference and homogeneity. Surely it may safely be conjectured that, whatever may be the nature of the normal form-determinants of the organism – be they material or dynamic – they are in some very real sense morphologically persistent in the germ.[11]

This did not mean that Wilson attributed all characteristics to heredity. In the same article on variation in mammalian dentition, in which he studied supernumerary teeth in the skulls of an

143

Australian Aboriginal and a New Caledonian, he supported the view of the Scottish anatomist Charnock Bradley that an extra molar in the human jaw could well be explained without reference to ancestry, as 'merely a variation resulting from a more than usually extensive backward prolongation of the dental lamina, and the formulation from it of one dental germ in excess of the normal number'. The fortuitous certainly had a role in development. Wilson favoured the outlook of most American embryologists in the 1890s who believed that neither the epigenetic nor the preformationist arguments could be fully in the right. They sought to reconcile the two principles.[12]

American embryology, which soared to spectacular heights of achievement in the 1890s from a slender biological footing, was primed directly and through the Naples Zoological Station by German research and nurtured every summer by gatherings of bold young scientists like E B Wilson, E G Conklin, T H Morgan, Ross Harrison, Jacques Loeb, Charles Minot and C J Herrick at the Marine Biological Laboratory at Woods Hole, Massachusetts, under the direction of C O Whitman (1842–1910) of the University of Chicago, who focused attention on unsettled biological questions including the revived controversy about preformation and epigenesis. Whitman edited the widely-read first seven volumes of *Biological Lectures* (between 1890 and 1899) delivered by scientists in residence as Friday evening lectures. Wilson read them carefully in Sydney.[13]

But if Whitman was the father of American embryology he soon found himself, as an evolutionary zoologist opposed to the reductionist implications of experimental biology, at odds with his offspring as it developed. The concept of epigenesis better suited American pragmatism. Impatient with descriptive morphology and suspicious of predeterminism in all its forms – this was the land of the free – the American school showed a distinct preference for experiment. It produced tangible results with prospects for practical application. But one American who consistently opposed the claim that biology would be advanced by experiment alone was E B Wilson (1856–1939) of Columbia University, New York City, whose book *The Cell in Development and Inheritance*, published in 1896 'to bring the cell-theory and the evolution-theory into organic connection', strongly influenced J T Wilson's thinking. E B Wilson sought to reconcile the problems of heredity, variation and differentiation through a better understanding of fundamental processes at the cellular level.[14]

Edmund Beecher Wilson, like James Thomas Wilson, was a naturalist from boyhood, and first pursued embryology by the descriptive method in cell lineage studies. In 1891 he turned to experimental embryology, concluding in 1894 that, while at the base of every developmental step lay an inheritance from the past, too much influence had been attributed to inheritance and not enough to the physiological conditions of development and how they operate. He was a broad-minded mechanist, convinced that while experimental embryology would yield deeper insights, the descriptive comparative method or what he called 'the study of phenomena where nature is the experimenter' would 'always form the very framework of biological science'.[15]

This was the state of embryology when early in 1900 Wilson and Hill in combative partnership set out to chart the embryological development of the platypus, one of the most phylogenetically interesting animals in the world. Wilson was the senior partner, senior in years and research experience by more than a decade; he was more proficient in German so he had the job of translating and summarizing material like Keibel's major work of 1893 on the embryology of the pig, and Gaupp's huge tomes on neurology; and he had a firmer grasp of the broad biological conceptions that framed their working assumptions. But Hill was no longer the 'raw youth' of eight years before when he had joined the Wilson household. He left philosophy to Wilson but he was an enthusiastic collector and a tough 'pushful' investigator. Both men studied their material intensively and independently, and in 'discussions' that according to legend could be heard a quarter of a mile away, wrangled like the pair of Scots they were over everything down to fine details like whether or not, in a graphic reconstruction, one individual cell should be included in the neural plate of a flat embryo. Wilson expressed his views 'in the most uncompromising, not to say dogmatic, fashion' said Hill, while Hill according to another colleague was wont to express his opinion 'with great finality'. Both had the voice of a Stentor. It was a matter of wonder to bystanders that they emerged from these sessions the best of friends. This abrasive working alliance served only to deepen their friendship and to secure for their work a very high degree of accuracy.[16]

It had taken them the best part of a decade to collect the material for this study. Though far from nearing extinction as many believed, the platypus unlike the echidna (the other Australian member of the monotreme class) was scarce and hard to find. Fur traders had decimated their numbers and since this animal breeds only once a year, the female usually producing but two eggs at a time, the restoration of their population was a slow process, even with the introduction of legal protection by the States and better control by the new Federal customs authorities over the export of skins. Furthermore the breeding season varies with locality and seasonal conditions, and the gestation period was unknown, so the results were somewhat hit-or-miss. Even when located the quarry is elusive. The pregnant female lays and incubates her eggs in the fastness of a well-concealed nest of grass, leaves and willow tree roots. The river bank entrances to their nests are conspicuous enough to the trained eye but between them and the nesting chamber the pregnant female tunnels a sinuous course 12 to 18 inches below ground and up to 60 feet long, a channel heavily guarded by tree roots. Penetrating these defences was hard labour – Caldwell used a team of navvies – and all too often there was no reward at all. Wilson and Hill caught six males to every female. Despite their persistent personal efforts they had to rely largely on the services of scientifically untrained collectors who required 'considerable inducement to carry on the work at all', so meagre were the prospects of success. All told they secured 12 suitable intra-uterine eggs, to which was added one more, a donation by Robert Etheridge, curator of the Australian Museum. The series was still far from complete for their purpose but because their campaign extended over several years and was better informed about localities and breeding times they collected more useable material than the expensive and rapacious expeditions of W H Caldwell in 1884 and Richard Semon in 1892.[17]

Converting these hard-won eggs into studiable form, on glass slides under a microscope, was a major technical undertaking and as much an art as a science. The objective was to get a picture of each specimen resembling as closely as possible its original state, and it required patience, skill and an understanding of the chemistry of various processes when applied to complex animal tissue. First each specimen had to be fixed by a reagent in order to maintain its original shape and to harden it for cutting into sections. For this procedure they used Kleinenberg's well known picric-acid mixture at the outset, but later they used a picro-corrosive-acetic fluid of their own devising. After rendering the material translucent by a clearing agent they proceeded to double-embed each specimen, first in cedar-oil-celloidin and then paraffin wax, to hold it firmly but without injurious pressure during the slicing process. Double-

146

embedding was indispensable they argued, for all embryological work of a critical character. Paraffin wax as an outer layer was also necessary to enable a ribbon of sections (joined by paraffin at the cut edge) to be produced by the cutting action of an automatic microtome. The accurate alignment of these serial sections on microscope slides was difficult, because the structure of eggs could give no common (axial) point of reference on the slides. To overcome this problem Wilson modified the system devized by two German embryologists (Born and Peter) by embedding blackened strands of human nerve fibres in the paraffin block to obtain accurate directing marks within each section. After slicing in the microtome the thin sections were floated on warm water to flatten them and then mounted by floating them onto glass slides previously treated by Mayer's albumen to hold them fast. When thoroughly dry each slide was coated with a thin solution of celloidin to ensure complete adhesion. The slides were then washed in a mixture of 90 per cent alcohol and 10 per cent chloroform. Staining was the final procedure. As a rule Wilson and Hill used only tissue-specific stains (rather than stains which coloured everything) like haematoxylin, a good nuclear colourant, or haematin (oxidized haematoxylin) and then counter-stained (or double-stained) with eosin; sometimes they used iron-haematin which produces exquisite nuclear detail, more often a dilution of Delafield's haematoxylin solution, or occasionally borax-carmine which is cytoplasm-specific; for certain purposes they used picric acid as a counter-stain to the haematin.[18]

Wilson and Hill employed no novel procedures but they did make modifications to some then current. Wilson's idea of embedding human nerve strands in the paraffin block to serve as directing marks is an example. He soon radically refined that method by designing a paraffin embedding chamber which made the whole process perfectly reliable and easier to perform. He also devized a simple method for making a stock of plates with directing strands of liver or cerebrum mounted on them; he found a way of making paraffin congeal faster, a way to keep the water-bath level when floating out paraffin sections of slides, and he hit upon a convenient and cheap expedient for suspending blocks of tissue and passing them through a series of different fluids.[19] He was constantly preoccupied with technique, forever experimenting with refinements and innovations. It is no wonder that the slides of marsupial and monotreme material that Wilson and Hill made around the turn of the century, now in the Hubrecht Laboratory in

Utrecht, are still consulted by students of Australian fauna. Their technique was superb.[20]

A unique feature of the uterine platypus egg presented them with a difficult technical problem in the intermediate or gastrulation stage of uterine embryonic development. While in the uterus the platypus egg has a parchment-like shell holding initially a large amount of inert yolk (i.e. as in birds, a meroblastic ovum), which restricts the cleaving cells of the embryo to a small disc-shaped area (or blastoderm) lying on top of the yolk mass containing the cells destined to multiply and differentiate. Its cleavage system is therefore called discoidal. During the gastrulation stage, when uterine fluid is absorbed to feed the embryo for the remaining period of gestation and incubation, the fluid rapidly enlarges the egg and progressively disrupts and liquefies the yolk, pushing the blastodermic and vitelline (gestative) membranes against the tough opaque shell which cannot be peeled away without damaging them. Five of their specimens were in this condition and they were the ones that held in their blastodermic membranes the secret of how the cells in the monotreme egg arrange themselves and differentiate to form the fundamental body plan characteristic of its species. Because of their opaque shells these eggs had to be opened in a random fashion, risking injury to the embryonic area, and the fluid evacuated, causing the membrane to crumple. This in turn made the correct orientation of the embryonic area highly problematical.[21]

Their careful scrutiny, greatly assisted by the use of Hill's Braus-Drüner binocular stereoscopic microscope, ultimately resulted in 134 pages of text with 32 illustrations, the first systematic and connected account of the development of the platypus from the eight-cell stage of segmentation through gastrulation and neurulation to the stage when the embryo has 19 or 20 pairs of somites and is about to be shed. It remains the most authoritative description of uterine platypus development but has, as they later acknowledged, 'a serious if localized error of interpretation'. This came from their reading of the fifth specimen in their series, which was at the early gastrulation stage which gave them much technical difficulty. They observed what they took to be two simultaneous manifestations of developmental activity in the blastoderm. The first was 'a small opaque area, somewhat oblong, but rather irregular', serial sections of which confirmed them in their opinion that it was a primitive knot with an early gastrulation cavity of 'tolerably typical' reptilian configuration. The second feature, quite independent and comparatively remote from the 'primitive knot' was an extensive area exhibiting a 'distinct linear primitive streak formation', a typically mammalian structure which establishes the longitudinal axis or spine of the embryo. The 'primitive knot' was actually a yolk navel or scar formed by the joining together of extra-embryonic ectoderm and endoderm layers when enveloping the yolk mass at the lower pole of the blastocyst, and played no part in embryonic development. Their interest lay in the apparent co-existence of these two structures in the monotreme blastoderm, one typically reptilian the other typically mammalian.[22]

This 'extraordinary fact' they deemed worthy of a brief preliminary paper, polished up by Hill in December 1902 on board ship bound for London and a holiday at 'home'. The Hills by this time had an 18-month-old daughter Katie to show their families and another on the way; and Hill was hoping to persuade his widowed father to join them permanently in Sydney. His old chief G B Howes at the Royal College of Science in South Kensington was 'marvellously delighted with the little paper' Hill reported to Wilson 'considers it the acme of platypus work so far and said right away this ought to go to the Royal. I handed it over accordingly and had a note yesterday [20.1.03] saying he had sent it in with a request that it be read while I am in here'. And it was, being published in the *Philosophical Transactions of the Royal Society* in February 1903 when Hill was on his way back to Sydney, alone this time – his wife having decided to stay with her family for the birth of their second daughter Mayna in July, and his father having declined his invitation – but with heightened enthusiasm for the work.[23]

For the next stage, which they termed post-gastrular, they had four specimens and the technical disability of being unable to detach the blastoderm from the shell without injury. To interpret surface observation they had to rely heavily on correlations with serial transverse sections. Studies of all these specimens confirmed them in their opinion of the co-existence of primitive knot and primitive streak which, they postulated, had joined up as a result of a remarkable elongation of the primitive knot's gastrulation cavity to form a typical embryonic area giving rise to the very long 'head process'. Their first mistake in interpreting a yolk navel as a primitive knot had led to this further misreading of the chain of events.[24]

From these observations they concluded that in all essentials the development of the platypus up to the early gastrular stage was the same as meroblastic (yolk-filled) ova of other amniotes (reptiles, birds, mammals) and thus disposed of Richard Semon's interpretation of amphibian affinity. The general character of the interior of the egg they homologized with the reptilian. Indeed they believed that *Ornithorhynchus* afforded 'an actual demonstration of the transformation of a Sauropsidan [reptilian] sub-germinal cavity into the cavity of a typical mammalian blastodermic vesicle', supporting Franz Keibel's view of the correspondence of those cavities. What continued most to fascinate them was the apparent co-existence of a reptilian structure (the primitive knot) with a mammalian one (the primitive streak). They believed they had discovered evidence of the origin of mammals, the 'link' between reptiles and mammals.[25]

To the modern biologist it might seem extraordinary that they should mistake a yolk navel for a primitive knot, notwithstanding the technical difficulty. What their mistake reveals is the all-pervading influence of the biogenetic law on evolutionists of that time, including Wilson who had a firm intellectual grasp of its invalidity. Unconsciously he was endorsing it. Questions of 'origins' and 'links' were topical. A preoccupation with the origin of mammals had led the Glasgow-trained medical naturalist Robert Broom to study the embryos of monotremes and marsupials in outback Queensland and New South Wales, before shifting his search to fossil reptiles in the Karoo region of South Africa. Baldwin Spencer of Melbourne and Richard Semon of Jena had made their separate expeditions to Queensland's Burnet River in 1892 to seek in the lungfish a link between fishes and amphibians. More extraordinary was the 20-year morphological search by the distinguished Cambridge physiologist W H Gaskell for evidence of the origin of vertebrates in the king crab and its forebears. Deeply impressed by the similarity of the segmental arrangement of the involuntary nervous system of vertebrates and the central nervous system of invertebrates, and transgressing basic morphological tenets relating to the alimentary canal, Gaskell pushed his theory from 1888 to 1908 when he published a book on the subject. Even August Weismann, whose theory of the continuity of germ plasm ultimately destroyed the biogenetic law, made persistent use of it.[26]

Far more interesting than gastrulation was the subsequent neurulation stage in the platypus embryo: the early processes of segmentation and differentiation of the central nervous system. This part of the investigation recruited all Wilson's fascination for neurology, his earliest and most enduring research interest. They had four specimens in this developmental stage, free of the technical difficulty of the gastrulation stage – the embryo and its membrane had achieved 'a definite and coherent condition' – and were able to follow the trail blazed by Hill and Martin with one embryo (specimen 'M') in 1894. There were gaps in their series but by using marsupial specimens at a corresponding stage they were able to trace development up to the point where the egg is about to be laid.[27]

They discovered a quite remarkable feature of early neural development in the platypus embryo: that the medullary (or neural) plates do not fold over to form a neural tube as in mammals but remain perfectly flat and exposed on the surface, thus affording a unique opportunity to study the process of neural differentiation without the complication and distortion of obscuring folds. They saw that the brain of the platypus is not formed into three parts as in mammals but two: a hind-part and a fore-part under which the primitive spine terminates. The fore-brain showed demarcations of four or five segments in front of the segment connected with the facial nerve (pre-facial neuromeres), with traces of subdivisions in some of them, and three segments behind it (post-facial neuromeres). Most important of all was their correct identification of neural (or ganglionic) crest: two strips of cells bordering the medullary plates which, in the region of the pre-facial neuromeres and between the ectoderm layer and scattered connective tissue cells, gives rise to an enormous growth of cells (relative to the rest of the neural system) on each side of the flat fore-brain. In 1895 Hill and Martin, influenced by Selenka's view of a similar structure in the opossum, had interpreted it as mesodermal in character, not essentially part of the brain. With the advantage of an embryo (specimen 'H') slightly younger than specimen 'M', Wilson and Hill detected that this cell mass was in fact continuous with the brain and that it was of predominantly ganglionic character: it was the beginning of the ganglion which gives origin to the sensory root of the trigeminal nerve, the largest cranial nerve (in Wilson's words 'the trigeminal ganglionic expansion of the neural crest'). Had they examined the next developmental stage of a marsupial, D M S Watson later remarked, 'they could not have escaped the conclusion that the mass not only produced the ganglion but also gave rise to the whole mesoderm of the mandibular arch'.[28]

This work took four full years of research and another year to write up. In between times Wilson turned out several smaller studies, all offshoots of this preoccupation with embryology. In one paper, on the snout of the monotreme mammary foetus, he amplified previous accounts of its cartilaginous skeleton, described for the first time the 'os carunculae' – a bony nodule that provides the young monotreme with a shell-breaker – and rounded off his earlier debate (principally with Johnson Symington) on the dumb-bell bone, satisfying himself that his view of its independent pre-vomerine origin was established as correct.[29]

Another paper on embryonic human development had a clinical source. He supplied a short commentary on a case encountered by the surgeon J B Nash, of a child with an unusual anatomical condition: absence of lower intestine (ascending, transverse and descending colon and sigmoid flexure). Wilson gave an account of the normal development of these structures in the foetus to explain how a range of congenital irregularities occur when the normal sequence of events is interrupted. The value of a precise knowledge of anatomy and the process of normal embryonic development in assisting the understanding of a disconcerted clinician is here clearly displayed. Though Wilson was more a biologist than a medico, he regularly paid his professional dues in contributions like this to triennial Australasian medical conferences.[30]

At the end of 1903 Anderson Stuart left for another trip to Britain, Europe and America. His main purpose was to inspect the latest equipment for installation in the Royal Prince Alfred Hospital's substantial extensions which he had master-minded. When the extensions were opened in October 1904 Prince Alfred's could claim to be the first modern 500 bed hospital in Australia and perhaps in the Empire. In England he recruited 'a model matron for his model hospital', called on King Edward at St James Palace and attended the 27th Congress of the Royal Sanitary Institute in York, representing the NSW Board of Health. He toured the Middle East in January 1904 and was entertained by Grafton Elliot Smith at the Cairo Medical School. In addition to his formidable programme in anatomical research and teaching Elliot Smith was engrossed 'for diplomatic reasons' in Egyptian anthropology. Stuart extracted from him the promise of various contributions to Sydney University's anatomical museum and Smith heard from Stuart the good news that Wilson would have a year's leave in 1905. Smith promptly communicated his pleasure to Wilson:

> I am delighted to learn that your long awaited leave of absence is at
> last in sight. It is just about time that you had some relief from the
> drudgery of teaching. I hope that you will make the most of your
> holiday and not hide your light under a bushel. You have so many
> pretty things to show and so much to say that people in England
> would like to hear... Do something with it... When are you going to
> publish some of your great accumulation of work?[31]

Notes

1. 'Johnson Symington': JPH to JTW 21.1.1903.
2. British embryology: Ridley, 35–50. Lankester: Ridley, 40, 50–1; Mayr, 535.
3. Scottish work and its inspiration: Keith 1912, 26–9; Ridley, 37.
4. German embryology: Mulvaney & Calaby, 136–7; Horder, 5; Churchill, 7–9 .
5. Embryos as material for cell theory: Horder *et al.*, 4. German advocates of mechanical approach: Mayr, Ch. 15. His: Maienschein, 85.
6. Experiments debate: Wallace, 338; E B Wilson 1893, 10 and 1896, 104–5; Churchill 1980, 121.
7. Weismann: Churchill 1986, 7–33. Suggestion by Driesch: Hamburger (in Mayr 104) notes that the Driesch model allowed for chemical interactions between genes and cytoplasm and the notion of feedback between nucleus and cytoplasm.
8. 'such an infinitely': CJM 1898, 411.
9. 'Weismann's theories': JSH to JTW, 3.1.1899. 'wholly to eliminate': JTW 1898, 827. 'mechanical imagination' and 'the future advance': *ibid.*, 835. 'either in its': JTW 1899, 25.
10. 'What a wonderful': JTW to J, 25.5.1938.
11. 'the new body': Bateson 1894, 33. 'It is obviously': JTW 1905c, 129. See also: Coleman 262, 306–7; Mayr 1982, 687, 701.
12. 'merely a variation': Charnock Bradley, quoted in JTW 1905c, 130.
13. American outlook: Horder, 87.
14. Americans & Woods Hole: Horder, 148; Mayr 1982. E B Wilson: 'the cell theory', quoted in *DSB* Vol. XIV 429.
15. 'the study of' and 'always form', E B Wilson's Sixth Lecture, 1894, 123–4.
16. Translation of Keibel: JPH to JTW, 30.1.01. Farewell speech for Hill: JTW 11.8.1906; DMS Watson *RSO* on JPH, 112. 'in the most': JPH in *RSO* on JTW, 655. 'with great': DMS Watson *RSO* on JPH, 113.
17. Platypus: Burrell 126–7; JTW & JPH in Burrell, 193. Specimens and 'considerable inducement': JTW & JPH 1907b, 33 and 34 resp.
18. Preparation of specimens: JTW & JPH 1907b, 34–6; Bracegirdle, ch 4; JTW & JPH 1903, 315. JTW 1900a.
19. JTW 1900a and 1910a.
20. Slides made by Wilson and Hill, in the Hill Collection held at the Hubrecht Laboratory: Boterenbrood.
21. 'a serious if': JPH in *RSO* on JTW, 648. JTW & JPH 1903a, 314–22 and 1907b, 34, 39–59.

22. 'a small opaque' and 'tolerably typical': JTW & JPH 1907b, 42 and 43 resp. 'distinct linear': JTW & JPH 1903a, 315.
23. 'extraordinary': JTW & JPH 1903, 316. 'marvellously delighted': JPH to JTW, 21.1.03
24. Post gastrular stage of study: JTW & JPH 1907b, 62.
25. 'an actual demonstration': JTW & JPH 1907b, 60.
26. Pre-occupation with origins: JTW, 'Some Phases of Mammalian Development', *Abstract of Proceedings, JRS of NSW*, 5.9.1900; JPH, 'The Monotreme and the Origin of Mammals': *ibid.*, 1906. Monotremes: 'Monotremata' in E P Walker, 1964. On Weismann: F Churchill, 1986, 30. On Gaskell: Geison, *DSB*.
27. Neurular stage: *Nature*, 24.8.1905, 401; JTW & JPH 1907b, 34, 92–101, 122, 138–54; Watson *RSO* on JPH, 107.
28. Watson *RSO* on JPH, 107.
29. JTW 1902b.
30. JTW 1905d.
31. Epps, 90–4, 148–9. 'for diplomatic' and 'I am delighted': GES to JTW, 1.2.1904 and 5.1.1904.

8

The Marks of Them That Know

After 18 years Wilson had a year off in 1905. A combination of family affairs and finances (and perhaps Anderson Stuart's programme) prevented it earlier, and even then funds were tight because, as was customary, he was obliged to make half his salary over to F P Sandes to act for him while he was away; assisting Sandes as a demonstrator was S A (Stewart Arthur) Smith, Grafton Elliot Smith's younger brother who had graduated in medicine in 1902. With his wife, four daughters and a nurse Wilson left Sydney on the *Moldavia* on 10 December 1904, arriving in London on 21 January.

Within two days of settling into a house in West Kensington Wilson was at work. London was his headquarters for the whole of 1905 but all told he spent only five months there. Interruptions were constant: to start with Jeanie had to be settled into St Paul's School and the three little ones with their nurse into a house at Maidenhead; there were gatherings with a multitude of Salomons and Wilson relations, and the Lorrain Smiths wanted as much time as possible with their 13-year-old niece Jeanie whom they now met for the first time. As well there were many reunions with old friends.[1]

In London there was Almroth Wright, building an Inoculation Department in the Pathology Laboratory of St Mary's Hospital in Paddington. Wright had left the Army Medical School at Netley in 1902 because the War Office rejected his anti-typhoid inoculation proposals during the Boer War. In 1904 C J Martin of the Lister Institute became an adviser to the War Office on that problem and was appointed also to committees of the Royal Society inquiring into tropical diseases. When the Wilsons arrived in January Martin was preparing to go to Bombay in March to set up field and laboratory studies of bubonic plague, then raging in India. Martin presided over the scientific work of the Second Plague Commission which fully endorsed Ashburton Thompson's findings of 1901–2 in Sydney on the etiology of plague and how to deal with outbreaks of it. The Lister Institute had begun its rise to distinction as an interdisciplinary biological research centre where a host of young Australian scientists were to get postgraduate training. In February Martin showed Wilson over the Institute, introduced him at dinner to Sir Michael Foster, the founder of the renowned Cambridge Physiological Laboratory, and took him along to a meeting of the Physiological Society where he met many other prominent physiologists.[2]

On a three day visit to Oxford in mid-February Wilson met more leading physiologists including Francis Gotch who had done important work on the mammalian nervous system. He found Haldane occupied with an enquiry on the ventilation of factories and workshops for the Home Office and the anatomist Arthur Thomson building the nucleus of an embryological collection. In W F R Weldon's laboratory he met J W Jenkinson, a comparative embryologist pioneering the experimental method in England. Wilson discussed the gastrulation stage of platypus development with him, noting dismissively 'He is determined to interpret in terms of Amphibian development.' In Manchester was Jim Smith, appointed the previous year to the Pathology Chair, busy equipping a pathological museum which involved the mounting together of specimens of the same individual as a basis for his new 'case method' of teaching pathology. He talked Wilson into subscribing to the journal *Museum,* and into giving a talk on the Australian Museum to a meeting of the Worcester Museum Society.

Wilson had four major assignments. The first was to become fluent in spoken German to better equip him for a tour of European institutions. The second was to make that tour, including also Britain's main research centres, inspecting current research and teaching in anatomy, embryology and neurology. The third was to write up two papers in final form. And the fourth was to attend in August the first international congress of anatomists in Geneva where he would display the embryological material he and Hill had educed on the development of the platypus. He needed also to take a real holiday.

On 2 March he set off for the *Institut Tilly* in Berlin, an establishment renowned for its efficient teaching of the German language. On the way he called at several anatomical institutions: at Amsterdam University he met A J P van der Broek to whom he had

156

sent some marsupial specimens in 1904 and saw a fine collection of skulls and skeletons and some of Vrolik's injection preparations; at Utrecht for an evening and a long day he discussed gastrulation with Hubrecht; at Giessen he examined Spengel's collection of mammalian osteology; on to Marburg's magnificent anatomical department where Disse demonstrated his sections of olfactory epithelium and he inspected the museum containing Zumstein's corrosion preparations of vascular structures of kidneys, lungs, liver etc.; then on to Göttingen's Anatomical Institute where he saw Blumenbach's collection, many of Henle's specimens, the nerve dissections used in Langenbeck's atlas, and he examined Kallin's reconstructions of wax models of the larynx, bronchi and lungs, models by Eternod and Keibel of human embryos and Wiedersheim's models of lower vertebrate brains; and then finally to Halle where he was not greatly impressed by Institute or Museum.

He reached Berlin on 9 March and the next day wrote in his diary '*Das Studieren fing an*' and for a month it continued without a word of English, except for one small lapse on 18 March: '*Der fünfte Gebürtstag von dear little Louise*'. A rule of the establishment was that no student speak, write, or read (except for home letters) anything but German. Even bi-lingual dictionaries were banned. William Tilly's teaching methods were phonetic and strict. Though Australian born and educated – he was related to the Clunies Ross family – his style was Prussian. Dapper, portly and vigorous, he ruled his institute and his large family as one. Whether the students were living in, or like Wilson living out, all took their meals at the family table where there was an embargo on salt. This Wilson found irksome, like most of the director's decrees. Mornings were taken up with lessons in phonetics, grammar, philology, literature, the history of music and art, liberally peppered with Tilly's 'philosophy': the evils of alcohol, the sins of the Latins, the virtues of the German people, the greatness of Goethe, the shallowness of America and the defects of Christian doctrine. Afternoons were occupied by walks with Herr Ingham, Wilson's *Konversationlehrer*. Practising the German Gothic script was an occupation for odd moments.

For the most part Wilson's diary entries were short, often '*Studieren und Spaziergang*' with the occasional '*Brief von Mabel*', but on 18 March he recorded in some detail a glimpse of the Kaiser driving along Unter den Linden to the Tiergarten. Displays of militant German nationalism and the servility of the German people to Prussian arrogance struck a chord of apprehension, though German science held his admiration. He emerged from the Institute

157

on 7 April and three days later met Mabel and Jeanie in Dresden. For the next six weeks business and pleasure were joined.

Before leaving Berlin Wilson visited Wilhelm Krause of the Anatomical Institute, whom he had met in Sydney in 1897 when Krause was looking for Aboriginal skulls; there he also met Wilhelm Waldeyer, the anatomist who in 1891 first clearly enunciated the concept of the neurone, and Rudolf Virchow's son Hans who showed him his method of preparing skeletal parts to study the relations of various components of the joints. At the Biological Institute he saw Oscar Hertwig's collection of embryological slides and negatives, and at the Leitz' Filiale an ultra-microscope showing molecules of a colloidal solution. Hans Held at the Anatomische Anstalt in Leipzig demonstrated a number of his neurological microscope specimens, including 'neurofibrillae of Apathy and connection or continuity of latter with so-called synapses' – excellent specimens, acclaimed both by the neuronists and their opponents, the reticularists, which even so did not resolve their long-drawn-out controversy on the fine structure of the nervous system. He also saw the His collection, Branne's vein dissections, and Gegenbauer's large embryological collection. In Jena, at the Zeiss workshop he inspected the latest microscopes, photo-micrographic and micro-projection apparatus, and 'the processes of lens grinding coarse and fine'. At the Vesalianum in Basel he met Johann Kollman who paved the way for the paedomorphic theory of human origins. Kollman showed Wilson illustrations for his atlas of embryology, George Corning demonstrated his splendid celloidin sections of both foetal and adult parts, and Wilson made notes of some clearing, injecting and staining techniques. In Strasburg University's anatomy department Gustav Schwalbe showed him his unequalled collection of skulls from foetal life to adolescence, Pfitzner's hand and foot collections and a skull collection of certain species of mammals for studies of variations. He noted that Schwalbe did not use formalin as a preservative because it interfered with maceration, preferring a mixture of glycerin, alcohol and carbolic acid.

In Freiburg in early May Wilson met Robert Wiedersheim the professor of anatomy, and the great August Weismann, now aged 71. He also met the embryologist Franz Keibel and the neurologist Robert Gaupp, both of whom were then working on marsupials and monotremes, so the work of Wilson and Hill was of immediate interest to them. Scientifically Wilson's four days in Freiburg were the highlight of his German tour.

Europe in spring was rich in diversions. First there was Weimar, the cradle of Goethe's poetry and Hegel's philosophy. In Nuremberg they wandered through the halls and chapels, the avenues of ancient lime trees, the houses of Dürer and Hans Sachs and the Germanic Museum. They spent Easter in Munich where Wilson met Richard Semon, whose interest in Australian lungfish and monotremes had given way to ambitious studies in cell memory and heredity, but he was interested to see Wilson's photomicrographs of early platypus development. Leipzig was suffused with memories of Jeanie's mother who had studied there more than 20 years before, and there they explored the scenes of her vibrant youth. On 13 April, the eve of his 44th birthday, Wilson took Jeanie for a long walk through the city. A weekend in Luzanne began with a thunderstorm but concluded with 'a splendid day' riding up the Sonnenberg by funicular railway and walking down. In Paris they had six days for shopping and art galleries before setting off for ten days of reunions and relaxation in Scotland till the end of May, picking up the young children and their nurse at Maidenhead on the way.

For most of June Wilson was at his West Kensington headquarters, working through the mornings, out and about in the afternoons, with the occasional full day of writing. In July the family went back to Scotland for a long summer holiday, taking a house in Firbank, Colinton, near Edinburgh. Cousin Hattie arrived from New York and from London came Aunt Lottie, a Salomons relation, and Annie and Maggie Lorrain Smith. Dr and Mrs A E Mills from Sydney arrived there about the same time, as did the touring Australian cricket team which lost that series to England. Golf figured prominently in Wilson's programme.

In Edinburgh there were reunions with former teachers: Turner, Cunningham, McKendrick, Symington, Crum Brown, Schaeffer and Beard, also Wilhelm Waldeyer who was over from Berlin to address the Royal Society of Edinburgh. They paid their respects to the Haldanes of Cloan in Perthshire, called on Anderson Stuart's mother in Dumfries and spent a long weekend with the Glovers at Gatehouse-of-Fleet. For their seventh wedding anniversary, on 14 September, Jim and Mabel were in Moniaive with Jeanie looking over the Mill House where Wilson was born and the school house where he grew up, taking a wagonnette drive up Craigdarroch Glen, Dalquhat, Castlefern Glen and then 'up linn', 'round the course' and 'up the throughgate', meeting relatives and friends of his youth. Old times meshed with the new during these long summer days, taking in a tour of the Highlands and Lowlands and lasting, with one significant interruption in August, till the end of September.

The first two weeks of August were taken up by a visit, with Mabel, to Geneva to attend the first International Congress of Anatomists. Over 200 delegates were from Europe, with only 23 British and four Americans. Though outnumbered by the Swiss and the French, the German delegates presented the largest number of papers, reflecting an established dominance of the field, against which one Frenchman registered a polite protest: '*Je ne comprends pas l'allemand*' he replied, bowing to a German critic of his paper. There were in fact quite a few sparks of non-German origin. The brilliant Spaniard Santiago Ramón y Cajal, and A Donnaggio of Naples, raised some Latin fire in a battle over microscopical evidences of the neuro-fibrillar network of the nerve cell. There were some remarkable embryological exhibits by the American George Streeter, among others by Europeans. 'If one may judge from the nature of several contributions to the Congress', concluded *Nature's* reviewer, 'there is a decided tendency to break down the barriers that separate the methods of the anatomist from those of the physiologist.'[3]

Few of the papers were on naked-eye anatomy considering that most contributors were teachers of medical students. Clinical interest was subdued. Nor was there much to interest the physical anthropologist. Comparative embryology and neurology attracted more attention and there was a strong interest in the embryology of marsupials and monotremes. Keibel contributed a piece on the urogenital apparatus of echidna, Bresslau of Strasburg an item on the marsupial pouch and Bardeleben of Jena and Gaupp of Freiburg got into an argument about the origin and nature of the mammalian lower jaw, using marsupial mandibles and human foetuses as evidence.

So the time was propitious for Wilson to reveal the results of several years work on the monotremes. On the morning of 8 May he read a short paper (speakers were limited to ten minutes and questioners to three) describing a pair of cartilaginous bars dividing the adult cranial cavities of echidna and platypus: facts of phylogenetic interest because they represent part of the original walls of the mammalian cranium, preserved only in the monotremes, though cartilaginous remnants are present in some other mammals. In 1902 Gaupp had identified them in the foetal crania of both species of monotreme, giving them the name *taenia clino-orbitalis*. Gaupp had surmised that, as in echidna (of which he had an adult specimen), these structures would be present in ossified form in the adult platypus. Wilson had evidence that in fact they differed and showed that, unlike the adult echidna, only the posterior part ossifies in the platypus, the forebrain part being represented by fibrous bands. This was an interesting contribution and Wilson was pleased to see it put on the list for publication.

Afternoons, reserved for demonstrations of material, were more lively and competitive. Wilson assembled an impressive display: stereo-photographs of wax models of a young mammary foetus of platypus illustrating his morning paper; results of work with Hill on monotreme dentition; photomicrographs of a definite and distinct group of neurones present in the medulla oblongata of the human brain, the subject of a paper yet to be completed; and, most important of all, his exhibition of photomicrographs of stages in the embryological development of montremes and marsupials, illustrating his major work with Hill. The last attracted a great deal of interest.

The Congress concluded on Thursday 10 August with a banquet at the Opera House, at which Wilson was flanked by Grafton Elliot Smith and the gentlemanly expatriate American, Edward Phelps Allis, a wealthy businessman who had invested heavily with money, time and effort in American scientific anatomy. In 1887 he had supplied funds to found the *Journal of Morphology*, the first American periodical devoted to anatomy and zoology, and in the same year he had established the Allis Lake Laboratory at Milwaukee. A friend and benefactor of C O Whitman, the first director of the Woods Hole Marine Biological Laboratory and editor of its *Biological Lectures*, Whitman had encouraged Allis to pursue morphological research himself. Poor health had induced him to live at Mentone in France, where he was engrossed in research into the heads and brains of fishes.[4]

Another American Wilson met at the Congress was the embryologist and neurologist George Streeter, then at Johns Hopkins Medical School who became a lifelong friend. In the British delegation were two Scottish acquaintances destined for larger roles in Wilson's life: Arthur Keith of Aberdeen, then at the London Hospital's Medical School whom Wilson first met in 1892 in Sydney when Keith was on his way 'home' from Siam; and R J A Berry, another Edinburgh man whose application for Melbourne's new anatomy chair Wilson was supporting, as he was also the application of F P Sandes of Sydney for the same appointment. Berry and Sandes were the 'home' committee's recommended candidates: in December 1905 Melbourne University opted for the Edinburgh-trained candidate.

In company with another Turner product, T H Bryce of Glasgow, the Wilsons left Geneva on 11 August to resume their summer holiday in Scotland. Two weeks later *Nature* proclaimed the success of the Congress. It was well organized, well attended and the 117 communications reflected anatomical developments around the world. Wilson's contribution was singled out for praise:

> The first place, both in importance of results and excellence of technique, must be assigned to the contributions made by Prof J T Wilson, of Sydney University, who placed before the congress the results of a prolonged investigation into the developmental history of ornithorynchus made by his colleague and collaborator, J P Hill, and by himself. With the material now at their command they will be able to write a full and precise account of the development of the monotremes and throw a great deal of light on mammalian morphology.... Most remarkable of all were the specimens and photographs showing the early developmental phases of the central nervous system. [5]

Wilson did not get his copy of *Nature* until 10 October, about the same time that this report was reproduced in Sydney under bold headlines in the *Sydney Morning Herald* and *The Australasian*. 'You seem to have taken the Congress by storm', wrote J P Hill who speculated that *Nature's* reviewer was Arthur Keith. Mungo MacCallum waxed lyrical: 'The news has given back to me for an hour or two the "light-winged spirit of youth" possessing which, one believed that recognition was proportional to desert. I have now for eighteen years been sure that you would, if you had a chance, command the acknowledgement of those "who are the marks of them that know".' And Mrs MacCallum wrote, 'I had not seen my professor so pleasantly excited for a long long time.' [6]

These messages and the arrival on 14 October of the binocular microscope he had ordered in June from an Edinburgh optician put Wilson in good heart as he settled down in early October to a heavy work programme. He had three papers to knock into final shape, beginning with the one he had delivered to the Congress on the *taenia clino-orbitalis*, and another long study, published in two parts in the *Journal of Anatomy* in 1906, on the morphology of the calamus region of the human brain. The latter was the result of marked discrepancies Wilson had noticed in anatomy textbooks and in the growing number of treatises on neurology. No authority he found could be relied upon. Henle's *Nervenlehre* of 1873 gave the most adequate description but was limited by the sectioning methods available at that time. So Wilson had prepared and studied a complete series of microscopical transverse sections of the adult human *medulla oblongata*, cut by the Minot microtome. He produced a highly critical and elaborately detailed account of this region of the human brain, describing for the first time the presence of a group of neurones in the *area postrema* of Retzius, which he called the *nucleus postremus*. Wilson read it to a meeting of the Anatomical Society at Barts Hospital on 24 November, one of five papers delivered that day and 'the only constellation in a sombre background of feeble twaddle' in Elliot Smith's colourful evaluation. Hill gave it high praise: 'by its critical acumen, no less than by its content of new facts and conclusions, [it] reveals the master hand of Wilson at its very best'. At his most relentless some might say, for the plethora of detail makes difficult reading. Wilson's passion for accuracy is a reminder of Turner's emphasis on the importance of minute detail, more detailed than ever in this case, probably because the morphological significance of his subject – the compelling purpose of such intricate quests – eluded Wilson at that time; he later suggested that the *area postrema* is a vestigial caudal continuation of the *tuberculum acusticum* of lower vertebrates.[7]

Wilson's success at Geneva landed him with more work: the onerous task of completing the big paper with Hill on the embryology of the platypus. Haldane was pressing him to submit it personally, together with a certificate of candidature for fellowship of the Royal Society. When he left Australia it was in a very rough state, even its general structure not having been decided. In letters Hill was liberal with apologies and exhortations. For Wilson the last three months in England were a hectic mix of festivities and writing, some of it on the move while he did a tour of current research in British universities, visiting Oxford, Sheffield, Manchester, Liverpool, Dublin and Belfast before making his final goodbyes in Dumfries, Moniaive and Edinburgh. His omission of Cambridge is curious, in view of the important and acclaimed work of its physiologists W H Gaskell and J N Langley on the involuntary nervous system. On 29 June he had spent some hours in Cambridge, noting in his diary 'visited nearly every college and the Backs' but presumably meeting no one.[8]

By 26 October he had finished the worrisome gastrular stage. He had consulted Jenkinson in Oxford, mulled it over with Hubrecht, Keibel and Gaupp in Europe and later with Arthur Keith, Ray Lankester and George Thane in London, consultations which suggest some uncertainty about the 'primitive-knot' interpretation of the 'lenticular mass of cells' in the early stages of blastodermic development. He finished the text in a 14½ hour stint by the early hours of Friday 1 December, left London by the noon train from Euston Station and from Manchester posted the paper to Sir William Turner to communicate to the Royal Society.

In Sheffield his attention was drawn to Professor McDonald's photos of granules in nerve fibres in the physiology department; in Manchester he was entertained by Jim Smith and his colleagues who included the expatriate Australian philosopher Samuel Alexander. In Liverpool he discussed the teaching of anatomy and its place in the science curriculum with the biochemist Benjamin Moore, and in the anatomy department he was shown some good models of the peripheral nerves as well as a fine series of bone preparations by A M Paterson, another Turner protégé. In the physiology department he met the eminent Charles Sherrington. A product of Michael Foster's Cambridge Physiological Laboratory, Sherrington was almost single-handedly unravelling the patterns of spinal reflexes and their interaction, just as his Spanish friend, the anatomist Ramón Y Cajal, was almost single-handedly unravelling the design of the vertebrate nervous system. In Sherrington's laboratory Wilson saw some of the many experiments Sherrington had performed on his 'Cartesian puppets' – animals with the upper part of their brain removed to deprive them of volition but not life – to work out his principle of reflex arcs and the integrative action of the nervous system, the subject of his Silliman Lectures delivered at Yale University in 1906 and published the same year, a landmark in the history of neurology.[9]

In Belfast on 12 December Wilson wrote an abstract of the platypus paper which on the 14th he delivered to the Royal Society at Burlington House in London after travelling overnight from Scotland. Lord Rayleigh was in the chair and among seven other Fellows in attendance were Martin just back from India, and Haldane. That business concluded Wilson took the 11.50 train for the north that night to rejoin Mabel for their Scottish farewells, concluding with a last visit to the University to see the physiologist Edward Schaefer's work on the diuretic action of pituitary extracts.

Back in London there was still work to be done, depriving him of Christmas relaxation: up to 12 hours a day for a week on the tedious job of preparing appendices and figures for reproduction, including hand-lettering for 17 plates. He was finally free of it when he saw the engraver's photographic proofs on 17 January, the day before leaving for Sydney.

The Wilson parents left London in advance of the rest of the family to spend a week with the Elliot Smiths in Cairo. Carefully packed in their luggage was the latest literature on microscopy and Wilson's prized new binocular microscope and camera, Zeiss stereoscopic equipment and sundry related items picked up second-hand in London and Edinburgh. In Cairo Wilson saw the medical school with its collection of Egyptian skeletons, mummies, ape skulls and brains, and at the zoo an excellent collection of lemurs. With Mabel he viewed the Sphinx and pyramids of Cheops and with Elliot Smith they both went by train and donkey to the Saqqara region to see the ruins of Memphis and the tombs of Ptah hotep, then to Mastaba to see some disinterred Egyptian skeletons. They left for Port Said to join their daughters and nurse on the *SS Mooltan* on 30 January with souvenirs of Egyptian brasswork and antiquities plus an ape embryo, an ape skull and a baboon skull to add to the prized microscope and its accessories.

On the voyage home Wilson at last had time to rest and reflect on the previous 14 months. He had left Australia feeling like a provincial on a pilgrimage to the centre of science and civilization but had found that his work, especially that on the platypus with Hill, was a focus of European interest. By concentrating on the unique opportunities of their geographic base they had made a significant contribution to revealing the secret of monotreme reproduction and early mammalian development. On monotremes they were the foremost authorities. His tour of European and British research centres, and the congress of anatomists, had provided invaluable opportunities to mix with scientists of the stature of Weismann, Keibel, Gaupp and Sherrington who till then had only been names. He felt better acquainted with American scientists like C O Whitman and E B Wilson for having met Edward Phelps Allis and George Streeter. And he saw, perhaps met if he did not converse with, the proud Spaniard, Santiago Ramón Y Cajal, the neuro-anatomist and self-taught neuro-histologist, whose name in later years was always on Wilson's lips. The impact of Cajal's work was delayed because it had to be translated from Spanish.[10]

Cajal was one scientist who flourished in isolation. As professor of histology in provincial Barcelona he felt as remote as Wilson from mainstream European research. In his case, however, isolation was partly self-imposed. A 'loner' by inclination, he was also intensely patriotic; he lived always in Spain and published exclusively in Spanish, determined that Spain should have a place on the scientific and intellectual stage. He recognized too that isolation had the advantage of 'distance' from the 'rich fantasies' of celebrated scientists, fantasies that become difficult-to-dislodge 'fads'. He preferred to trust his own ability to see and to reason. Though isolated, Cajal was in the vanguard of mainstream research.[11]

In contrast British anatomy was well behind the field. It had not experienced the great surge of interest in cell research stimulated by major advances in technique in the 1870s and 1880s, inducing an expansion in European and American anatomy to include microstructure. Fields like neurology and embryology were therefore relatively uncultivated by British anatomists. For when British physiology broke away from her anatomical parent in the 1870s 'the clever child took with her the microscope and the fine study of structure, leaving nothing but the cadaver for anatomy'. Histology in British medical schools – and in Australian medical schools by inheritance – became part and parcel of physiology departments, jealously guarded because in histology lay the best promise of research rewards.[12]

At Sydney University, Anderson Stuart lectured in histology but rarely practiced it for he had little interest in research. No doubt he served up what he had been served in Edinburgh as a student and assistant of William Rutherford, a histologist of distinction but again more an instructor than practitioner. Practical histology was taught by Stuart's physiology demonstrators Haswell, MacCormick, Almroth Wright, Charles Martin, Frank Tidswell, H Hawker, H G Chapman and J R L Dixon, the last two also lecturers in histology. Wilson's contribution to histology training as an anatomist, embryologist and neurologist was substantial. By means of his liberally illustrated lectures begun in 1895 – on the nervous system he would 'put on the screen one slide after another of every type of nerve cell ever seen in the mammalian body' – his research enterprise and his infectious fascination with technique made students familiar with microstructure and the technical proficiency required to study it. Still, histology lay formally in physiology's domain and it may well be that after observing the predicament of British anatomy Wilson resolved to reclaim it in Sydney as part of anatomy's birthright. The *status quo*, however, was preserved there till Anderson Stuart died in 1920. Melbourne made the change in 1910 during a major review of its medical curriculum. On the initiative of the physiology professor, W A Osborne, histology was handed over to R J A Berry's anatomy department and at the same time a course was established in neuro-anatomy.[13]

The SS *Mooltan* berthed in Port Melbourne at breakfast time on

26 February 1906, giving the Wilsons two days to see friends. They dined with the Berrys who had only just arrived in Melbourne themselves, and called on the Harry Brookes Allens, the Baldwin Spencers and the William Bridges. They also saw uncle James, as Wilson always did when in Melbourne, and he took Jeanie to visit her uncle Joseph, the roving member of the Lorrain Smith family. Three days later, on 1 March, the *SS Mooltan* docked in Sydney where Louis was waiting to greet and assist the Wilson entourage. The next day Wilson received a hero's welcome from staff and students of the Anatomy Department. At the first international congress of anatomists he had put the Medical School of the University of Sydney on the map. Anderson Stuart built the Medical School; Wilson furnished it with a reputation.

Wilson was soon back in his familiar groove, shouldering the yoke of his various offices and restoring his spirits in combat with Hill to reveal another secret of the wily platypus. This time they studied teeth development in two mammary foetuses, finding evidence of five quasi-permanent teeth in each jaw plus indications of vestigial representatives of deciduous predecessors to the front teeth. This paper was published by the prestigious *Quarterly Journal of Microscopical Science* in 1907, the year their big paper on platypus development appeared at last in the *Philosophical Transactions of the Royal Society of London*. Both papers were seen through the press by Hill who had left Sydney in August 1906 forever, to take the Jodrell Chair of Zoology and Comparative Anatomy at University College, London.

With growing responsibilities – by 1906 he had three children, a son having been born in January – J P Hill had to look to his future. In 1903 he had applied for but did not get the new Chair of Biology at Victoria College in Wellington, New Zealand. In October 1904 Sydney University created a new position for him, lecturer in embryology, increasing his annual salary by one hundred pounds, to 450 pounds. But it was still only half the salary of the biology professor. In 1905 Haswell's indulgence in the latest fashion for motor cars starkly demonstrated for Hill the distance between the two:

> Haswell is the latest victim – he now drives up with his chauffeur like a bally lord and says he saves an hour a day – Big car representing my entire screw.

In London Hill's father-in-law Mr Steele, Chief Inspector of Inland Revenue, was bothered perhaps more than Hill about Hill's

167

circumstances. Opportunity came in 1905/6 when three zoology chairs fell vacant in England: at Oxford, the Jodrell Chair at University College, London and, through the death of Hill's former teacher G B Howes, at the Royal College of Science, South Kensington. Hill's claims were promoted by Wilson while he was in England, as well as by the eminent scientists who had supported his application for the chair at Victoria College in Wellington in 1903. 'Frankly I don't wish for it – it's a bit elevated for my humble taste' Hill had confided to Wilson on 21 May 1905 concerning the South Kensington post, but 'to keep the peace' he had submitted an application which proved successful. By then, however, he had accepted the Jodrell Chair.[14]

On 11 August at a formal farewell Wilson paid tribute to Hill's great research abilities, his prodigious energy and patient undeviating perseverance. Skilled though he was in the laboratory, it was the naturalist, the collector in him, said Wilson, that was basic to his success. Australia had given him great scope for this propensity and Hill had acquired 'a collection of marsupial embryological material which might lead to international complications with Germany if the versatile Kaiser were to become interested in Zoology'. The loss to the university was considerable and it was not the first:

> Our university has been fortunate in the acquisition to its junior staff of a series of brilliant young scientific investigators, but surely unfortunate in her lack of ability to retain them. I will not attempt to discuss the policy which has this necessary effect. I will only say that the scientific reputation of the University of Sydney – and she does possess one in spite of what her calumniators may say – her scientific record and reputation owe not a little to the contribution of men like Wright and Martin, Elliot Smith and J P Hill. It is surely one of the problems of the future if not of the present, how to keep men of this stamp amongst us when we have got them. We are still Colonies even though we name ourselves States. Can we afford to colonise the scientific institutions of the old world with the young blood of our scientific investigators? It is true that in most cases the mother country gave what the mother country has taken away but is our need not the greater?

Again and again, publicly and privately, Wilson criticized the University's short-sighted policy of not funding the research of her promising scientists.[15]

Hill left Sydney with feelings of regret and trepidation. 'I feel very much like a lost soul and can't help regretting this move', he wrote to Wilson from Adelaide en route on 23 August. 'How the deuce I'm to go thro' with it I don't know – I'll have to try to however – no doubt my fear and dislike of the place will go in time but meanwhile I am pretty miserable – I could do anything to be rid of it.' In London he found Martin thin and careworn 'overburdened with routine & he says quite frankly he would sooner be in Melb! Just my sentiments!' Hill buckled down to his new and onerous administrative and teaching tasks, fearing at times that he would forget what a marsupial looked like. He taught junior students, as well as advanced students in vertebrate embryology, using lantern slides liberally. Though not a good lecturer he transmitted his own enthusiasm so effectively that many zoology students stayed on to work at embryology and half of those took the DSc. He secured the services of a personal technician (the first zoologist to do so in Britain), a lad called F J Pittock whom he trained as Wilson had trained Louis, in photography, photomicrography and plate-making. In 1907 Hill made an inspection of German science similar to Wilson's tour of 1905, including the standard dose of Dr Tilly.[16]

By April 1908 Hill was beginning to pick up the threads of his marsupial work again. He began a study of the early development of the marsupial cat *Dasyurus viverrinus* using the great collection of eggs he had garnered from breeding these animals in captivity between 1899 and 1904. In 1910 he produced a fourth major contribution to the embryology of marsupials with a magnificent description revealing that at cleavage two rings of four cells appear, the embryo developing from the upper ring, the lower ring forming only an enveloping placental membrane. He drew the conclusion that, so far as the scant knowledge of early mammalian (eutherian) development permitted, early marsupial development represented an intermediate position between monotreme and eutherian forms. With this 'very important and illuminating contribution to the problem of mammalian development' Hill was launched independently on his life's work. He was to become the world's leading authority on marsupial reproduction and embryology.[17]

Wilson did miss Hill. They made an effort to continue joint work on platypus heads – each of them working with half a head – but separation put an end to the collaboration of Wilson and Hill. They published only one more joint paper, to correct their error of interpretation about the yolk-navel, wrongly identified as a primitive knot in their big paper on platypus development. Richard Assheton of Cambridge and Keibel of Freiburg had triggered doubts in Wilson's mind, and in 1911 he raised the question with Hill:

> ...I admit having been impressed by [Assheton's] suggestion that our early primitive knot in platypus is not identical with the primitive knot of our post-gastrular stage, but is rather of the nature of a yolk-blastopore structure, and, probably quite extra-embryonic. What do you think of his view? His criticism would only really affect the appearances of that particular stage which we called gastrular, though, of course, some of our deductions and inferences therefrom, would require considerable modification.[18]

They published their correction in 1915 in the *Quarterly Journal of Microscopical Science.*

Now the sole representative of the Fraternity of Duckmaloi in Sydney, Wilson began a period of reappraisal. Less certain of his research direction, he was more easily distracted by medical, university and civic affairs in which increasingly he was called on to take a leading role. His domestic responsibilities were growing too. At the age of 45 he took great pride in the birth of a son, Thomas Douglas Glover, on 10 December 1906; a second son, John Julian Glover, on 19 November 1909 further secured the Wilson line and expanded the household to eight. By spring 1908 Wilson was building a holiday house in a little wilderness on the coast 20 miles north of Sydney. The Wilsons were firmly tied to Sydney.[19]

In the laboratory as he cast around for direction Wilson explored the boundaries of his new binocular microscope and broadened his command of technique. He published three technical papers during 1910–11: one recorded modifications to his paraffin embedding method using nerve strands and other animal structures as directing marks, with tips on floating out paraffin sections and a simple expedient for suspending blocks of tissue in fluid; a second supplied a method, with recipes, for obtaining a fine, but not too fine, colour-injection of the arterial system of cadavers for dissection; and a third described an improved method for mounting frozen sections of the cadaver in the anatomical museum. He was never happier than in the laboratory, making things with his hands.[20]

He also returned, after more than 20 years, to the question of the innervation of the achselbogen muscle in the human armpit, prompted by two German critics of his 1888 paper, G Ruge of Zurich and his pupil L Tobler. For the Australasian Medical

Congress held in Sydney in 1911 he delivered a paper describing 20 new cases he had investigated over the intervening years, while for the *Journal of Anatomy* he reviewed the now extensive literature on the subject and replied to his critics. He stood by William Turner's view that the true achselbogen in humans is a vestige of the muscle that moves the skin in loosely-skinned mammals (the *panniculus carnosus*), but indicated that there are other muscular slips whose morphological value had not been determined; and he agreed with Ruge and Tobler that the achselbogen was usually innervated from anterior thoracic (pectoral) nerves. Wilson's disagreement with Ruge and Tobler was simply that they pushed the doctrine of nerve-muscle correlation too far. There was a degree of individual variability in the innervation of the achselbogen just as there were reciprocal size-relations in man between the intercosto-humeral nerve and the nerve of Wrisberg, as Cunningham had proved in 1877. Nerve segments did not always perfectly coincide with muscle segments.[21]

As President of the Anatomy, Physiology and Pharmacological Section of the Australasian Medical Congress held in Melbourne in October 1908, Wilson addressed the subject of recent advances in neurology. The history of modern neurology was short but impressive. By 1908 it had, in Wilson's judgement, 'almost won rank as a distinct branch of biological science'. For him and many others at that time no domain of biology surpassed it in general or special interest. His interest in embryology was promoted, if not prompted as in the case of Ramón Y Cajal, by the advantages of using embryonic instead of adult material to study nervous structure: the nursery stage was much less complex than the fully grown forest.[22]

The bewildering complexity of nervous tissue had long resisted all efforts at understanding. It awaited a breakthrough in histological technique, and the eyes of a biologist who could correctly interpret what was revealed by it. Both happened in the 1880s. The Italian Camillo Golgi with his chrome-silver impregnation method and the German Paul Ehrlich with his methylene-blue stain supplied the technique to silhouette just a few nerve cells with all their thread-like fibres, showing also their relationship to other structures against a white or yellow background. 'All was as sharp as a sketch with Chinese ink on transparent Japan paper', wrote Ramón Y Cajal to whom belonged the discerning eyes. He demonstrated that the nervous system was an agglomeration of discrete and definable cells or neurones which made contact but did not fuse with other neurones: there was a space or synapse between them. The neurone was the basic structural and functional building block of the entire nervous system.[23]

This neurone theory was at odds with the then-prevailing idea of the nervous system as a reticular process, a tangled network of interconnecting and interlacing fibres with nerve cells positioned at connecting nodes. The battle between the neuronists and the reticularists continued well into the twentieth century, even after the American anatomist Ross Harrison proved the neurone theory by conclusive experiments, showing for example in 1907 a living nerve fibre growing out from its cell body in tissue culture. Wilson in his 1905 European tour had met proponents from both sides: Waldeyer (who had coined the word *neurone* in 1891) in Berlin and in Leipzig Hans Held, a reticularist; and at Geneva he had witnessed a skirmish between Ramón Y Cajal and the Italian A Donnagio, a colleague of the leading reticularist Camillo Golgi.[24]

The neurone doctrine gave coherence to many areas of neurological research, transforming and correcting much that had preceded it. Wilson briefly reviewed several such areas pioneered by clinicians and pathologists, including the diverse forms of peripheral sensibilities and the localization of brain functions. On his own particular interest at that time, the histogenesis of the vertebrate nervous system, he offered observations based on his detailed study of neurular development in the platypus embryo. Recounting the development of this system from its origin as a circumscribed area of ectoderm on the surface of the blastodermic vesicle he drew attention to the proliferating cells on the margin of the neural plate (especially prominent in the cephalic region) which were ganglionic in prescriptive significance and were not involved, at least in higher vertebrates, in the subsequent formation of folds and closure of the medullary tube (spinal cord). In this configuration Wilson discerned the two basic components of the nervous system: the main if not the entire sensory apparatus derived from the original ectodermal *neural* plate including the marginal ganglionic strips (supplemented perhaps by some more outlying patches of sensory neural ectoderm); and the main if not the entire mass of the cerebro-spinal axis and the peripheral motor nerve apparatus derived from medullary plate. The traditional terms 'cerebro-spinal' and 'sympathetic' for these two divisions were misleading archaisms he argued, and for them he proposed to substitute 'ganglionic' and 'medullary' to distinguish the leading elements of 'the most fundamental subdivision available on morphological grounds'. While acknowledging that the two divisions subsequently interlock in the formation of mixed nerves, he maintained that 'in a most significant sense they remain distinct structural and functional complexes in the permanent organisation'.[25]

The interest of this lecture, never published, is in Wilson's grasp of the rapidly accumulating and broad advances in neurology and in his evaluation as a *morphologist* of the fundamental plan of the vertebrate nervous system. For in the British world it was the physiologists who were making the important pronouncements, as the Anatomical Society of Great Britain and Ireland had acknowledged in 1900. Basic to Wilson's clarification of the most fundamental division in the vertebrate neural arrangement, as he acknowledged, was the widely acclaimed achievements of Cambridge physiologists H K Anderson, W H Gaskell and J N Langley, and Cambridge-trained Charles Sherrington, on the origin and composition of the 'sympathetic' system (renamed *'involuntary'* by Gaskell and *'autonomic'* by Langley), work which had a distinct anatomical orientation. Gaskell's research over 30 years veered from pure physiology to pure morphology with a mixture of the two in between, while Langley was caricatured as a 'neuroanatomist who flirted from time to time with physiology', and Sherrington's genius lay, according to modern authorities, in his ability 'to convert anatomical data into physiological fact'. C J Martin's ideal – it was also Michael Foster's – of bringing biology's two great divisions together in one enterprise, of bringing cell theory into intimate association with evolutionary theory, was here realized; but at the expense of scientific anatomy. Physiology flourished as never before in Cambridge while Cambridge anatomy, dispossessed of histology, languished.[26]

On 25 February 1909 Wilson was unanimously elected a Fellow of the Royal Society, an event that had been on the cards ever since his acclaimed performance at the Geneva Congress in August 1905. At Haldane's suggestion in October 1905 he had submitted a certificate of candidature and had read his paper before the December meeting of the Society. His election was to await publication of the paper but after that was done, in 1907, it seems to have been forgotten until Haldane and Elliot Smith decided in 1909 to bring the matter to a satisfactory conclusion. Signatories to the original certificate were Fellows resident in Britain, so Elliot Smith arranged with Haswell for a supplementary one to be sent, signed by all the Fellows in Australia. This was somehow lost in the post but the knowledge of its existence had the desired effect. Jim Smith was also elected a Fellow at the same meeting. 1909 was Haldane's first year on the Council of the Royal Society.[27]

Congratulations poured in, including one from D J Cunningham who had succeeded William Turner in the anatomy chair in Edinburgh in 1903. 'I don't think the honour was ever more worthily bestowed' he wrote. A few months later Cunningham died, setting in motion the chair-filling game that periodically rippled around the Empire. Wilson's friends in England set up another chorus for him to come 'home'. Elliot Smith, who always got excited at such times and was about to take the Anatomy Chair at Manchester, wrote with dramatic flourish:

> At any moment now the whole Anatomical world in G.B. may be thrown into a cataclysm. In case of emergency if I see a reasonable opening may I push your candidature for Glasgow, Edinburgh or Oxford?... It is your simple duty to British Anatomy to come over to the old country for there is no one but yourself to take the lead.

Martin cool-headedly urged Wilson to consider Oxford – and so did Haldane – if Arthur Thomson got Edinburgh, arguing that the Edinburgh position carried too heavy teaching and administrative loads, whereas Oxford would admirably suit Wilson's style. Martin acknowledged however that the 900 pounds per year at Oxford might not be enough for Wilson with his large family, and emphasized 'You would *have to apply* for Oxford I understand', adding 'it would be awfully good to have you back, but I don't suppose you'll come'.[28]

Wilson responded with restraint. He cabled Hill to the effect that he would consider the Edinburgh opening if invited. Hill therefore proposed to bring Wilson's name forward 'quietly and unostentatiously', and no doubt he did, but nothing came of it. Wilson had no strong desire to leave Sydney. Apart from feeling that Australia had recently lost to England too many good scientists, he suspected that his scientific interests would take a back seat in Britain's halls of learning. As he had told the Melbourne University Medical Society plainly in 1907,

> those who are entrusted with the working of these great institutions are really groaning under the bondage of ordinances which have been long outgrown, practices which are more or less effete, and vested interests which hamper and restrict, even if they are powerless to suppress, the full development of the modern academic spirit.[29]

Besides, a move just then would not have suited the family. Sir Julian Salomons had recently died and it would have been a severe wrench for Mabel to leave her mother at such a time. Also, Mabel was expecting her fifth child.

Notes

1. General source material on JTW's sabbatical activities in Europe and Britain: Diaries and 'Scientific Notes' for 1905, in Wilson Papers. SUA.
2. Wright: Colebrook in *RSO* 1948, 297–314. CJM: Chick in *RSO* 1956, 174–208.
3. *Nature* review, 'First International Congress of Anatomists', 28.8.1905, 400–3, probably by Keith.
4. Congress of Anatomists: JTW Diaries and 'Scientific Notes'. Allis: De Beer, 238–9; Evans & Evans, 8, 9; *Who Was Who in America* Vol. IV.
5. *Nature* 28.8.1905, 400–3
6. 'You seem to': JPH to JTW, 12.10.1905. 'The news has': WM to JTW, 10.10.1905. 'I had not': Mrs MacCallum to JTW, 15.10.1905.
7. JTW 1906b. 'the only constellation': GES to JTW, 23.11.05. 'by its critical': JPH on JTW, *RSO* 1949, 649.
8. JTW Diaries and 'Scientific Notes'.
9. Sherrington's work: Stevens, 71–83.
10. *Ibid.*
11. Cajal: *DSB;* Hamburger 1980, 600–11; Cajal (Trans. by A D Loewy) 1971, 7–35 . 'rich fantasies': Cajal, in *Perspectives in Biology and Medicine,* 1971, 15. Cajal on JTW's lips: JMGW to author.
12. British anatomists and neurology: Mayr, 469; Geison, 331. 'the clever child': Osler, quoted Cushing, 92.
13. William Rutherford: *Centenary Book,* 303–4; Geison, 138–9. Critique of histology lectures: *Hermes,* Aug. 1914, 45. JTW's illustrated lectures: *Hermes,* 17.7.1896, 11; 'put on the screen': SAS, 7. Histology at Melbourne Univ.: Russell, 110.
14. Hill's salary: Senate Mins 10.10.1904. 'Haswell is' and 'Frankly I don't': JPH to JTW, 21.5.1905.
15. 'a collection' and 'Our university has': JTW speech to farewell Hill, 11.8.1906.
16. 'I feel very' and 'overburdened with routine': JPH to JTW, 23.8.06 and 19.4.07.
17. Hill's work: Watson, *RSO* 1955, 101–17.
18. 'very important', and 'I admit': JTW to JPH, 12.5.1911.
19. Family papers.
20. JTW papers: 1910a, b, c.
21. JTW papers: 1912; 1913.
22. JTW 1908 (unpub).
23. 'All was as': Cajal quoted in Sherrington, *RSO* 1935, 430.
24. Harrison: Abercrombie, *RSO* 1961.

25. 'the most fundamental' and 'in a most': JTW 1908 (unpub).
26. Anatomical Society's observation: *J of A* 1900, in congratulating GES. [See also Keith, *J of A* Vol. 62, 242.] Gaskell & Langley: Geison, 334 and entries in *DSB;* Stevenson in Brooks & Cranefield, 69. 'neuroanatomist who': Fulton (*ibid.*), 68. 'to convert': Clarke & O'Malley, 370. See also Liddell, *RSO* on Sherrington, 247.
27. JTW's FRS: GES to JTW, 26.3.1907 and 3.3.1909; JSH to JTW 25.2.1909.
28. 'I don't think': Cunningham to JTW, 18.3.09. 'At any moment': GES to JTW, 19.6.09. 'You would *have to*': CJM to JTW, 1.7.09.
29. 'quietly and': JPH to JTW, 2.7.09. 'those who are': JTW, Address to Melb. Univ. Med. Students, 1907 (unpub).

9

Practical Idealist

Wilson could hardly have been more of a contrast to his 'senior colleague'. Anderson Stuart was the public face of the Medical School. Forceful, egotistical and autocratic, on campus he was a conspicuous figure: tall, always in morning suit and carrying a cane, a cravat at his chin and top hat over a strong Roman nose, he came and went in a hansom cab even to the Prince Alfred Hospital which was only about a five minute walk from the school. A good concise lecturer, if as some claimed 'over-didactic', he had presence and a good voice and what he regarded as the one essential for good teaching: 'the gift of orderly thinking in the presence of others'. Though by 1902 he had conceded some value to more personal methods of teaching like the tutorial, he robustly defended the lecture: 'No, we lecturers are not going to be wiped out just yet!' His lectures featured good blackboard diagrams but no use of the epidiascope because in his experience a darkened room put discipline at risk. He was inclined to wander the corridors and in and out of classes to see that all was as it should be. Anything unseemly was summarily penalized: 'Smoking in my Medical School? Two pounds! Pay it to the Registrar in the morning.' Neither teaching nor research attracted him; physiology he advanced little. He found his metier in building and organization, administration and politics. As Dean of Medicine and Fellow of the Senate Stuart wielded considerable power in the government of the University. Students lampooned him as 'the boss of the Varsity' and 'the Lord High Panjandrum of Camperdown'.[1]

Wilson they caricatured as a 'swot [who] Learned everything compulsory and everything that's not.' Tall and spare, with a scholar's stoop, dressed usually in a nondescript three-piece suit and invariably a red tie, sometimes awry, he arrived by tram every morning at ten to nine, walked up the private stairs to his office, exchanged his jacket for a long white coat and entered the Vesalian lecture theatre at exactly nine, his assistant Louis at the door checking the attendance roll. 'There was,' said one student of the early 1900s,

> something of the mastiff about him in his keen scent for research. His lean sallow face with its high cheekbones seemed always tense with concentration. His eyes burned with a fierce enthusiasm for the subject in hand. No one dared, even if he had wanted, to disturb *this* professor's lectures.[2]

Outwardly aloof and severe, and becoming more so as student numbers and his responsibilities increased with the years, the initial reaction of most students was one of fear. One former student recalled the occasion when Wilson mounted an interesting demonstration of bones on a long table protected by a guard rail, over which he, a timid first year, ventured a curious hand and was suddenly stunned by 'Jummy's' large voice: ' "Leave those bones alone!" I jumped about a foot in the air , and then "Jummy", seeing how abashed this young man was, melted, looked conscience-stricken and then said in a kindly way, "I'm sorry, but you know I really must not allow those bones to be touched".' Students played on Wilson's tender conscience. It was said to be a good ploy to manipulate a stern rebuke from 'Jummy' during the year so that in reparation 'Jummy's' feelings would be favourably disposed at examinations.[3]

Students laughed – or many did – at Wilson's foibles like his outrage at dissecting room disturbances. Wilson laid heavy emphasis on dissection, requiring every student to dissect the human body at least once. Occasionally pent-up emotions – for every student experienced some disquiet doing this work – erupted in 'meat fights' which would escalate from the surreptitious throwing of a piece of fat or skin to hurling 'parts' and even all out fisticuffs. Wilson would storm in, castigate them for this 'horror of desecration' of their 'brothers and sisters' and deal out to all involved the maximum penalty, a two pound fine. In lectures they could be startled by a sudden attack on slavish note-taking – 'I said *luke* at it not write! Use the eyes the guid God gave you!'; or bemused by his occasional injunction to pursue Truth and Beauty; or join with a chorus of stamping feet when he used his favourite word 'tolerably', to which

practice Wilson sometimes responded with humour: 'He stopped
and he looked and, of course, everybody froze and he said,
"Gentlemen! You seem to take exception to my use of the word
'tolerably'. And I say that I shall use it as often as I please because it
expresses tolerably well what I mean."' Students respected him as a
hard worker, an eminent scientist and a just authority 'whom no
amount of stamping would ever frighten and would fulfil to the last
letter any threat he found necessary to make'. 'You just *knew* that he
could *never* do anything out of expediency.'[4]

'Gentlemen', was Wilson's invariable form of address to his
classes, though almost from the beginning there was a female
presence in them, which grew very slowly with the years. Anderson
Stuart had raised no barriers to the admission of women on equal
terms with men. His one female student, he testified in 1887, had
had a good effect on the men, and if a teacher felt embarrassed, the
fault probably lay with him. As for ward work, if female nurses could
do it, why not female medical students? This was a remarkably
'advanced' view for that time, but his attitude, as he said at the time
and later, was really much more equivocal. He neither encouraged
nor discouraged, he claimed. Women did experience marked
difficulties with examinations – perhaps due to inappropriate
secondary schooling or, as one woman believed, to discouragement
by 'continued failure' – and in getting clinical experience: it was not
until 1906, after a public outcry, that a female graduate was accepted
for a year's residency at Royal Prince Alfred Hospital.[5]

'Wilson did not like women', complained former women
students many years later. Always seated in the front row, they felt
totally ignored as he directed his lectures over their heads to the
main body of the class. 'I was afraid of him', was another complaint,
but then so were they all. Like Anderson Stuart Wilson equivocated.
He certainly espoused the female cause for university education and
he experienced no difficulty teaching 'certain subjects', for he was no
prude; indeed he believed that the fashion for keeping young
women ignorant of the facts of human sexuality to be highly
reprehensible. But like most of the population he thought that in
general medicine was not for women: to succeed in medicine, he
argued, a woman must be very highly motivated; and there was 'no
great call for them' outside certain areas like the diseases of women
and children, for which he conceded they were 'admirably suited'.
He gave both help and encouragement to the Sydney Medical
Mission established in 1900 by women graduates to alleviate the
medical problems of the poor in the inner city areas. That enterprise

chimed in with his idealist conviction that the good citizen had a duty to exercise his or her 'practical social sympathies'. In the dark days of June 1918, when the Allies faced defeat in France and the Australian Government removed the embargo on the enlistment of medical students, Wilson himself issued a call for 'capable young women' to fill the places of men students in the medical school. It was their 'public duty'.[6]

Most students harboured some resentment about his lectures. Anatomy was dull. 'Jummy *made* it dull' complained one former student with umbrage that had survived 60 years. 'He was dull, dour and humourless', said another. Wilson kept anatomy too strictly within arbitrary bounds said medical vocationalists, squandering the natural interest of most students in clinical references. Yet there were those – a rarefied few perhaps – who were impressed by his 'dry but precise and very clear descriptions ... the hard workers certainly thought he was marvellous... He thought as an evolutionary zoologist'. Osteology may have bored most students, but neurology lectures were in another category, as one of his stronger critics conceded: 'I have got to admit that he could by his method of teaching neurology make it sensible. Neurology was a difficult subject unless one got the concept of tracts ascending to the brain and he could demonstrate with his epidiascope the various tracts and make it sensible.'[7]

Wilson made exuberant use of the epidiascope (operated by Louis) from 1895 when he introduced it to illustrate embryology lectures. He overused it to the point of student bewilderment complained S A Smith, Grafton's younger brother, throwing on the screen 'one slide after another of every nerve cell ever seen in the mammalian body'. Wilson's urgent whisper, 'Focus, Louis, focus', parodied down the years by generations of students commemorated this routine. Around 1900 he introduced frozen sections as a useful method for showing the comparative position of all parts of the body before they were disturbed by dissection: a cadaver was frozen and then sawn into cross sections, each one inch thick, then set in plaster of Paris in two-inch-deep trays before being filled with spirit, covered with a glass plate and mounted in sequence. Another familiar procedure featured Wilson with a skull under his armpit poking a long knitting needle at the characteristics he meticulously described. 'I have the tip of my probe in the foramen of Magendie' he would intone, to the exasperation of those students seated too far away to see, which was most of them. 'I doubt if those in the second row could have seen it, let alone us up in the back', said one aggrieved student 60 years on.[8]

Student dissections yielded more illustrations. In 1890, if not earlier, he instituted prosectorships: the six best dissectors of second year were recruited to the prosectory, a special room where they dissected one body simultaneously with the rest of the class, and another to display various parts for lectures; the best of these became reference material in his museum mounted in the early years around the walls of the Vesalian Theatre, later collected together in the Hunterian Museum. The brilliant T K Potts, a prosector of 1911 and 1912, contributed some exquisite specimens including one of the sympathetic nervous system as seen from the back, with the bones removed from half the brain so that all the spinal nerves could be seen, more especially the vertebral chain of ganglia, down to the thigh. The fat and genial Barney Coen, a demonstrator from 1911 and later in charge of the dissecting room, contributed specimens on his specialty, the 'Hedaneck'. For other museum specimens Wilson searched far afield: from New Guinea in 1914 after difficult negotiations came 40 skulls, the product of head-hunting, while from the Maison Tramond in Paris he acquired some very fine wax models of embryos.[9]

Wilson was at his best in the laboratory, 'advising, criticizing and, above all, encouraging, all with great vehemence'. Quite often it was as a collaborator that he guided a young protégé through the literature, procedures and techniques of research, quick to step aside as with Grafton Elliot Smith who registered very early his emphatic independence; watchful and protective as with Johnny Hunter in whom he recognized physical frailty; or tough as with Grafton's younger brother S A Smith who 'had an indolent streak in him'. 'No one will obtain from me a doctorate of medicine unless he is truly *doctus*', he told Smith 'in the tones of a military commander', proceeding then to outline a work programme for the MD examination, the very idea of which overwhelmed S A Smith's aspirations.[10]

In spite of the University's negative policy on research, Wilson, by precept and example established in his own department a tradition of research which drew international respect. It had a strong leaning to his own dominant interest, neurology. Elliot Smith and Hunter were the star products of this informal school but it raised many other teachers and researchers of no mean stature – Raymond Dart, Joseph Shellshear, Una Fielding, H J Wilkinson, Neville Burkitt – as well as medical practitioners like G H S Lightoller who was so bitten by the research bug that he combined it with a busy practice. To these students Wilson communicated also his spiritual convictions. While undergraduates in their irreverence might scoff at Wilson's high-minded injunctions, those who worked close to him absorbed them as a sort of ethical code. 'His influence on me was so great that even today', wrote Raymond Dart in 1959, 'I often find myself guided by the standards he implanted in my young mind.' Student obligations to Wilson were far deeper than solid knowledge, observed MacCallum: 'the spirit of his teaching .... helped them to realise the ethics of their profession, its dignity, its responsibility, its value for the service of man.' As a teacher Wilson seemed closely to resemble his father with his vigour, piety and references to things of the spirit, a style bolstered and codified by the idealist creed.[11]

In general Sydney's Medical School was all the better for the differences of its two leaders, at least in the first two decades. They directed their gifts and energies to different spheres, one advancing and protecting the school outwardly, the other nourishing it inwardly. Their representations in the broadening scientific community were also divided, especially in the early years, probably to deploy efficiently their limited time and energies. For example Stuart, who was elected a Trustee of the Australian Museum in March 1890, resigned in March 1893, making room for Wilson's election in May 1893 to that position which he held until 1920. Stuart took a high profile in the Royal and (Royal) Zoological Societies of NSW, while Wilson played a prominent role in the Linnean Society of NSW. Both worked to promote the Australasian Association for the Advancement of Science and intercolonial medical congresses: Stuart as administrator, Wilson as contributor. But as an 'obsessive, even compulsive, organizer' Stuart's outside interests expanded increasingly into bureaucratic, quasi-political areas like public health, hospital administration, civil ambulance and transport, the Red Cross and British immigration. Wilson's interests in civic affairs also expanded with the years, exemplary citizen that he was, but they never attenuated his commitment to the medical school; as a practising scientist he was particularly concerned with curriculum development and the needs of research. Stuart retained his power within the University, but from 1903 when he became heavily preoccupied with the Prince Alfred Hospital, delegating more and more of his university duties to his protégé H G Chapman, Stuart's influence within the medical school waned – his mornings only were spent there – and Wilson's grew. That Stuart early apprehended in Wilson a challenge to his own

182

authority is suggested by the fact that Wilson never became dean of the medical faculty till after Stuart's death. Nevertheless by the early years of the new century Wilson's authority was paramount in the school. 'Meat fights' broke out only when Wilson was believed not to be in the building. His presence was felt rather than seen, like that of God Almighty.[12]

In university affairs Wilson was emerging as an authority. On 6 April 1908 he was elected Chairman of the Professorial Board whose members were the Chancellor, Vice-Chancellor and professors of the four faculties (arts, medicine, law and science), and whose duties were 'to manage and superintend the discipline of all students in the university, and ... to determine all matters concerning the studies and examinations which affect the students of more than one Faculty.' Little more than a disciplinary board at its inception in the mid-eighties, when much inter-faculty business was conducted informally, by 1908 the Board found itself grappling with academic, organizational and administrative matters of considerable weight, matters which required sound and prompt resolution during the university's rapid expansion in student and staff numbers and in the range and diversity of its educational purpose. This was a time of educational quickening: between 1900 and 1912 new faculties, departments or courses were established in dentistry, pharmacy, massage (physiotherapy), public health, veterinary science, agriculture, psychology, education, economics and commerce, military studies and astronomy, with departments of botany and applied chemistry shortly to follow. The Board faced the problems of fitting these new activities into the university's academic and administrative structure, their staffing, accommodation and funding as well as the ways and means to promote research, which all agreed was essential for good teaching. Wilson presided, except for the period 1913 to 1915, from 1908 until he left for Cambridge in 1920. Over this period the Board assumed the full scope of its responsibilities as the highest academic authority in the university which was, claimed the Board in a 1911 report over Wilson's signature, 'the highest authority in the State on matters of education'. The NSW Department of Public Instruction thought differently.[13]

However, the Senate, as the all-powerful governing authority of the University, controlled the effectiveness of the Professorial Board as an educational authority, and the Senate at that time was the creature of its president, Chancellor Sir Normand MacLaurin, and Professor Anderson Stuart. Close friends since their first association in 1883 – without MacLaurin's support Stuart would never have realized his ambitions for the Medical School – they had completely dominated the Senate from 1896 when MacLaurin became Chancellor. In circumstances where the position of Chancellor carried a heavy executive responsibility and there was no full-time administrator apart from the university Registrar, the 'political' combination of MacLaurin and Stuart was 'almost unstoppable'. Every Sunday morning at MacLaurin's home in Macquarie Street they held informal counsel. 'They were an admirably adapted pair', said Sir Charles Bickerton Blackburn, 'for when Stuart's forceful pertinacity met with a check the persuasiveness of his suave more crafty partner often won the day.' But a political battle was brewing which they were destined to lose.[14]

The Senate was the target of a growing number of critics. It was lethargic, conservative and unrepresentative *Hermes* complained perennially. Of its 20 members, four were ex-officio representing the four faculties, while the remaining 16 were elected by convocation and appointed for life, all but three appointed before 1890. In 1907 the Annual Conference of the Labor Party resolved to liberalize the structure of the university by abolishing life tenure for senators and widening the franchise for their election. In 1908 similar recommendations came from the conservative and influential *Sydney Morning Herald* as well as the Women's Progressive Association of NSW and in 1909 from Convocation, Francis Anderson and Peter Board. The thrust from the last two, who were in the vanguard of State education reform, had both professional and political weight.[15]

In 1901 Professor Francis Anderson had opened a crusade for the reform of New South Wales' public education system; by 1903 Peter Board had emerged as a man admirably equipped to guide the reform movement. An Australian-born Scot and a passionate democrat, this 'quiet, clearly-spoken, wiry, bearded inspector' was 44 years old when appointed under-secretary and director of the Department of Public Instruction in 1905. The combined efforts of Anderson and Board radically reformed primary and teacher education. By 1906 they were joined by Alexander Mackie, an imported Scot and principal of the new Teachers Training College, who in 1910 became Sydney University's first professor of education.[16]

By 1909, when secondary education came into the reformers' sights, the University was drawn into fierce debate touching on the role of the University in the State. Board and Anderson attacked the University's control over secondary education through its external

184

2° education for uni, or for life

examinations and matriculation standards and conditions. Secondary education was confined to an academic straitjacket, they argued. 'The secondary school', said Anderson in 1909 '... is more than an anteroom to the University. It is a stage in the education of the citizen'. Board proposed that an independent council be established to regulate the affairs of secondary education. Opposing this at the University was another pair of Scots, Mungo MacCallum the dean of the faculty of arts and H S Carslaw the professor of mathematics, who proposed that examinations and the inspection of schools be under the control of the (yet to be appointed) professor of education. But Peter Board could not countenance a university professor having authority over Department schools: stalemate.[17]

The constitution of the University Senate, especially the life tenure for elected members, was seen by the reformers as the main obstacle to bringing the University 'more into touch with the requirements of the age'. The *status quo* was stoutly defended by the Senate's president, Chancellor Sir Normand MacLaurin (who was also a member of the Executive Council) and Professor Anderson Stuart. Life tenure for senators, as with judges, was a very good system said MacLaurin for otherwise 'control would fall almost entirely into the hands of professors'. Stuart was incensed by the proposition of senators having to contest their positions at elections every five years as in South Australia: 'The Chief Justice of the Commonwealth might be defeated by a sucking barrister'.[18]

The first Labor government in NSW, elected to power in October 1910, gave Peter Board solid support and in November, among other proposals to improve the university's efficiency and accessibility for the less privileged – like more funds to worthy students and to the University and better adult education provisions – announced its intention to reconstitute the Senate. Tension rose in the University and the Professorial Board, the main forum for debating the University's control of secondary education, was exposed to more public interest than usual. On the Board sat all the prominent parties to the argument over Senate reform, except Peter Board: MacLaurin, Anderson Stuart, MacCallum, Carslaw, Francis Anderson and Alexander Mackie. These six combative Scots were refereed by a seventh, Wilson, who was much exercized. The irrepressible Carslaw claimed that when Wilson took to jumping on him in Board meetings his voice could be heard in the quadrangle a quarter of a mile away. To the press Wilson expressed the view, as Chairman of the Board, that the University's urgent problems of development and efficiency had little to do with the constitution of

JTW referees th senate education debate

Wilson's voice

185

the Senate, and that there should be an 'inquiry into both the structure and the working of the present University machinery'. It was extraordinary he said that the government should be looking at cut and dried proposals without such proper investigation 'as would be called forth by the proposal to alter the workings of a coal mine', and that 'those who look for a solution of the real University problems in mere changes in tenure and election of the Senate are barking up the wrong tree'. The issue then receded into the background during 1911 while Peter Board was overseas.[19]

The machinations of MacLaurin and Anderson Stuart in the Senate were neither edifying nor conducive to good government. They were an open secret, breeding resentment, frustration and cynicism. Wilson must also have had in mind the restrictions placed on the Professorial Board's advisory jurisdiction by law – to 'matters affecting more than one faculty' – and by custom – to only those matters referred by the Senate. The Medical Faculty for instance never sent its reports to the Professorial Board, but always direct to the Senate. To members of the Board, who carried a high degree of personal responsibility for the administration, teaching and research work of their separate departments, it seemed natural and right that they should be entrusted with a collective responsibility for advising the Senate on all matters pertaining to the work and development of the University, a function performed by professorial boards in most universities. To establish this practice at Sydney would involve Bye-law amendments to remove the legal restriction and to provide that reports of faculties and other academic bodies be sent as a matter of course to the Board which could then if it thought fit make comments or suggestions to the Senate. To these recommendations the Senate turned a deaf ear; this situation was to remain unchanged until 1936. The Board's answer to this impasse was to report on issues anyway, not only at the Senate's request but on its own initiative. Another recommendation, that a Proctorial Board be constituted as a sub-committee of the Professorial Board to deal more efficiently with student discipline, was effected in 1914.[20]

The undergraduates added their mite to strained relations. Discord between the Senate and the undergraduates was longstanding, aired annually in May during the week-long festivities for the Commemoration of Benefactors. The official Commemoration ceremony was a public function marked by speeches and the conferring of degrees in the Great Hall. Popular interest, however, focused on the student procession of floats through Sydney's streets caricaturing public figures and current

186

events, and on the evening Reunion Meeting: two occasions for the release of student exuberance which overflowed from time to time to disrupt the more serious proceedings. In 1908 the undergraduates misbehaved more exuberantly than usual at Commem, targeting according to established tradition, the Chancellor for his longwinded and frequently inaudible speeches and the dean of medicine for his arrogance. In 1909, when three senators proposed the exclusion of undergraduates from Commem, the undergraduates turned to Wilson to discuss the problem. On the eve of Commem, Friday 30 April in the Great Hall, Wilson, according to an arts student F W Robinson, 'called us to our senses by letting us see – for the first time – what Commemoration really meant'. As a result, so said both sides, the festivities stayed within the bounds of decorum. Wilson was a 'true and sympathetic friend of the undergraduates', said *Hermes*, while MacLaurin's son wrote two days later to thank Wilson for his efforts which had resulted in the Chancellor enjoying an unusually serene Commem.[21]

In 1910 student behaviour at the Commem ceremony reverted to its customary rowdiness and the Senate accordingly abolished future student participation in the official proceedings. For Commem in 1911, therefore, the students hired the Sydney Town Hall to conduct their own festival on Saturday 13 May. Proclaiming 'the triumph of green hearts over sere' they sang disparaging songs about MacLaurin (*an ancient Scotchman/ Who's tough and very wily/ Who's seen his prime in ancient time/ But works on slyly*) and Stuart (*Who cries aloud/ For a title proud/ To a deaf regality*) – and others which, incidentally, gave an honourable mention to 'Louis and Jum'. They then demonstrated outside MacLaurin's home in Macquarie Street with behaviour that amounted in Wilson's view to 'insult and molestation' of the Chancellor. Anderson Stuart, who had caught sight of the programme of songs before the event, wanted all participants sent down for a year. On 15 May a special meeting of the Professorial Board ruled to summon the student representatives to answer charges of 'molestation of the Chancellor'. Wisely and temperately MacLaurin intervened to request that the charges be withdrawn. So the matter was resolved by summoning the student representative, reading the charges and the Chancellor's letter and requesting an apology for 'breaches of discipline and decorum' in certain songs sung at the Festival. The President of the Undergraduates Association duly apologized. The exclusion of undergraduates remained, however, though the Senate solved nothing by it. Commemoration was a dull thing without the undergraduates while the student Festival, readily established, continued to hold university dignitaries up to public ridicule. In 1914, with a new Senate governing the University, the traditional Commem was re-established but then suspended for the next four years because of the war.[22]

By 1911 relations between Wilson and Anderson Stuart had deteriorated markedly. There was no shortage of aggravations at the school. Another revision of the medical curriculum in 1910 bore the marks of pressure from the clinical sector of the profession. A Senate committee comprising MacLaurin, Anderson Stuart and medical senator Sir Philip Jones initiated a move, later endorsed by the faculty of medicine over Wilson's protest, to reconstitute materia medica as a single subject in the medical curriculum. On Wilson's advice in 1902 it had been replaced by integrating its three disparate elements – pharmacognosy, therapeutics and pharmacology – into relevant areas of the curriculum. This arrangement had not met professional needs said the committee which moved to abolish special therapeutics, a clinical elective in the fifth year since 1902, and to substitute two compulsory courses, materia medica and therapeutics in third year and posology (dosage) and prescription writing in the fifth year. By 1914 there was pressure to establish a chair in materia medica, pharmacology and therapeutics.[23]

Wilson continued to resist the sustained clinical push to abbreviate the 'introductory foundation' of the medical curriculum for the building of a more elaborate clinical edifice aimed at giving 'our students an education of such character that they become sensible practitioners – the destiny of seven eighths of them'. That was the 'craft' or 'trade' idea of medicine which, on its own in Wilson's view, deprived medicine of its right to a place in a university. In a speech at the annual dinner of the University Medical Society in July 1912 he gave his audience 'abundant food for reflection on a subject in which there is nowadays a tendency towards neglect, viz thorough instruction in the elementary sciences'. Of the four speeches delivered on that occasion, 'it must' ran the report, 'be given the palm'. Wilson was pitting his strength against a powerful force. As one observer wrote:

The spirit of commercialism which has laid such ruthless hands on the community in general in the present age seems to have also snared in its toils the majority of the members of the Medical School, both graduate and undergraduate. The opportunities offering in the medical

188

profession today are such as lead the great majority away from the rugged path of scientific achievement on to the more easy but crowded road leading to money making, comfortable living and self indulgence.

Good opportunities for research in all branches of medical science at the University, at graduate and undergraduate level, were not being taken up.[24]

Then there was the contention over histology (microscopical anatomy). Wilson strongly believed that this important subject, as part of the domain of structure, belonged in anatomy departments as in Europe and the United States. In Britain a peculiar conjunction of circumstances had lodged it in physiology departments and Australia's two Medical Schools had followed suit. In 1910, however, Melbourne's Medical School transferred histology to anatomy, very likely on Wilson's advice, but his efforts to do the same in Sydney met with no success. In Wilson's view histology was neither welcome nor comfortable in physiology departments, and would be taught and studied with greater depth of appreciation and imagination by anatomists. Certainly there were reports that histology was poorly taught with very poor material in Sydney's physiology department and some students sought the assistance of a coach. Histology in Wilson's view was not important to physiology which, more appropriately, was expanding in a chemical direction, but it was vitally important to anatomy securing equal rights with physiology in the province of the cell. As Martin had said in 1898 the understanding of the cell would require their joint efforts. The opposition of physiologists, in Sydney as in Britain, to histology's return to its natural parent had more to do with academic power and prestige than what was right for either teaching or research.[25]

And student numbers were higher than ever: medicine was by now the largest faculty at Sydney University, and arguably the third-largest school in the Empire. Stuart with his customary skill secured government funds in 1908–9 and again in 1910–13 for major extensions to ease the accommodation problem. The Medical School building increased threefold. But there was no easing of the shortage of teaching power. Teachers were critically overtaxed by student numbers, advancing science, demands for more practical work and the special teaching required for the university's new courses in public health, dentistry, veterinary and agricultural science and massage (physiotherapy). More teaching staff with more technical staff to support them, better remuneration and better conditions were all urgent necessities.

189

There was a climate of weariness, unrest and uncertainty at the school.[26]

A more potent source of antagonism between the two medical leaders was Stuart's reaction to Wilson's growing prestige. Now an FRS, Chairman of the increasingly influential Professorial Board, something of a favourite with the students, and incidentally a prominent figure in NSW military affairs, Wilson was in demand as a speaker at student conferences, medical congresses, university functions, inter-university functions like the inauguration of the University of Queensland in 1911, as well as to the community at large, especially on defence and the Empire. Speech making became a familiar burden. Never comfortable on the public platform Wilson was none the less an attractive speaker, fluent in his 'rugged Scotch burr', and one of four university leaders – the others were Edgeworth David, Francis Anderson and Mungo MacCallum – who in these turbulent early years of the new century interpreted the university's various interests to the public outside its walls. A visiting British philosopher described Wilson in 1908 as a 'charming man .... a great power in the university here, and much interested in philosophy'. Wilson was eclipsing Stuart in most arenas and Stuart was not one to tolerate a rival. Early in 1911 he cancelled Wilson's plans to visit Europe and Britain in 1912 to be formally received as a Fellow of the Royal Society during the celebration of its 250th year and to attend in June/July the first Congress of the Universities of the British Empire, in which Wilson had taken a close interest. Stuart decided that he would represent the University of Sydney at those functions. Wilson released his anger in a letter to Hill on 12 May 1911:

> I told you that I hoped to be home about the end of the present year; but, owing to certain action on the part of my senior colleague, which I greatly resent, my visit will have to be delayed for another year, at least. I consider that Stuart has treated me abominably in this matter, and at last, after all these years, we have reached a condition of tolerably definite hostility.

So Stuart sailed off at the end of 1911, just as Peter Board was returning from overseas after attending the Imperial Education Conference in London and investigating other education matters for the government. [27]

In March 1912 the Labor minister for public instruction, Mr A Campbell Carmichael, an Australian-born Scot like his departmental

190

head Peter Board, directed Board to draft a Bill for the reform of the University according to the government's stated policy. Board declined to consult either the parliamentary draftsman or, apparently on Francis Anderson's advice, the University Senate. There was, however, much behind-the-scenes manoeuvring. Anderson Stuart was away for much of this but MacLaurin, outraged at Board's cavalier treatment of the Senate, maintained a stubborn opposition to the whole idea as did MacCallum whose trenchant criticism of the crudities of the draft Bill, read in confidence to the Senate only three days before its introduction into the Legislative Assembly on 26 September, guided the University towards constructive debate. By the time it came before the Professorial Board on 14 October MacLaurin had moved to Wilson's position of November 1910, calling for a full inquiry prior to legislation, while Wilson the practical idealist was disposed to accept the Bill if certain amendments were made. Carslaw had become an enthusiast for the Bill while MacCallum continued to carp at the government's astonishing levity.[28]

The Bill's most radical provision was for the annual award of 200 open exhibitions giving exemption from matriculation, tuition and degree fees on the merit of passes in the new Leaving Certificate examination. Exhibition scholarships were to be awarded at the rate of one per 500 of the NSW population aged 17 to 20. This raised questions of standards: on current figures nearly all new entrants to the university would be 'scholars', most of mediocre scholastic attainment, and a disproportionate number would enrol in the professional schools, especially medicine, at the expense of arts and science which, argued Edgeworth David 'hold the keys to the highest kind of university education'. Another provision to further widen the university's gates was the establishment of evening tutorial classes open to unmatriculated students, to which teachers' college students and government schoolteachers would be admitted without payment of fees. (The long-established evening classes were deemed to be dilettante and lacking in purpose.) And what of the cost? To make good the university's loss in fees the government proposed to raise its annual grant from 10,000 pounds to 20,000 pounds. Not enough, calculated MacCallum, and, recalling the funding cuts in the 1890s during the depression, how secure was it anyway? And what of accommodation, equipment and staff, he added: 'The first necessity is not an increase in undergraduates, but an addition to the teaching power. Most departments are undermanned.'[29]

In the end result the University was to lose little – even its control of matriculation remained intact – except the traditional

Senate. But that was the issue which had aroused the passions of MacLaurin, Anderson Stuart and like-minded colleagues, whose attitudes in turn aroused the passions of the undergraduates and their allies. There was much debate on the constitution of the Senate and much adjustment to the Bill. The Act that was passed at the end of 1912 abolished life tenure by limiting Fellows to five-year terms; the government was to be represented by four Fellows appointed by the Governor, the university teaching staff by five (one each for the four faculties and the chairman of the Professorial Board), the graduates of the university by ten, and three were to be elected by 'the aforesaid Fellows'.[30]

Wilson played a key role in securing amendments which promoted the workability of the resultant Act and its acceptance by the University. At the Professorial Board meeting of 14 October he had proposed a deputation to the Minister for Public Instruction to put six amendments, which the Board unanimously endorsed: substantially increased funding; representation of the four faculties and the Professorial Board on the Senate; retirement of Senate Fellows in rotation to maintain continuity; safeguards to university authority over educational standards and scholarship tenure; and avoidance of any barrier to scholarship holders doing arts/science studies before going on to vocational courses. Anderson Stuart, back from his trip and a member of the deputation, was presumably aligned with Wilson in accepting the Bill if so amended.[31]

Two matters – representation on the Senate for the Professorial Board and the retirement of Fellows by rotation – the Minister reserved for further consideration. (The government later agreed to the first and rejected the second.) The other issues relating to the university's authority on educational standards, scholarship conditions, and increased funding he agreed to immediately. The financial concession was generous. Mr Carmichael undertook to introduce a Bill to increase the university's statutory endowment to 30,000 pounds a year and to provide annual sums on the estimates for its other needs.[32]

MacLaurin's dour opposition persisted until Carslaw was able to persuade him to accept the reforms gracefully along with the money: 'once MacLaurin saw that Board's ideas for reform were safe, and included much increase in the annual grants,' said Carslaw, 'he became its advocate'. Opposition vanished. The University (Amendment) Act 1912, which Carslaw hoped would, in Lord Haldane's words which he quoted, 'secure for our national endeavours the help of our best brains', received Royal assent on 3

December 1912. Peter Board then saw to it that Chancellor MacLaurin and Vice-Chancellor Judge Backhouse were appointed Fellows of the Senate for life, a graceful gesture closing a bitter contest. And in 1914 Professor Anderson Stuart was made a knight of the realm.[33]

No such honours came Wilson's way but his influence, if little known to the general public, was growing to impressive proportions and pervading the whole University, whether in deliberations with his colleagues or in direct contact with students of all faculties as chairman of the Professorial Board. It was not attained by 'ordinary methods of intrigue and wire-pulling, of "hustling" and push', but by the 'sheer momentum of his personality', wrote MacCallum who took the trouble to analyse Wilson's influence. Deriving its source from what MacCallum dubbed his 'practical idealism', held with utter conviction and dedication, Wilson quite simply served justice and truth with no bias of self-interest, no preference for his own or kindred studies and with few prejudices or preconceptions. He had moral authority. To this he added the rare intellectual qualities of the true scholar: grasp of thought and breadth of outlook. His own impulse to know and understand and the pressure of his manifold interests and duties gave Wilson 'comprehension of and insight into ... many subjects'. He was no orator though the depth of his passion often lent eloquence to his utterances. Wilson's 'trade', said MacCallum, was 'to think, to know and to do' and his distinctive gift was his critical faculty, steadily built over the years, which MacCallum described in these words:

> One cannot but be struck by his firm and complete hold on any question under discussion. It is possible to disagree with him; it is impossible to deny that he has looked at the matter in its various aspects, that he has sought to discover the elements of truth in contrasted views, and that in his solution he has tried to reconcile them, or, failing that, to give preference to what after careful consideration seems to him of most importance. There is nothing of one-sidedness in his deliverances; but as little of the opposite fault, inconsistent compromise. He gets to the heart of the matter, and works out from that to a coherent and consequent body of principles. None challenges a pronouncement of his; one finds that one has to combat not a single unit but a whole army of reasoned convictions.

The greatest value of Wilson's critical gift, MacCallum believed, lay not in debate but in the authority it gave to his 'whole scheme of thought'. If not well known to the general public – his admirers regretted that he did not speak in public more often – by 1912 Wilson had emerged at the University as a leader of energy, vision and integrity.[34]

'Universities are a more valuable national asset than Dreadnoughts' the Right Honourable George Reid had declared in May 1909, alluding to another major public issue in which Wilson took a keen interest: the building of Australian defence. The question of whether it should be structured around a national or imperial perspective was the central issue of the time. From May 1905 when Japan defeated the Russian navy at Tsushima and simultaneously Britain withdrew five warships from the Pacific to meet the German challenge in Europe, the long-feared 'yellow peril' began to dominate the Australian imagination. It dawned on the more thoughtful that Australia would have to adopt defence and foreign policies independent of the mother country. However, Imperial patriotism was strong in the Australian people and when in March 1909 it was revealed that Germany would soon have seven to Britain's projected four battleships of the HMS *Dreadnought* class (17,900 tonnes, 21 knots) public feeling was aroused, to hysteria in some quarters. New Zealand had offered to pay for one, even two, dreadnoughts for the Royal Navy; Australia it was proposed should do likewise. The Fisher Government held to its resolve to create an Australian navy rather than subsidize the Royal Navy, a policy the Admiralty itself endorsed a few months later with the decision that the Dominions could create their own fleet units and control them in their regional waters. The Australian fleet unit was to have one armoured cruiser, three light cruisers, six destroyers and three submarines. The seal of independence came in 1911 when the King granted the title 'Royal Australian Navy'. But it was not full independence. In foreign waters Australia's navy would take orders from the British Government and in time of war it would be integrated with the Royal Navy under Admiralty control. This state of interdependence met the realities of the Australian predicament and reflected the ambivalence of Australian allegiances, but it did not satisfy Captain C R Creswell, first Commander of the Royal Australian Navy.[35]

In the wake of Tsushima Britain renewed and strengthened her alliance with Japan as a means of safeguarding her interests in Asia and the Pacific, but this did little to allay Australian fears. Voluntary organizations sprang up to alert the general public to Australia's vulnerability and to push the politicians into addressing the nation's security. Some, like the Millions Club which Wilson addressed in

1906, aimed to stimulate British and European migration (to double Sydney's population, to over a million). Others, like the Victoria League to whose NSW branch Wilson delivered an inaugural address in 1906, aimed to promote 'closer union between British subjects living in different parts of the world'.[36]

The most important voluntary organization, the National Defence League founded in Sydney on 5 September 1905 by Wilson's colleague Lieutenant-Colonel Gerald Campbell, then commanding the NSW Scottish Rifles, brought under review the Australian Army, a ramshackle amalgam of former colonial garrisons comprising in 1901 1,544 regular soldiers, 16,105 part-time militia and 11,361 volunteers. While never large the League fielded an impressive assembly of Sydney's leading citizens: Sir Normand MacLaurin was its president until 1908 when Sir Julian Salomons replaced him; Gerald Campbell and the Hon. W M Hughes were joint secretaries; and on its general council were professional luminaries, politicians of all persuasions, the wealthy and the learned, including Sydney University professors MacCallum, Edgeworth David, Anderson Stuart, Warren – and Wilson when he returned from his year in Europe early in 1906. Its clear objective was compulsory universal military training on the Swiss militia model, fiercely espoused by Gerald Campbell who stumped the country for the League, edited its influential quarterly journal *The Call* and badgered successive prime ministers and defence ministers until provision for it was enacted in the Defence Act of 1909. To the November 1906 issue of *The Call* Wilson contributed an article titled 'The Urgency of the Defence Problem', critical of 'the comfortable reliance on a mother country for protection'. In Sydney's education centres, his particular sphere of influence, Wilson campaigned with Campbell from the same platform.[37]

For Wilson in 1906 there was no contradiction between strengthening the bonds of Empire and advocating an independent Australian defence system. He was both a staunch imperialist and an alert nationalist. For Australia he wanted 'unity in membership of that curious political and social organism we call the British Empire', meaning probably no more than an informed cooperative association with the various dependent and independent States of the Empire. Race patriotism was not enough, as the American colonies had long ago made plain. He also wanted Australians to confront three facts: that their defence system was virtually non-existent, that their 'aspirant nation' was strategically vulnerable, and that the Immigration Restriction Act of 1901 had given offence to her neighbours, especially Japan, the dominant power in the region.

> Were we in no sense provocative ... there might be colour ... for an
> optimistic view. But with 'white Australia' – No! We must be
> prepared to defend our policy or abandon it. And if the mistake of
> abandoning it were made, we should then still require to be
> prepared to assert the supremacy of our civilisation, customs and
> institutions against the ever-increasing danger within the
> Commonwealth.

There was no reproach in looking to the mother country in time of
need 'so long as we are honestly striving to do our best to help
ourselves, and the mother country too when we can'. Bearing arms
was the duty of every able-bodied man. Universal military training
would not, as critics argued, instil militarism in the Australian
psyche nor endanger civil liberties and neither would it conscript in
the sense of converting a citizen into a professional soldier. But it
would, Wilson argued, in a more fundamental way than anything
else protect 'the freedom and very existence of the Commonwealth'.
As to style, the spartan simplicity of the militia model, well suited to
both the Australian style and the Australian purse, was the most
efficient means of building an army.[38]

The ambivalence of Australians regarding Imperialist and
national (or Australianist) views of defence strategy bedevilled the
building of the Australian defence forces as one side or the other
pulled policies and plans. The Royal Australian Navy could in 1914
only operate as a unit of the Royal Navy. The army on the other
hand, built by compulsory training on the militia principle and with
no provision for overseas service, lacked the professional officer
training standards and the imperial purpose envisaged by its first
commander Major General E T Hutton, who in defeat had left
Australia at the end of 1904. However, his imperial outlook had
been implanted in many of his junior officers, preeminently Colonel
W T Bridges. The Australianist view was represented by another
highly capable professional officer, Major J G Legge. In 1905 both
Bridges and Legge were involved in an interesting initiative in
military education undertaken by the University of Sydney.[39]

In November 1904 the British government had proposed that
graduates of Australian universities whose courses included certain
subjects of military value be eligible to compete for commissions in
the British army. In April 1905 the University Senate adopted a
proposal by the Professorial Board to establish a Department of
Military Studies which would serve not only candidates seeking
British commissions, but those seeking commissions in the

Commonwealth permanent and citizen forces. In July 1906 Colonel Hubert Foster, a British regular officer who had served with Hutton in Canada, was appointed Director of Military Science under a Board of Military Studies which, not surprisingly, was made up of those university men who supported the National Defence League: Chancellor MacLaurin, Vice-Chancellor Renwick, Professors Carslaw, Edgeworth David, MacCallum, Warren and Wilson, Mr S H Barraclough and Major R C Simpson of the University Volunteer Rifles as well as Colonel Foster; on behalf of the Commonwealth there were Colonel Bridges and Major Legge. Wilson was the most consistent attender at Board meetings. A three-year part-time diploma course 'suited to the University spirit' commenced in Lent term 1907 with studies in military history and science, military engineering, military topography, military law and administration. The Commonwealth Government, in support of this venture, made available qualified officers to give certain lectures, placed officers as students, recognized the examinations as qualification for entry to or promotion in its permanent military forces and supplied equipment and facilities for the practical work. By August 1910, 102 militia or volunteer officers had completed the course, a result which Foster claimed justified the creation of a military chair at the University. The Commonwealth Government, however, had already decided to establish the Royal Military College at Duntroon near the propsed federal capital city, which opened in 1911 with Colonel Bridges as its first commandant. Wilson, an early guest there, unreservedly approved it: 'I greatly admired the whole scheme of the College both in aim & in actuality and always maintained that it was *the most efficient* Australian undertaking of any kind whatsoever, that I had any knowledge of', he wrote years later.[40]

The Bridges and the Wilsons were family friends (Mabel was godmother to one of the Bridges' daughters) and whenever Wilson went to Melbourne he paid them a visit. When he did so on Sunday 9 June 1907 Bridges probably discussed his latest plans for a militia corps with a full range of intelligence functions, as an affordable means of repairing the army's appalling lack of information about the topography and military resources of Australia and neighbouring countries. He saw the corps as both an interim intelligence authority pending the establishment of such a body within the regular army and a precursor of a General Staff, another pressing need in the army's structure that Bridges and the British War Office – which wanted Dominion military staff representation on its new Imperial General Staff – were urging. (The Imperial General Staff was one of a package of army reforms introduced in 1907 by Lord Haldane as Secretary for War; he saw it as a bond of Empire which, if the need arose, could readily concentrate the scattered military forces of the Empire into 'a really homogenous Imperial Army'.) On 6 December 1907 the Corps came into being with Bridges, as Chief of the General Staff, directing the work through its commanding officer Colonel J W McCay, a lawyer and former defence minister. There was no clear distinction between intelligence and staff work, and when the militia, through the Australian Intelligence Corps (AIC), began infiltrating staff ranks, senior regular army officers, who had no formal staff training, became restive. McCay's tendency to argue, as lawyers are wont, did not help.[41]

Wilson transferred from the NSW Scottish Rifles, which he had commanded since 1 January 1907, to the new appointment of Officer Commanding, Intelligence Corps, NSW District, on 26 May 1908 and from the beginning it was clear that he would have problems with the regular army command. Accommodation sparked the first contest, requiring the intervention of the Military Board in January 1909 to direct Commandants to provide suitable premises at all district headquarters. Nominally based at the University until April 1909, when temporary quarters were allocated at Victoria Barracks, Paddington, it was not until the end of February 1910 that the NSW Intelligence Corps moved into permanent offices, which even then were not fully equipped.[42]

The status of the Corps gave rise to another long-drawn-out wrangle. McCay insisted that Commanding Officers of the AIC have direct access to District Commandants, bypassing their staff. On this issue the Board ruled that as 'senior officers of a Branch of the District Headquarters staff' they had the right of direct access to the Commandant on the work of their Corps; only on administrative matters were they to communicate through staff officers. By March 1911 McCay was arguing that the AIC was not purely an Intelligence Corps: AIC officers needed to have knowledge of the Operations Branch of the General Staff in order to carry out their intelligence work in the field. The Board agreed to this, but stood firm against giving the AIC officers equal status with General Staff Officers.[43]

By late 1909 Wilson had his full establishment of 14 officers meeting regularly on Thursday evenings for the systematic study of military questions and to report on their various work projects. Some officers, especially those doing topographical work, made frequent weekend field excursions. Also involved were 'various gentlemen outside the Corps – both military and civilian – [who] ... rendered valuable assistance in the work of the Corps.' Wilson's second-in-command was Major H C Manning, three years Wilson's senior and an ex-rifleman. Captain T H Kelly, an artilleryman and in civil life a Sydney city alderman prominent in the metals industry, was promoted Major in April 1910 when Wilson became a Lieutenant Colonel. Four of the six captains had a Sydney University background: Associate Professor S H E Barraclough (mechanical engineering); A J Gibson a civil engineer with extensive knowledge of NSW road and rail systems; J M C Corlette a civil engineer on the staff of the Hunter District Water Supply and Sewerage Board; and H G Edwards an Arts graduate who held the Diploma of Military Science of Sydney University, the Section's Staff Officer responsible for the proper compilation of records. Captains E S Vautin and W S Sherbon were public servants in military administration. Three of the six lieutenants also had a Sydney University background: J B Wilson was a mining engineer (later a lawyer) and lecturer; A W Freeman had trained there as a mining engineer; and G A Taylor an engineer/architect and promoter of the new sciences of air and radio-telegraphy communications. Lt A W Jose was a journalist and correspondent for *The Times* of London, Lt R E Hale was a draftsman with the NSW railways and Lt W G R P Nordmann a veteran of the South African war. The ages of these men ranged from 22 to 50, most of them over 30 and all but one well-established in careers relevant to military intelligence work. They were not the raw recruits of military colleges. They required not so much to be trained in the practical skills of intelligence work as to be deployed to duties which exploited their expertise for military intelligence purposes. Wilson's role was to coordinate their skills and provide instruction and field experience in military organization and procedures, with the necessarily strict attention to detail.[44]

Early in its existence the Corps participated in an exercise testing the efficiency of Australia's warning system of surprise attack or invasion. In January 1909 Wilson with four of his senior men attended the first week-long Intelligence Course of Instruction, held in Melbourne and at Easter the whole Corps took part in the Annual Training Camps in each State, when it was noted that General Staff Officers made little use of them for intelligence purposes. In June Wilson and eight others attended Colonel Foster's first advanced course in General Staff work and shortly afterwards he took part in a District Staff Ride. Several of his officers attended other special courses.[45]

199

Organizing the wide range of information gathered by the Corps was a major task. A monthly intelligence diary was established, military handbooks prepared and data on such matters as supply, transport, communications, regional employment and population collected from government authorities, Public Works, Lands, Customs and Navigation Departments, the Water and Sewerage Board, the Observatory, the Statistician, and the Tourist Bureau. For information on foreign countries, especially in the Pacific, foreign newspapers were systematically examined, bibliographies of relevant literature prepared and confidential enquiries about foreigners and foreign activities pursued. Compiling and recording all information with the necessary readiness for immediate use was Wilson's special interest. In January 1911 he produced a classification system entitled 'Standing Orders relating to Correspondence and Records'. It drew criticism in the Inspector General's report of 7 March 1911:

> These orders ... are evidently the work of an expert, but I must confess to the misgiving that they are too elaborate for the work of this Corps. Altogether they require the maintenance in each District, as well as at Head Quarters, of four (4) separate card indices, one register, and one catalogue, and the scope of the headings embraces subjects ordinarily dealt with in the Central Registries... My enquiries showed that some Intelligence Officers do not understand the system, and I suggest ... such simplification as may be possible.

At the time of inspection the officers had scarcely had time to understand the system, retorted McCay, and it was necessarily elaborate since it related 'mainly in substance to indexing the Corps records, which indexing is essential'; but he agreed to consider simplification. By early 1912 it was reported that 'the system of indexing is now understood'. It proved a ready tool in the amalgamation of AIC and District Headquarters libraries, commenced on 1 July 1912, a task largely borne by the AIC.[46]

However, with the main business, mapping, it was clear by late 1909 that this was a job of enormous dimensions, well beyond the resources of this part-time militia force. McCay therefore recruited the services of full-time mapping staff including four British NCOs of the Royal Engineers who in April 1910 were allocated to the AIC. Mapping gradually moved outside AIC control, though the Corps continued its efforts and achieved some notable feats: in Wilson's sector Captain Corlette and his team in 1910–11 topographically surveyed and mapped 750 square miles around Newcastle. In 1912 areas north of Port Jackson and at Liverpool were surveyed and the

Easter Camp held that year near Pymble included a survey camp of five AIC officers with a detail of University Scouts getting topographical work experience. Shire engineers assisted the Corps by updating about 40 parish maps.[47]

Kitchener's whirlwind visit in the summer of 1910–11 invigorated Australia's makeshift army and glamorized the military life. He did what the government had hoped: he won public support for compulsory military training, the basis of the new defence scheme recently passed into law. Kitchener endorsed it and built on it: the main issue was how to meet the much expanded requirement for military training. The government adopted his proposal for 215 carefully selected and highly trained 'area officers' responsible for training and administering the citizen forces (including cadets from the age of 12) in their defined areas. Until graduates from the new national military college at Duntroon became available to fill these positions many AIC officers were appointed to them, including Captains Hale and Nordmann from Wilson's section. Another, E O Milne, was recruited from NSW Government railways to investigate the problem of Australia's uncoordinated railway networks, which Kitchener highlighted as a serious impediment to mobilization.[48]

In late 1911 Wilson was busy organizing a major Intelligence Staff Tour (or Ride) – a training exercise in strategic, tactical and administrative work, from the Officer Commanding down to the patrol leader, in simulated war conditions – to be held in the Parramatta-Penrith-Liverpool districts west of Sydney in the last week of January 1912. Such exercises required a thorough grasp of the military craft and meticulous planning. This tour which was immediately to follow the AIC's second week-long January course of instruction in Melbourne involved the provision of railway warrants, billets, horses and saddles for officers at various country centres, as well as literature, work syllabus and rough maps of the theatre of operations which extended over 1000 square miles. One reconnaissance of the area by Wilson with McCay, by then a family friend, was done in a style which much impressed Wilson's nine-year-old daughter Dorette, a privileged passenger. She recalled

> setting off in this marvellous open touring car with bright shining brass fittings, all gleaming in the hot sun. Of course we were driven by a chauffeur and it was a very hot day, and we toured around the countryside of NSW. When lunch time came we stopped at a country hotel for lunch. To my dismay there was no room for us in the dining-room and we were told we could eat in the servants' hall

downstairs, with the chauffeur of course and lots of other people.
My childish snobbishness was black affronted, but neither the
General or my father turned a hair!

And in late January when the whole family visited Wilson in camp
at Liverpool she was 'very impressed with his grand tent which was
lit by a very small electric light bulb'. Wilson's characteristically
sharp reaction to a failure to 'chart up the maps' was an event
caricatured and commemorated on the menu of a dinner at Paris
House on 16 November 1912 to mark Wilson's effective retirement
from command of the AIC 2nd Military District. His command did
not formally end until mid-1913, but he was soon to depart on 15
months sabbatical leave. For the same reason he resigned from the
NSW Council of the United Services Institution.[49]

· By the end of 1912 the Intelligence Corps was under new
management. McCay had finally fallen out with his superior officers
in the regular army at headquarters and took leave overseas on 5
December, until the expiry of his 5-year term (30 March 1913),
when his position at headquarters in Melbourne was abolished and
the six AIC sections were placed under the control of the General
Staff Officers of the six military districts. Inevitable though the
conclusion of the Citizen General Staff may have been, it gave
McCay much distress. In his view the General Staff should have
included citizen soldiers. In January 1912 in response to army
headquarter's carping, dismissive criticisms of the AIC he had
written to the Secretary, Defence Department:

> It must be remembered that if Australia fights, it will be with a
> Citizen Army led largely by Citizen Officers and some Citizen
> Officers must have some knowledge of Staff work or Staffs will be
> insufficient in numbers in war.... I venture to hold the view that for
> many years to come the Commonwealth must rely largely on
> Citizen Officers for General Staff work.

Of course he was right. McCay himself was to become a
distinguished commander of Australian troops at Gallipoli and in
France, as also did his friend John Monash, Wilson's Victorian
counterpart. And there were not a few others whose AIC training in
staff work qualified them to serve as Brigade Majors, Staff Captains
and the like. They won something of a reputation for the AIC in the
field of war. On the home front many of them gave valuable (if less
esteemed) service in more reclusive occupations.[50]

Debate in the general community on defence, foreign policy and

Imperial relations was lifted by the Round Table movement established in Australia by Lionel Curtis in 1910. Wilson was recruited to the Sydney group by Mungo MacCallum with an invitation to dine at the Australian Club on 26 October 1910.

> It is to meet a man Curtis, from S. Africa, who is very much interested in the problem of Imperial Defence & who had a good deal to do with the Unification of the African Colonies. He is on a quasi-secret mission here, & has, practically, asked me to invite some likely persons to discuss matters.[51]

Lionel Curtis was not a South African, nor had he a quasi-secret mission except in his own eyes. He was a zealot for imperial federation with 'a habit of mystification'. He probably laid down the rules that gave the Round Table an undeservedly clandestine, even sinister, reputation: membership was restricted, secret and by unanimous invitation, and articles in its journal were anonymous. The movement was founded in London at the time of the 'dreadnought' scare in 1909 by a group of influential men congregated around Lord Milner and three of his South African 'kindergarten': Philip Kerr, Robert Brand and Curtis. Curtis then embarked on his mission to establish similar groups in the dominions. In Australia groups were founded in Sydney, Melbourne, Adelaide, Brisbane and Perth.[52]

The Sydney group was notable for the breadth of its political representation (the NSW Governor Lord Chelmsford and a former Labor prime minister J C Watson were supporters), its labour sympathies and its strong academic contingent. Of the original 18 members five were professors – MacCallum, Wilson, Peden (Law), Edgeworth David, E R Holme (English) – besides Sydney University's Vice-Chancellor W P Cullen, R F Irvine who became Sydney's economics professor in 1912, Andrew Harper the Principal of St Andrew's College, Dr Norman Kater a former student of Wilson's; MacCallum's son Mungo was the first honorary secretary. Colonel Hubert Foster the Director of Military Studies at Sydney University became a member in 1912. In the original Melbourne group were more of Wilson's colleagues: Brigadier-General William Bridges, the biology professor Baldwin Spencer and the physiology professor William Osborne. They were men of intellectual status and proven ability – 'men of weight ' to use Curtis's phrase – with a strong commitment to the Empire, meeting for enlightened debate on current affairs and to write articles of high quality for *The Round Table*, published in London.[53]

Australian Round Tablers, however, did not support Curtis's

design for an imperial parliament above the British and Dominion legislatures with absolute power over defence and foreign affairs. With careful and sophisticated arguments they consistently backed their politicians in putting Australia's national security ahead of imperial interests, even reiterating the idea which had deeply offended British sensibilities when Deakin proposed it in 1908–9, of approaching the United States for protection. *Hermes* in July 1911 applauded these 'singularly dispassionate' discussions of local affairs in the context of the empire as a whole, but by 1913 'the Australian view' of the Empire's naval policy and the Pacific question was giving embarrassment to the editors of *The Round Table* in London.[54]

For Wilson this new intellectual forum gave his abiding philosophical interest fresh stimulus. Here was another evolving 'organism' – a favourite metaphor in the discourse of the times – with its set of relations to probe and explore: of one government with another in the British family of nations, the centre with the periphery, the citizen with the State and the Empire. He was fulfilling too in greater measure the citizen's duty, which in T H Green's code of ethics was placed high: the welfare of the State depended on its citizens performing the duties of their station to the best of their ability. British Idealists were very public-spirited but not paternalist. By pursuing the 'common good', T H Green taught, the citizen cultivates his 'best self'.

Wilson was a very busy man, immersed in the practical ideals of daily life, his commitments ever expanding. 'In a modern society', he wrote in 1906, 'the sphere of civic duty and responsibility is a wide one'. His strongest commitment, however, was to his family where he found refuge, refreshment and recreation. In his social philosophy the family occupied an important place, indeed it was society's dynamic core:

> Home & married life in a well matched union are God's greatest gifts
> to us.... From the home as centre one's interests reach out into the
> social circle – the community – the church & the State with all its
> varied interests political social intellectual & aesthetic. Human life is
> a big thing and in spite of much that is petty & ignoble it is full of
> noble aims & ideals which require cultivation and claim devotion.

There was nothing new or peculiarly Idealist in this idea of the home and family, though it was by long tradition peculiarly British. Almost all Britons subscribed to it, especially those concerned with moral reformation like the Wesleyans and Evangelists.[55]

At the end of 1912 the Wilsons and their six children moved from 'Apheta', to 'Eurotas' in Edgecliff Road – an imposing white house with a central tower of three storeys, verandah and balcony in front, tiled entrance hall, ten rooms, two bathrooms, tower rooms and a tennis court. Jeanie, now 21, was an arts graduate, Louise aged 12, Dorette ten, Katharine eight, Douglas six and John three. All in turn attended Shirley, a model school and kindergarten in Edgecliff Road run by two influential educationalists, Miss Harriet Newcomb and Miss Margaret Hodge, who had, in Wilson's words, an 'extraordinary sympathy with the ways and whims of children'. With a broad curriculum and all sorts of supplements to formal classes they contrived to develop individual powers and wide sympathies, while insisting nevertheless on discipline and earnest concentration. Only in religious instruction was the curriculum feeble. Shirley's religion was undenominational Protestantism, a sort of pantheism which, if it agreed with Wilson's general philosophical stance, did not admit his personal witness for Christ. Empire tended to take the place of God. Science was accommodated as 'nature studies', botany, and geology excursions, and from 1906 more exact teaching for senior students in a laboratory and kitchen, opened in September by Wilson with a eulogy to science that Archibald Liversidge would have applauded.[56]

Wilson was a devoted father though to his sons, in particular, he appeared somewhat remote and unbending, for he was well into encumbered middle age when they arrived. He was really a passionate man and naturally demonstrative, but strictly self-disciplined. In general he was tolerant of the naughty world while working always for its improvement, but for his children as for himself he set high standards. He kept a dutiful, sometimes exasperated, eye on their education and moral development. At one period he deemed Sunday School standards to be deficient and took over that part of the three youngest children's education. John landed himself in difficulty over the pronunciation of 'charity': try as he did it would only come out as 'charitee'. Wilson campaigned long and hard against the Australian accent. Like most Victorian fathers he dealt out the serious punishments, usually a verbal pasting but on one occasion a thrashing that caused misery all round. 'Really' recalled Katharine, 'Father only had to look at you and flash his bright blue eyes in anger and that was quite enough for anyone.'[57]

He had a deep personal need for order. The natural disorder of small children he found difficult to tolerate and he insisted on punctuality: such was his horror of being late that he sometimes caught an earlier train than the one he intended. He explained this foible as a consequence of his father's lack of punctuality, which often in his boyhood had thrown him into a frenzy. Occasionally he went on a rampage to impose better or tidier habits and then Mabel calmed the troubled waters. Like most mothers of large families she was more matter-of-fact about domestic management. With the assistance of a cook and two maids (a nurse as well when there was a baby), a weekly laundress and a weekly gardener. Mabel presided over a large, lively and very hospitable household. She was the perfect antidote to Wilson's simmering anxieties.

In their first decade of married life the Wilsons took regular holidays in the Blue Mountains, to escape the sticky summer heat of Sydney which gave Mabel migraines. But late in 1908 the venue shifted to a little wilderness north of Sydney. Wilson bought a block of land from Francis Anderson at Bayview, on Pittwater, where supplies arrived by boat once a fortnight. The narrow sweep of Pittwater up to Lion Island was like a Scottish loch, and their style of life there had a Scottish flavour: back to bare boards. Wilson designed a simple cottage consisting of a large living room which doubled as a children's dormitory, with a kitchen at one end and parent's bedroom at the other and verandahs front and back. Furniture was basic, with bunks containing storage compartments lining two walls of the living room while another wall was shelved to hold crockery, cutlery, books and games. In the centre was a large deal table. It was a plain and functional arrangement given a touch of class by Mabel's tough bunk-covers printed in a William Morris design of muddy greens and muted reds. Straight from Wilson's boyhood came the insulated 'hay-box', into which saucepans were placed after coming to the boil so that meals would cook slowly overnight or while the family was at the beach.

Bayview was altogether different from the grand establishment at Woollahra. There were no servants and Mabel did the cooking, for which she trained at the Technical College. The children had their regular chores, going in pairs to fetch milk from the Anderson's gardener and vegetables from a cottage about a mile away. Wilson built a carpentry shed, made and installed a wood lathe and later added rooms to the house. He enjoyed his Bayview labours and the ritual of coming in hot and sweaty after a hard morning's work for a well-earned beer. He planted masses of interesting shrubs and trees but rejoiced most of all in the crops of pears, peaches, passionfruit, melons, guava figs and 'improved' isabella and muscatel grapes:

abundant fruit was his idea of the exotic. Children's interests took priority and usually it was their friends, not the parents', who were guests. Wilson made kites for them and they had a large rowing boat named 'The Marnie', after Marnie Masson the daughter of Melbourne's chemistry professor (later Marnie Bassett the historian) who was a frequent visitor. He read them the tales of Scott, Dickens and Kipling and on Sundays *Pilgrim's Progress*. Through their grandfather's treasured telescope, ensconced in a special fitting on the front verandah, he taught them something of the moon, Jupiter, the rings around Saturn and the names of stars. For all Wilsons Bayview remained forever a kind of Eden.

Notes

1. TPAS: *Centenary Book*, 242–3; Chisholm, 43; Epps, 156. 'over-didactic': Bickerton-Blackburn, 123. 'the gift of': TPAS quoted in Epps, 39. 'No, we lecturers': Stuart, 86. Epidiascope and discipline: Epps, 5. 'Smoking in my': Davies, 208. TPAS' metier: *RSS,* 286. 'the boss of': Sydney Univ. U'grads Assn, 1910.
   Personal recollections on JTW as a teacher, by former Sydney students to author: Malcolm Britnell Fraser (12.6.78); Ian Mackerras (3.10.78); Sir Douglas Miller (29.5 and 20.6.79); Sir Kenneth Noad (30.5.79); Raymond Dart (6.1 and 15.3.80).
2. 'swat [who] Learned': Sydney Univ. U'grads Assn, 1911. JTW activities: *Hermes*, 29.10.98, 3. JTW's appearance etc.: Fraser to author. 'There was something': Moran, 8, 9.
3. 'Leave those bones': Noad to author. Use of rebuke: A G S Cooper to J, 6.1.1964.
4. 'horror of desecration': Miller to author. 'I said *luke*': Money to author. 'he stopped and he', and 'You just *knew*': Mackerras to author.
5. Women medical students: Russell, K F 1977, 75 (for TPAS' views); *Centenary Book*, 220–7.
6. JTW and women students: *Centenary Book*, Ch. 6; interviews with Dr Edith Clement, Dr Grace Cuthbert Browne and Lady Murray. 'no great call': JTW, quoted in *The Age*, 30.6.1930, on arrival by ship in Melbourne. 'capable young': JTW, *SMH* 22.6.1918.
7. 'Jummy *made* it': Noad to author. 'He was dull': Miller to author. Squandering of interest: GES quoted in SAS. 'dry but precise': Mackerras to author. 'I have got to': Fraser to author.
8. Epidiascope from 1895: *Hermes* Oct. 1898, 3. 'one slide after': SAS, 7. 'Focus, Louis': Mackerras to author. Frozen sections: Granville Sharp to J, 1.6.1962. 'I have the' and 'I doubt if': Noad to author.
9. Dissection and prosectorships: Fraser to author. Barney Coen: A N B,

'Bernard James Coen', *SUMJ* Vol. XXI, June 1927, 29. Specimens from
New Guinea and Paris: Mackintosh, *History of Medical Museum*, SUA.

10. JTW as adviser, collaborator: SAS, 6; Dart 15.3.80, to author. 'had an
     indolent': Noad to author; Oliver Lancaster to author Oct. 1992,
     regarded SAS as very clever but intellectually lazy. 'No one will': SAS, 11.

11. Anatomy dept and research: *Centenary Book*; SAS, 6. 'His influence
     on me': Dart 1959, 28. 'the spirit of': MWM in *SMH,* 5.6.1920.

12. TPAS and JTW and Aust. Museum: Board of Trustees, Minutes of
     meetings. TPAS's activities: Young, TPAS entry *ADB*; *Centenary
     Book*, 191. JTW's authority: Moran, 9. His presence: Fraser to
     author. Deanship of Medical School: JTW was acting dean in 1890.
     Thereafter during his absences Stuart appointed a medical senator
     (e.g. Dr Philip Sydney Jones) to act for him. Wilson was thereby
     excluded from the Senate until 1916 when he became an ex-officio
     member as chairman of the Professorial Board.

13. 'to manage and': *Calendar* for 1893, 408. 'the highest authority':
     Professorial Board Report of 28.4.1911, SU Archives, Report Book,
     G1/14/4, 52.

14. Criticisms of the Senate: Crane & Walker, 153; Anderson 1909, 23;
     Hermes, 15.5.1907. MacLaurin & TPAS: Ann Mitchell, *ADB* entry
     on MacLaurin. 'almost unstoppable': *Centenary Book*, 185. Sunday
     counsels: C B Mackerras to M C O'Connor, 17.10.1968, in
     possession of author. 'They were an': Bickerton Blackburn, 132.

15. Crane & Walker.

16. 'a quiet, clearly-spoken': Crane & Walker, 18, 19.

17. 'The secondary school': Anderson 1909, 21. Peter Board proposal:
     Crane & Walker. Counter proposals: Carslaw, *Hermes* Dec. 1909,
     116–19; *Hermes* Dec. 1910, 111–14.

18. 'more into touch': Crane & Walker, 157. 'control would fall' and
     'The Chief Justice': report in *DT*, 31.3.1911, of evidence given
     before the South Australian Commission on Higher Education in
     Sydney.

19. Carslaw on JTW: SAS, 6. Professorial Board: *Calendar,* 1911.
     'inquiry into both': JTW reported in *DT*, 5.11.1910.

20. Report of the Professorial Board, 14.5.1913, and Board Minutes.
     Senate rejection: Minutes, 13.10 1913. Situation unchanged to
     1936: Emeritus Prof. W M O'Neil, Ch. of Prof. Board 1965 to 1975,
     n.d., SUA. Proctorial Board adopted: Senate Minutes, 2.6.1913.

21. Students and Senate 1908–9: *Hermes* July 1910, 27–9. 'called us to':
     The Union Book of 1952, 85. 'true and sympathetic': *Hermes* May
     1909, 5. H N MacLaurin to JTW, 2.5.09.

22. 'the triumph of': *Hermes* May 1911, 5. Songs: Undergrad. Assoc.

Cttee, *Programme of Songs for Student Festival, 1911.* Professorial
Board action: Minutes, 65–70, and items in *DT* and *SMH* for May
1911. Result: *Hermes* May 1912, 3–4 and Aug. 1912, 48; *Senior Year
Book* for 1922.

23. JTW's protest: Faculty of Medicine Minutes 8.7.09, 18.10.09,
    26.4.1910; Editorial, *SUMJ* Nov. 1912, 1. Clinical pressures for
    curriculum change: *Hermes* Dec. 1909, 122 (TPAS invites
    comment); May 1910, 19–20 (Pres of Med Soc asks for more time
    for clinical work); Barron, *SUMJ* Nov. 1910, 22. Curriculum changes
    1910: *SUA Report Books* (G1/14/4), 24.8.09, 87–95; Location of
    materia medica and histology: *Centenary Book* for 1901, 118–120,
    196. Pressure for materia medica etc.: *SUMJ* Oct. 1914, 3.

24. Push by clinical sector: editorials and articles in *SUMJ;* clinical
    evenings instituted in 1908 (Nov. 1910, 10, 12); G H Barron, Pres.
    of U of S Med. Soc. 1909 (Nov. 1910, 17–23); 'our students...'(Nov.
    1912, 1–2); Cecil Purser, in favour of clinical work from 3rd year
    (Nov. 1912, 17); further items to 1914. JTW response: 'abundant
    food' etc., *SUMJ* Nov. 1912, 5–6. 'The spirit of commercialism':
    SUMJ Dec. 1913, 1.

25. Melbourne school: Russell. Histology teaching: JTW memo on Chair
    of Physiology, adopted by Committee of Faculty of Med. 20.4.1920,
    Minutes April 1920; JTW Inaugural Address, Univ. of Cambridge,
    1921. Reports of poor teaching: *Hermes* Aug. 1913, 45. Martin: Pres.
    Address, AAAS, 1894. Opposition in Sydney: Barron, *SUMJ,* 22.

26. Growth of Sydney school: Bickerton Blackburn, 126–7; *Centenary
    Book,* 175. Increased pressures: *SUA Report Books* (G1/14/4), 126–7.

27. 'rugged Scotch burr': Portus. 'charming man': Henry Jones to his
    family, 26.7.1908, quoted Hetherington 211–12. Congress of Univs
    of the Empire: Naylor 1913 and Congress Reports. 'I told you that':
    JTW to JPH, 12.5.1911. Peter Board overseas: Wyndham, *ADB* Vol.
    7, 329.

28. MacCallum criticisms: *SMH,* 7.10 and 9.10, 1912. Carslaw on
    inquiry: *SMH,* 19.10.1912 (to which JTW responded in *SMH* and
    DT, 21.10.1912, to clarify position of Prof. Board). Carslaw an
    enthusiast: article in *The University Review* June 1913.

29. Education Bill's provisions: Carslaw 1913, 46–50. Leaving
    Certificate: according to Carslaw 1913, 48–9, NSW Dept of Public
    Instruction had from 1911 promoted adoption of the Scottish system
    of Intermediate and Leaving Certificates. 'hold the keys': TWED in
    DT, 11.10.1912. 'The first necessity': MWM in *SMH,* 22.12.1912.

30. Carslaw 1913.

31. Changes recommended to Minister: Prof. Board Minutes,

14.10.1912.

32. Increase in Univ. funds: Carslaw, *SMH*, 19.10.1912.

33. MacLaurin and Education Bill: Crane & Walker, 159–60. 'secure for our': Carslaw 1913, 52, quoting Lord Haldane speech at the Univ. of Bristol 17 Oct. 1912.

34. MWM in *SMH*, 5.6.20.

35. 'Universities are': Quoted in *Hermes* July 1909, 37. Action in Pacific: Meaney, 266. Naval policy: Souter, 136–46.

36. Australian fears: Meaney, 127. JTW's 1906 addresses (unpub.).

37. National Defence League: Barrett, on Campbell *ADB* Vol. 7, 548; members named in *The Call*, 8.8.1906; Foster, 81. 'the comfortable': JTW, 1906e.

38. 'unity in' and 'Were we in' etc.: JTW, Address to Women's Political League, 1906 ms.

39. Bridges & Legge: Grey, 75–83; Coulthard-Clark 1988. Initiative with U of S: *Calendar* 1907, 432.

40. Military Studies at Sydney Univ.: Coulthard-Clark 1986, 5, 9. Hutton's idea of military studies was first supported by the Senate in Dec. 1893: U of S *Calendar* 1894, 256. U of S scheme: Report of the Committee on Military Ed., Senate Minutes for 6.11.05, 4.12.05, 109–11. Comm. Govt support: *Calendar* 1906, 403. Board members: *Calendar* 1907, 432. JTW attendance and activities: Minutes, Bd of Mil. Studies, SUA, G3/26. Curriculum etc.: Report of Bd of Mil. Studies, Senate Minutes 214–16, 3.12.06; Coulthard-Clark 1979. Attendances by 1910: AAM, 1862/7/155. 'I greatly admired': JTW to LH, 12.8.1940.

41. JTW visit to Bridges, 1907: JTW Diary. Intelligence Corps: Coulthard-Clark 1976, Chs 1 & 2. 'a really homogenous': H Foster, 26. Intelligence and Staff work: G Serle, 169–70; *ADB* on Bridges; P Serle, *ADB* entry on McCay; Pedersen, 22.

42. Accommodation problems: MBM 22.3.09, AAM, 1907/7/47A; MBM 29.1.09. Also Coulthard-Clark, 23, 28(f.n.), 29, 31.

43. 'senior officers': AAM, 1849/2/162. March 1911 decision: AAM, MP84/1902/7/137.

44. JTW's establishment: Coulthard-Clark 1976, 22 and App 6; MO 222/09. 'various gentlemen': 2MD Commandant's Report. Leadership task: Pedersen, 22.

45. Intelligence officers not used: Pedersen (quoting Monash), 31. Advanced course: Coulthard-Clark 1976, 27; *ADB* Vol. 7, 559 on Foster; G Serle, 170.

46. Intelligence Corps activities: AAM, MP86/1907/7/47A; Coulthard-Clark 1976, 31–2. JTW on classification: McCay to Mabel,

27.12.1911; A W Jose to J Bowie Wilson, 6.6.1916, Jose Papers. 'These orders' and McCay retort: AAM, MP84/1902/7/137. 'the system of': AAM, MP84/1, 1849/2/258.

47. Survey camps: AAM, MP84/1, 1849/2/258.

48. 'area officers': C-Clark 1976; for Milne see *ADB* Vol. 10 and W S Sherbon to JTW, 23.8.1937. Aust. commitment: G Serle in *Monash*, 171.

49. Staff Ride: AAM, MP84/1902/7/137; C-Clark 1976, 37. 'setting off' and 'very impressed': DC Notes. JTW retirement dinner menu, Wilson papers.

50. Intelligence Corps: new management, Pedersen, 31–2. 'It must be': McCay, AAM, MP84/1902/7/137. Monash's opinion: G Serle, 192–3.

51. Round Table: Foster. 'It is to meet': MacCallum to JTW, 26.10.1910.

52. *The Round Table*: JTW to J, 18.10.17; Portus, 232. Curtis: Rowse, esp. 339.

53. Sydney Round Tablers: Foster.

54. 'singularly dispassionate': *Hermes* 1911, 49. Australian viewpoint: Meaney, 163–9; Foster, 76.

55. 'In a modern': JTW 1906e, 6. 'Home & married life': JTW to LH, 30.3.1927. British tradition: Himmelfarb, 54–7.

56. 'extraordinary': Munro, 7. Philosophy of Shirley: Mackerras 1991, 31–7. JTW (unpub.), 1906.

57. [Final paragraphs] Wilson family, Woollahra and Bayview: LH and KR to author, 15–17.3.1983.

10

Second Sabbatical

Sabbatical leave evolved in Australian universities as a way to overcome the debilitating effects of isolation from their cultural roots. Any brief periodic leave of absence, as established in Britain, did not meet the case of the Antipodes. Distance alone imposed a two-month travel period. And more substantial leaves were required by colonial academics who bore more than the responsibility for teaching and research: there were libraries and laboratories to build; faculties, curricula and standards to establish; staff to recruit; a corporate life and community relations to foster, all without adequate manpower and funds. Establishing the university ideal in practical frontier communities required enormous energy, push and dedication. Of all the needs that pioneering professors might have listed, the need to be 'in vital touch with their fellows elsewhere' was paramount. Wilson went so far as to argue that 'Professors should not merely be given leave to go – they ought rather to be periodically hunted out of their chairs, for the health of their own souls, and hence of those committed to their care'. In the first decade of the century, when Empire ties were being strengthened, a periodic full year's leave for professors became accepted practice at Sydney University. Till 1914 the cost of his replacement fell on the professor, but after the war one year's leave in seven on full pay became an established professorial privilege.[1]

The cost of Wilson's leave overseas in 1913, however, was not the major financial drain he had expected, for the fortuitous reason that Lady Salomons had died in 1912 leaving Mabel a substantial inheritance. They were able to travel first class – a luxury much appreciated by Wilson since the extra facilities made all the difference to his seasick-prone family. On Saturday 16 November 1912 the

212

Wilsons boarded the *Moldavia* for a year in Europe, a party of nine: four adults, including 21 year-old Jeanie and a nurse, and five children ranging in age from 3 to 12 years. The trip had required a great deal of planning and preparation – and the last-minute quiet assistance of omnicompetent Louis to cope with children, luggage, transport and tickets. Hardly were they under way when a sense of devastation visited Mabel. At 38 and recently bereaved of her mother, with a strenuous year in Europe ahead of her, she found in Melbourne that she was pregnant. For once her spirits flagged and she railed against Woman's lot and flat-footed Fate. Wilson consoled her. Under the pressure of myriad mundane affairs he was apt to blow a fuse, but on large questions he was fortitude itself. Their programme had to be modified somewhat but, he said with calm decision, 'we shall do exactly what we planned to do'. On Boxing Day they disembarked at Naples and the next day Mabel took Katharine and the two boys with their nurse Belle by train to Neuchatel in Switzerland to install all four at Villa Blanche where they were to learn French. That done, she rejoined Wilson, Jeanie, Louise and Dorette in Naples to start a three-month tour of Italy.[2]

In Naples Wilson took up a book on Greek architecture in preparation for their excursions and in his diary, concisely and systematically, he recorded his impressions – this for example of a visit to Pompeii:

> Note fine Doric pillared market-place or old forum, triangular with temple of Hercules along its base opposite entrance. Pillars of this forum of stone (in drums). Pt of entabulature complete & typical Doric.

On the back pages of his diary he recorded all of the family's expenses down to the last ice cream. A two-week tour of Sicily elaborated his understanding of civilizations that had left their marks on that island: Greek, Roman, Islamic, Byzantine and Norman. In the anatomy department at the University of Palermo he was appalled to find there were '*No bodies at all available at the time*' for dissection. On to Rome for two strenuous weeks with Tacitus for bedtime reading. In mid-February the party swept north through Perugia and Assisi to beautiful Florence where, despite freezing temperatures, they were willing captives to its art treasures; on the last day there Wilson returned alone to the Church of Santa Maria Novella 'to look again at Orcagna's altar piece & frescoes in the Strozzi Chapel'. Then it was on to Siena, Pisa and Bologna where he paid his respects to Professor Valenti, admired his fine new anatomy building and beautiful equipment, his collection of African crania and wax models, but 'otherwise nothing *very* striking'. In Padua Wilson was frustrated at not gaining admission to the old anatomy theatre, where three centuries previously Fabricius of Aquapendente had pioneered the comparative approach to embryology. In Verona the fine Romanesque church of San Zeno took most of his attention. On to Venice, another city they were reluctant to leave, and as the finale to their Italian holiday, Milan and the opera at La Scala. On 20 March Louise and Dorette joined the French classes at Villa Blanche and four days later Mabel and Jeanie set off for Paris and the pleasures of new maternity clothes, *haute couture*, in compensation for Mabel's unwanted pregnancy. Wilson headed for Monaco as the University of Sydney's commissioned delegate to the Ninth International Congress of Zoology. A letter from Barff had informed him of it in Rome. He had bought a dress suit in Florence.[3]

The Ninth International Congress of Zoology was a splendid affair – the largest of its kind ever held – hosted by His Serene Highness the Prince of Monaco, a marine biologist who had founded in 1910 the Oceanographic Museum where the Congress was held: it was to become an important centre for oceanographic research. Wilson arrived in time for the opening address at 6 p.m. on 25 March by the Prince who stressed the value of marine zoology to research on the origin of life and concluded with a panegyric to science which gave 'dominion to creative force over the vain rivalries of man'. This important meeting was convened to settle a vexed question in zoological nomenclature: the 'priority' rule, which for the last 70 years had required newly discovered organisms to be known by their first-published name, even when this did not make scientific sense. Any incompetent researcher by this ruling could name a species. Much acrimony resulted and the stability of international nomenclature was threatened. The Monaco Congress found a solution in the 'plenary powers' rule which provides that exceptions to strict priority may be granted by the International Commission of Zoological Nomenclature acting under its plenary powers if a later name becomes so widely accepted that its suppression would sow confusion and instability. This new rule found 'the fulcrum between strict priority and proper exception'. Wilson did not participate in the formal debate on nomenclature but talked it over with some who did: Dr J A Allen of New York, Prof. S W Willeston of Chicago, Dr Hoyle of Cardiff. As for gossip, while lunching with his friends the Hubrechts and Dr Forsyth Major he learned that J P Hill had been nominated for the FRS.[4]

Wilson's subsequent report on the nomenclature debate to the Anatomical Society of Great Britain and Ireland injected some short-lived stimulus into its long-standing but much-postponed committee on anatomical nomenclature. In 1893 German anatomists had produced a revision of anatomical terminology known as the Basle Nomina Anatomica, or the BNA, which was rejected by Britain and France though acclaimed in America and the British colonies and dominions. Wilson had introduced the BNA system in his department soon afterwards. While Macalister of Cambridge after weighing the pros and cons felt that acceptance of a revised BNA was inevitable, it was strenuously opposed by others led by D G Thane of University College London who argued in 1917 that, 'if changes in our current nomenclature were desirable, they should not be based on a formulary which may be adapted to German usage and requirements, but entirely at variance with ours'. British anatomy's independence and self-respect demanded adherence to the old terminology he believed. Clearly the time for international settlement of anatomical nomenclature was not yet[5]

By its fourth day the Congress was winding down and early on the fifth Wilson left for Paris to join Mabel and Jeanie. He and Mabel inspected the osteological and wax model collection at Tramond's Warehouse and the fine old Anatomy Museum at L'Ecole de Medecine, while at a neighbouring bookseller they picked up a set of 10 plates of frozen sections that were going cheap. Post-impressionist painting and the music of Berlioz were their main diversions before crossing the Channel on 2 April. Maggie and Annie Lorrain Smith met them at Charing Cross Station and deposited them at their rooms at 127 Queens Gate, Kensington.

London in the spring: but it was a different London from 1905. A note of hysteria in the air and petty violence in the streets intimated a new and deep disharmony in British society, and this at a time when Europe's strongest military power was challenging Britain's naval superiority. Nevertheless the London season was as brilliant as ever. The Wilsons had a feast of opera, theatre and art, including Forbes Robertson in Hamlet and Caesar and Cleopatra, plays by Galsworthy, Arnold Bennett and Synge, performances by Melba and McCormick in La Bohéme, Caruso in Tosca, Percy Grainger at the Albert Hall and, at the Palace Theatre, Harry Lauder, who unexpectedly delighted Wilson. Works by Burne-Jones, Rossetti and William Morris were on exhibition at the Tate Gallery and by Rotherstein and Sickert at the New English Art Club. Wilson joined St Stephen's Club and on Martin's recommendation the Savile Club where he entertained various friends and colleagues. He saw John Haldane who had much business in London, quite frequently. He said a few convivial words at a dinner for the Sydney University Wanderers at the Comedy Restaurant in Panton Street. At Queens Gate the Wilsons entertained family friends like the Norman Katers, the Murray Priors, Mrs Bernhard Wise and the Ashburton Thompsons, who were house-hunting. 'Atty' was about to retire from the NSW Board of Health, and he and Lilian with her three children Brian, Julian and Norah Simpson had decided to settle in London. Mabel would then have no relatives in Australia.

But for Wilson London meant primarily the society of Martin and Hill. By 7 April he was at work on platypus embryos with Hill in his laboratory at University College where two days later Elliot Smith and Jim Lorrain Smith dropped in from Manchester to see him. Hill's laboratory was his business address until Hill left on 20 June to collect marsupial material in Brazil. At University College he met D M S Watson, a vertebrate palaeontologist working on marsupial and monotreme skulls, also MacGregor who was working with Hill on *Dasyurus* and Max Poser with whom he discussed optical apparatus. He walked and talked with Martin, looked over the Lister Institute and Martin's long work on bubonic plague. Wilson was coming to grips with the work of his closest research colleagues. By contrast his own work, bereft of these peers and besieged by 'extraneous work', had withered or at least not blossomed in print. Only five short papers published since 1907, three on technique and two review papers on the achselbogen muscle. Did Wilson perhaps hope that he might re-establish himself within the Fraternity of Duckmaloi? Did Martin? They did discuss futures. In 1913, as was not the case in 1909, the Wilson family was eminently transplantable.[6]

In May, Robert Broom, whom Wilson had not seen for about 17 years, walked in to Hill's laboratory and Wilson soon found himself deep in the morphology and palaeontology of fossil reptiles; he reexamined the evidence of reptilian affinities in his platypus embryos. Broom was a keen reminder of the halcyon research-focused days of the early 1890s in the bush of NSW and he had stayed in close touch with Elliot Smith to whom he had sent a considerable amount of research material over the years. Broom was in London to deliver his Croonian Lecture on the 'Origin of Mammals' to the Royal Society, an honour probably engineered by Elliot Smith who, in characteristically ebullient style, also gave him sound advice on how to 'sharpen his claws' for the effort: 'always remember to sugar your most heretical pills with a deferent (though confident) statement of them' and 'dont assume any knowledge on the part of your hearers or offend their conceit of themselves by telling them it is non-technical'. Elliot Smith was a seasoned controversialist – he had been contending with established authority all his life – and required his troops to perform well.[7]

The Royal Society at Burlington House was a familiar rendezvous over the next few months. After lunching with Hill and Elliot Smith, Wilson was admitted formally to its fellowship at 4 p.m. on 24 April, Sir Archibald Geikie (the Edinburgh geology professor of his student days) and his 'Australian' peers Martin, Liversidge and Arthur Dendy being among the illuminati to greet him. On 7 May he attended the Society's soirée at which Elliot Smith and Arthur Smith Woodward demonstrated their controversial reconstruction of the fossil human skull and the ape mandible presumed to be from the same individual – a splendid 'missing link' – found the previous summer by Charles Dawson at Piltdown in the Weald of Sussex. Almroth Wright entertained Wilson and Bishop Frodsham of North Queensland to dinner at the Royal Society's Club on 29 May before delivering his lecture on 'The Physiology of Belief'. Arthur Balfour was there and spoke up in criticism. Present also was Bernard Shaw who said nothing. Wilson confided his opinion to his diary: 'characteristic of Wright but awful stuff as philos[ophy]'. On 5 June he attended Broom's Croonian Lecture, and on 11 June Mabel, in her Parisian finery (and seven months pregnant), accompanied Wilson to a conversazione at the Royal Society where they joined Martin and Harriette Chick of the Lister Institute, Liversidge, Robert Broom, Mrs Elliot Smith, the physiologists Halliburton and Starling (friends of Martin from his student days), A B MacCallum of Toronto and Schäfer of Edinburgh, the biologists McBride, Bateson and Poulton, Mrs Hooper and the geographer Griffiths Taylor of Sydney, and the anatomist C J Patten of Sheffield.[8]

Wilson, Mabel and Jeanie spent nine beautiful days in May with the Haldanes at Oxford where they explored, picnicked, watched the boat races, sketched and photographed. Precocious Naomi, aged 16, had written a play then being performed in Oxford while her brilliant brother Jack, aged 21, was busy with Mendelian experiments on guinea pigs, besides rowing in the eights for New College. The Wilsons met a number of Oxford notables including the Gilbert Murrays, Warden Spooner of New College and Rait the historian, attended an exquisite music recital in New College Chapel and an exhibition of paintings by Reynolds, Gainsborough, Turner and the

Pre-Raphaelites at the Ashmolean. Wilson met the biologists E S Goodrich and G C Bourne at the Museum and had several sessions with the experimental embryologist J W Jenkinson and his old friend Arthur Thomson with whom, besides anatomy and embryology, he discussed Vitalism and university politics in Oxford, Edinburgh and Sydney. No doubt he also discussed academic politics with Haldane whose strong claims to the prestigious Waynflete Chair of Physiology were passed over in that year in favour of Charles Sherrington. Haldane resigned his Readership, bringing an end to his teaching career, but remained a fellow of New College till the end of his life and 'Cherwell' remained his home. His work-base shifted to the Coal Owners Research Laboratory at Bentley Colliery near Doncaster, of which he had become Director in 1912, moving in 1921 to Birmingham University. Haldane's output of original research, now at least partly yoked to the welfare of miners, suffered no setback. Predictably Wilson and Haldane also discussed Vitalism into the small hours of one morning. Possibly they also discussed defence: Haldane was then advising the Admiralty on the ventilation of battleships and submarines.[9]

One afternoon Wilson had tea with the historian Reginald Coupland at Trinity College to meet Lionel Curtis again. In 1912 Curtis had been appointed to a Fellowship of All Souls and to the Beit lectureship on the History of the British Empire, at Oxford. He was at the height of his influence in the Round Table movement and working at a relentless pace to shape its philosophy and policy on the imperial question. In his view there were four possible principles for future imperial relations – the *status quo*, independence, cooperation and organic union – and the only real alternatives were independence or union. Curtis was an Either-Or man. He became a missionary for organic union and the gospel of citizenship, a distinctively British formulation which owed much to the mystique of the British constitution and the philosophical Idealism of Oxford and T H Green. These ideas were probably the focus of a seminar in colonial history then being conducted by Curtis at All Souls. Curtis invited Wilson to dinner that same evening at Trinity College where he met the seminar members as well as the historian Professor George Wrong, a prominent Round Tabler from Toronto, Richard Jebb, a leading analyst of the empire, and Edward Grigg of *The Times*, who was then also the editor of the *Round Table*.[10]

As a pragmatic Australian Round Tabler, Wilson represented the reality of the defence issue in Australian politics. The Japanese threat to Australian security had sharpened Australian concern for national defence while maintaining a commitment to empire. Australians had dual loyalties which did not sit well with Curtis's view of the British Empire as a State which alone had full sovereignty. Some of Curtis's closest colleagues like Coupland disliked it too, as retrogressive politics dangerous to the cause of freedom. Curtis was really no scholar. Concerned entirely with the future, he was a propagandist who bent history to his thesis. Wilson recorded many years later his admiration for Curtis's intellectual and moral qualities but added 'I do not consider him well grounded from the strictly philosophical point of view'. The Round Table was highly active in 1913. Moots were held frequently at various places and dominion members, usually Canadian, often attended. But Wilson had no more contact with them that year. Curtis just then was preoccupied with the reception of his ideas in the Empire's senior dominion, Canada, where he spent most of October and November.[11]

Defence was on Wilson's mind. At Earls Court with crowds of others he and Mabel viewed a military and naval exhibition of model ships, guns of all sorts, fortifications, signalling apparatus and mimic naval warfare. They saw something too of President Poincare's visit to London in late June demonstrating Franco-British solidarity. The national mood was bellicose and it was directed at Germany. Wilson's preoccupation was imperial naval policy, reflecting Australian concern over the Admiralty priority of concentrating naval forces in the North Sea at the expense of the Pacific. In September 1912 the Melbourne Round Tabler Frederic Eggleston had severely criticized this and other British policies and suggested that the fleet units contributed to the Royal Navy by dominions bordering the Pacific be controlled by an authority which, while not divorced at all from British naval authorities, would give the governments of those dominions a direct say in overall policy. He called for an immediate imperial defence conference on the issue. Eggleston's views gave rise to heated controversy throughout 1913 among the Australian groups, and with the London editor, who resisted publication of 'The Australian View', the product of group discussions on the question. It was published 'only after great pressure' was exerted in June 1914, and even then only in summarized form. In Sydney, while MacCallum approved the article as stating 'the position admirably', Colonel Hubert Foster in arguing the British case rejected Eggleston's views emphatically. He was supported by Sydney's Arthur Jose and Melbourne's Professor Harrison Moore who attacked the principle

219

of local navies. However, Admiral Creswell, a Melbourne Round Tabler and commander of the Commonwealth Naval Forces, supported Eggleston and persuaded the Fisher government to denounce the Admiralty's policy in March 1913.[12]

In London on 18 April at the Commonwealth Offices Wilson had 'a talk' with Captain Collins who had charge of large defence orders and naval intelligence. Collins, a former head of the Commonwealth Department of Defence, was, like Creswell, a 'navalist' from way back. What they talked about Wilson did not record in his diary. But he did expand a little concerning an interview on 25 June with Julian Corbett of the Royal Naval War College at Greenwich, an authority on naval history and naval strategy. Wilson recorded that they talked over Australian and Imperial defence problems. Corbett, he noted in his diary, 'had seen Col. Foster & been greatly impressed. Ideas pract. identical with Fosters... Wd. not undertake an article for Aust Natl Def Annual because might have to say what might tend to discourage Aust feeling with wh. he is after all sympathetic.' Evidently Corbett appreciated the dilemma. The following October Admiralty control of the Australian station formally ceased, only to revive during the war when the Australian fleet was dispersed into various British squadrons. The situation became anomalous and attitudes continued ambivalent.[13]

By late June 1913 the Wilson family base had shifted to 25 Cluny Drive, Edinburgh, but only rarely were they all in residence over the next three months. Friends relieved the parents of their children for much of the time: Jeanie went to her Lorrain Smith cousins in Annan, Dumfriesshire, Louise and Dorette to Aunt Lottie in London and then to the Haldanes at Cloan in Perthshire, while Katharine and Douglas holidayed with the Hills at Elie in Fifeshire. For the birth of the youngest Wilson, James Maxwell Glover on 31 August, the whole family was at home though as a coming event it could not have been much discussed: Louise, aged 13^1/$_2$, was utterly astonished. In holiday mood over these three months – with a couple of interruptions – Wilson played golf and talked philosophy with Haldane and Lorrain Smith, the Seths, the Glovers and Samuel Alexander; he dropped in on Edward Schäfer at the university, visited friends, paid his respects to Sir William Turner now aged 81, and took the whole family on a four-day pilgrimage to Dumfries and Moniaive. The new baby imposed little restraint on family movement.[14]

On 5 September Wilson went south to London to represent the University of Sydney at the 17th International Medical Congress, at the Albert Hall, 'the greatest scientific congress ever held in the metropolis' according to *Nature's* reviewer. William Bateson addressed it on heredity, Laveran on tropical medicine, Harvey Cushing on surgery of the pituitary body and Paul Ehrlich on the treatment of syphilis with salversan. Among those specially honoured was Almroth Wright for his work in bacteriology, over which section Martin presided.[15]

Arthur Thomson of Oxford presided over the Anatomy and Embryology Section attended by distinguished scientists from Britain, Europe and America. There were several sessions of special interest to Wilson. To one, led by Eternod of Geneva on recent work on the early development of the human ovum, Wilson showed a number of stereoscopic photomicrographs through a human embryo with nine pairs of somites, its tissues 'beautifully fixed'; to another on the morphology of the sympathetic nervous system led by Carl Huber of Michigan, Wilson advanced a view that he might also have put to the nomenclature committee of the Anatomical Society: that the terms 'sympathetic' and 'cerebro-spinal' were not morphologically appropriate for the two divisions of the vertebrate nervous system and that 'sensory ganglionic' and 'medullary' should replace them.[16]

On August 12 Wilson chaired the final session on cerebral localization of function (the mapping of brain locations concerned with body functions) and the significance of sulci (brain fissures), a large but comparatively new field to which Grafton Elliot Smith had made enduring fundamental contributions. Ariens Kappers of Amsterdam, the star performer on this occasion, delivered a 'brilliant' comprehensive review of the literature interpreted in the context of evolutionary biology. Elliot Smith in 'entire agreement' regretted only that 'there were no representatives of the rival 'Brodmann' school' for the discussion.[17]

This reference to a rival school is interesting. Smith and Kappers were studying brains at the macroscopic level, seeking to correlate brain conformation with the particular attributes, needs and functions of different species. The German anatomist K Brodmann and the Edinburgh-trained Australian clinician A W Campbell (under the influence of Charles Sherrington), attacking the problem with microscopes, sought to correlate body functions with different patterns in cell structure; they produced monumental histological surveys of the mammalian cerebral cortex. A third group led by the neuro-physiologist Charles Sherrington and clinicians like Henry Head, David Ferrier and Victor Horsley sought the answers from experiments. All three groups were working in the field of anatomy properly defined but, in Britain where histology had been appropriated by the physiologists, British anatomists (being confined to gross structure) were scarcely involved. Elliot Smith in Manchester was exerting himself to re-assert the anatomist's jurisdiction over the whole domain of structure. On the question of cerebral localization of function he had already done this. Using fresh brains and equipped simply with a razor and a hand lens he had produced in 1907 his celebrated topographical map of the whole of the human cerebral cortex, at once simple and comprehensive, integrating the findings of the three disparate research groups.[18]

That last session was, in the opinion of the section reporter F Wood Jones, 'perhaps the most important of all', but another issue dominated the interest of anatomists at the Congress: the developing row between Elliot Smith and Arthur Keith over the cranium of Piltdown Man. It had been introduced to the public in December 1912 at a meeting of the Geological Society by the palaeontologist Arthur Smith Woodward who described the skull, and Elliot Smith who gave an account of the endocranial cast. Smith Woodward, however, had made an error in the reconstruction of the cranium, giving it a simian appearance and an unusually small cranial capacity. Elliot Smith endorsed Smith Woodward's view, saying that Piltdown Man possessed the most simian and primitive human brain ever recorded. Arthur Keith, however, had detected the error and during the Congress publicly demonstrated that the skull, when correctly restored, was not significantly different in general appearance and endocranial characters from the skull of a modern man. Had he not done so, Keith claimed, visiting German scientists would have done. Keith had, in July 1913 at a private demonstration of the reconstructed skull, swayed Elliot Smith's opinion. But by the time of the Congress in August, and through the following months of controversy in the pages of *Nature* concluding with a paper to a crowded meeting of the Royal Society on 19 February 1914, Elliot Smith managed to convince himself that his first judgement was right. At this meeting Keith again pointed out 'the glaring errors in the reconstructed brain-cast [Elliot Smith] exhibited', and, concluded Keith, Elliot Smith 'must have felt I was in the right, for he never published the paper he had read to the Royal Society'; a subsequent reconstruction by Elliot Smith and Dr John Beattie did not differ materially from Keith's. This public disagreement ended a long friendship. Elliot Smith, a Royal Medallist of the Society and its Vice-President in 1913, carried conviction while Arthur Keith, elected a fellow only that year, won the reputation in that company of being a 'brawler'. In public Keith pushed his argument no further, which was a pity, Wilfrid Le Gros Clark pointed out many years later, for if taken to its logical conclusion the incongruity between the cranium and the mandible might have led to an early exposure of the Piltdown fraud. In 1914 Arthur Keith was elected President of the Royal Anthropological Institute.[19]

That the Piltdown skull and mandible did not fit together was in fact argued at the time by David Waterston, the Edinburgh-trained Professor of Anatomy at King's College London in a letter published by *Nature* on 13 November 1913, immediately following one by Elliot Smith. Waterston was satisfied that the cranial fragments of the Piltdown skull were essentially human in all details but that the mandible, as shown by radiograms published in *The British Journal of Dental Science* on October 1913, was practically identical with that of a chimpanzee. It seemed to Waterston 'to be as inconsequent to refer the mandible and the cranium to the same individual as it would be to articulate a chimpanzee foot with the bones of an essentially human thigh or leg'. But the controversy did not follow up questions of authenticity. It became stuck on the contest between two titans on the technicalities of skull reconstruction. Had Elliot Smith admitted error in his reconstruction – as Keith believed he did privately – the argument might have reached the right conclusion at the time. But his reputation was at stake.[20]

Wilson witnessed this contretemps at close quarters. He attended the main events, read the *Nature* articles and warmly entertained both parties at 12 Vicarage Gate, Kensington, the family residence from early October. His old bonds with Elliot Smith were unimpaired while new ones with Arthur Keith strengthened. He must have had opinions but, unusually, they were not confided to his diary. He was probably discomforted by this unseemly public wrangle between two thoroughly congenial friends whose interests, convictions and careers ran remarkably parallel. As anatomists they were schooled in the Scottish tradition – Arthur Keith was an Aberdonian trained by Sir James Struthers, Turner's great contemporary – and their inspiration was Charles Darwin, the source also of their compelling interest in anthropology. By 1913 they were both distinguished scientists, prolific contributors to scientific literature, attractive writers in the popular press, great communicators who were drawn to broad issues, challenged by controversy. Both revelled in the Darwinian drama of human history. With all that in common, joined in both cases to a strong competitive instinct, it was probably inevitable that a disagreement between them would become a public spectacle.[21]

In 1913 the established medical order in London was changing. For a decade the medical curriculum had been under debate. 'The cry of course is more time for clinical and other work of the later years', Hill had informed Wilson in 1908. 'We are simply evolving along your lines only here it is a much more prolonged and cumbrous process'. Two important contributions to the debate accelerated that process. Hot on the heels of the American critic Abraham Flexner's report of 1912 on medical education in Europe, which condemned London's proprietary system (it was in the hands of 19 hospital medical schools) for producing inefficient teaching, low standards and poor science, came supporting evidence from the Haldane Royal Commission into University Education in London, published in April 1913. Set up merely to incorporate Imperial College within the university structure, the Commission's report was a manifesto for revolutionary change in the constitution of the university and in medical education. The time had come for London to give precedence in its medical curriculum to scientific (or laboratory) medicine, essentially a German invention, over clinical medicine around which English medical education had evolved. British medical scientists like the physiologist E H Starling and the anatomist Arthur Keith who had experienced the vitality of learning in German medical laboratories and had fought the difficulties of trying to reproduce it in two of London's poorly equipped medical schools where as science teachers they had the status of salaried officers, fuelled the argument for change. So too did the Canadian William Osler of Johns Hopkins, then teaching at Oxford, who urged the need for the 'hospital unit' to treat, teach and research; this was as necessary to the medical professor as a staffed laboratory to a chemistry professor. Richard Haldane hardly needed convincing of the merits of the German system. His report brought London medical schools within the sphere of influence of the university and led in the 1920s to the introduction of the professorial system and other features of university-based medicine as practised in Scotland, Germany, America and Australia. Funds for the necessary laboratories came from public and private sources.[22]

Wilson's interest focused on the devalued status of anatomy in the British medical curriculum, eclipsed by the younger disciplines of physiology and pathology. Flexner had criticized British anatomy as too much drilled into students by systematic lectures and demonstrations, too little communicated by practical work. In the opinion of Grafton Elliot Smith the problem lay deeper than that: anatomy had ceased to keep pace with the times. In Manchester since 1909 Elliot Smith, with missionary zeal, had raised a standard for the revival of British anatomy by expanding the undergraduate syllabus and promoting original research – in which he included clinical work – by his staff. Wilson fully agreed that the best teachers are active researchers, and by example had demonstrated. He had more difficulty with another of Elliot Smith's convictions, that 'the teaching ... should be directed towards the needs of the practice of medicine'. Anatomy in Wilson's view served nothing but scientific truth. It belonged to biology. Medicine's right to a place in a university rested, he argued, on its cardinal commitment to science, not vocation. Elliot Smith, like Wilson, was not clinically inclined – they were both primarily morphologists – but he did recognize the incentive value of clinical interest, giving the anatomy student his 'first glimpse of the promised land' of medical practice. He used clinical reference to illuminate anatomical data, instituted a course in applied anatomy for fourth and fifth year students and fostered easy relations with clinicians. Elliot Smith was persuaded, as were Starling, Haldane and Arthur Keith, that England's traditional clinically-oriented medical course, if short on science, did produce excellent practitioners.[23]

Other features of Elliot Smith's programme also gave Wilson pause. Lectures were limited to the important introductory course and to subjects like certain parts of the nervous system which were not adequately covered by textbooks or dissection. Systematic lectures were drastically cut, including emphatically the whole 'antiquated' osteology class, respecting which Elliot Smith bore his old master a grudge:

> Looking back to my own student days, when, full of enthusiasm for the subject, I first began anatomy and sat at the feet of one of the most clear-sighted and inspiring teachers, I have the most vivid recollection of the manner in which those first two terms of osteology rapidly killed all interest in the subject. It was not merely that I ceased to learn anything from the lectures, but a positive and intense repugnance to the business of acquiring a knowledge of the bones took possession of me.

The anatomy course should not be hung on the skeleton, he declared. Ever the iconoclast, it is arguable that such radical surgery of systematic lectures achieved very much. This brilliant public lecturer who 'could expound in the clearest possible manner the most intricate and involved problems to a lay audience', was not a success as an undergraduate lecturer. Perhaps, conjectured a member of his staff, he over-rated the abilities of the average student, or maybe 'his lectures were not sufficiently systematic and lacked the necessary sequence and co-ordination'. Whatever the reason, only the most able students with a good background in biology could follow Elliot Smith's erudite, free-ranging expositions.[24]

Dissection was also reduced, an unthinkable idea for Wilson who to the end of his life maintained that 'One can never have too much dissection.' Sydney students in 1912 dissected the whole human body at least once. For Elliot Smith dissection remained important as the chief means of enabling the student to find his way about the human body, but he paid little attention to detail which for Wilson was a principle of William Turner's to which he remained faithful. Elliot Smith introduced other methods of investigation like X-rays and the live model, revolutionary innovations in Britain at that time. He argued that every device of investigation in the biological and clinical sciences should be exploited by the anatomist. He tried but did not succeed in having histology transferred from the physiology department to the anatomy department. That historic event occurred after he left Manchester in 1919.[25]

Elliot Smith's aims were to shift the attention of the anatomist from the cadaver to the living human body, to bring anatomy into closer relationship with physiology and clinical experience and to make anatomy a vital part of the medical curriculum, indeed to reinstate anatomy as 'the real basis of medical education'. In adjusting the teaching of anatomy to medical needs Elliot Smith was also bending over backwards to appease the powerful medical corporations.[26]

He was therefore enraged by the decision of the Royal College of Surgeons in October 1913 to appoint three surgeons, 'whose energies are necessarily devoted to work other than mere anatomy' and only one 'professed anatomist', as examiners in anatomy for its Fellowship, the only major incentive in the country for advanced work in anatomy. The College, as the custodian of 'the greatest anatomical museum in existence' which its conservator, Arthur Keith, was presenting in a brilliant series of lectures and demonstrations to highlight the importance of scientific anatomy to clinical medicine, was hardly serving its best interests. On the contrary, by this decision it was 'driving students to the crammer and the textbook monger, and paralysing the work of those teachers who are endeavouring to instruct their advanced students in a knowledge of the whole structure of the human body and its real significance'. This was the substance of a letter of protest Elliot Smith wrote to *The Lancet*.[27]

The importance of scientific anatomy to clinical medicine! This proposition, which Wilson could heartily endorse, was discussed during a long weekend visit to the Grafton Elliot Smiths in November with other medical men like Lorrain Smith and A E Boycott. In London the following week Wilson too drafted a letter of protest to *The Lancet*. He addressed the contradiction between the College's ideal and its practice. If the FRCS was merely to be a higher *professional* qualification there could be no quarrel with the examination being conducted predominantly, even exclusively, by masters of the surgical craft. But if, as recent examination papers revealed, possession of the FRCS was also to guarantee a certain competence in *scientific* anatomy – and Wilson applauded that ideal – then fuller representation of professional anatomists on the examining board was essential. This could require breaking the tradition that only Fellows could examine for the Fellowship, as the physiologists had done some years ago. In typically thorough fashion Wilson elaborated his argument with four possible designs for the FRCS course. But he did not send the letter. A very deliberate question mark beside the diary entry indicates that second thoughts prevailed, but what they were he did not record.[28]

Wilson's Sunday in Manchester did not include church. 'Spent day in talking shop' begins his diary entry for Sunday 23 November and then lists a group of physicists including Ernest Rutherford with whom he spent that day. It is likely that among other things they discussed imperial university relations which Rutherford, like Wilson, was keen to promote. In June–July 1912 among the delegates of 53 universities Rutherford had attended the first Congress of the Universities of the Empire, at which Anderson Stuart, by overruling Wilson's sabbatical plans, had with H E Barff represented Sydney University. The Australian universities led by Sydney had been instrumental in the establishment of a central bureau with a permanent committee and secretary to supply information on the courses and conditions, resources and specializations of the various universities, and to facilitate the interchange of university teachers. A decision was also made to hold Congresses every five years.[29]

At the end of 1913 Rutherford was preoccupied with another coming intellectual and imperial event: the 84th meeting of the British Association for the Advancement of Science to be held in Australia in July–September 1914. Rutherford, with Arthur Dendy,

J W Gregory, Archibald Liversidge, C J Martin and William Bateson, was on the 'Australian Committee' of the British Association which from mid–1912 had concerned itself with the funding of invited members, the selection of those members, the enrolment of the 300 British, European, American and Dominion scientists who applied to attend, and the arrangement of the sectional programmes. First canvassed at the 1884 meeting in Montreal at which Caldwell's telegram on platypus reproduction had made a dramatic impact, Liversidge had never let the idea of an Australian meeting die, and by 1913 it was cast as the coming of age of Australian science and in the words of the Australian Prime Minister an 'additional step towards imperial unity'.[30]

Virtually all of Australia's scientists and scientific institutions were in some way involved. Led by Professor David Orme Masson of Melbourne it was brilliantly organized by his protégé David Rivett as a grand procession through Australia's six States and New Zealand's two islands. Rivett spent the last half of 1913 in London attending to arrangements at that end. He returned to Australia in December just as Edgeworth David, the president of ANZAAS and head of the NSW Committee for the British Association meeting arrived in London to confer with the British authorities. Like Wilson and all travelling Australian academics, David had in one short month a number of briefs to fulfil, one being to advise Shackleton on his next expedition to Antarctica. But when he dined with Wilson at the Savile Club on 28 December, together with C J Martin and Professor Lyle of Melbourne, the forthcoming meeting of the British Association was probably the main topic of conversation.[31]

Adult education, then experiencing a revival in England, was another matter which claimed the attention of Edgeworth David and Wilson. A new experiment, involving the collaboration of the universities with the Workers Educational Association founded by Albert Mansbridge, was organizing tutorial classes at university standard for working people willing to pledge themselves for three years to regular course work including the writing of essays. This was an earnest effort to deliver 'real education' to the educationally deprived, an ideal which the university extension scheme had not fulfilled. The demand for such classes spread quickly. Commenced in 1908, by 1914 there were 145 in England and Wales, and 3,234 students.[32]

As with so much else, this new idea was transported to Australia. Peter Board had seen the Oxford WEA scheme in operation in 1911 and it was this kind of organization he had in mind when drafting the provisions for adult education in the University (Amendment) Act of 1912. With a disciple of Mansbridge, David Stewart of the NSW Labor Council, Board prepared the ground in NSW for a visit in July and August 1913 by Mansbridge who was able to overcome resistance at the University. He persuaded the Senate and the Professorial Board to set up a Joint Committee for Tutorial Classes consisting of three members each from the University and the WEA of NSW, founded by Stewart in November 1913. As lecturer and organizer Mansbridge recommended Meredith Atkinson, a young Oxford graduate then conducting a tutorial class at Durham University, and Sydney University concurred. Atkinson was appointed after Wilson and Edgeworth David interviewed him in London. Peter Board arranged government funding for the project and Atkinson arrived in Sydney in March 1914.[33]

The Meredith Atkinsons dined with the Wilsons, Edgeworth David and Henry Barraclough (who had arrived quite unexpectedly on the Wilson's doorstep on 31 December) one evening early in 1914 at 12 Vicarage Gate. For Jeanie it was a remarkable occasion:

> Long ago as it is, I remember that evening well, sitting on a footstool by the fireside, listening in silence ... while these men, rich in University knowledge and experience, mellowed with wisdom, lightened with humour, drew a picture of what awaited him for the younger addition to their number. I remember the thin, eager face of Meredith Atkinson, shining with enthusiasm, eagerly questioning, hungrily accepting such satisfying food for hope and thought, his doubts smoothing themselves out. His last words of farewell that evening were 'I'm sure I shall like it', which meant, I think, 'I'm sure I can do it'...[34]

Great expectations were lodged in adult education especially by Idealists, many of whom were teachers. They had an enormous faith in the efficacy of education, not only as a way to lift working people 'to higher works and higher pleasures' to quote Mansbridge but as he added to 'bring about rational action upon municipal, national and imperial affairs'. *The Round Table* and the Congress of the Universities of the Empire debated and supported the WEA movement as did Richard Haldane, a friend of Mansbridge from about 1907 and a lifelong evangelist for adult education. The hearings of the Royal Commission on London's education were good publicity. 'We think', concluded the Commissioners, 'the University should consider the work it is doing for these men and women one of the most serious and important of its services to the metropolis.'[35]

Wilson had always supported enterprises which exercised university people's 'practical social sympathies', like the University Boys' Club, the Toynbee Guild, the Sydney Medical Mission and the University extension lectures. He worked hard for those organizations, as he was to do for the WEA. He saw it as an 'audacious' enterprise, attempting 'nothing less than the intellectual & spiritual awakening of the masses. They have attained political power & self-consciousness of it. The future of the country depends on the spirit in which that power is exercised'. Education would make democracy safe.[36]

A re-invigorated Hill had returned from Brazil in late November with, among fresh marsupial material to add to his vast collection, some prized *Didelphys* embryos: his field trip by happy chance had coincided with that animal's breeding period. Wilson's routine for the last two months of his sojourn returned to the rhythm of Hill's laboratory, working away at platypus embryos. Most likely this was when he and Hill put together the paper acknowledging the error in their 1907 paper on the development of *ornithorhynchus* relating to the 'primitive knot'. It was published in 1915 in the *Quarterly Journal of Microscopical Science* – the last spark, did they but know it, of their fiery collaboration.[37]

Wilson's instinct for research was as keen as ever, his work and judgement esteemed: the technical quality of his human embryo photomicrographs had made an impression at the Medical Congress; Broom had enjoined immediate publication for his recent work on platypus embryos; the Anatomical Society had accorded him the status of a vice-president. Research was his first love, but it was unlikely to find fulfilment in utilitarian Sydney by any contrivance within his power. He had surveyed the prospects in the UK of a post more accommodating to research and the indications were that Oxford, to Wilson's eyes, was the most attractive. There were signs of growing intimacy with the Haldanes and Mabel and Wilson returned twice to Oxford in the closing months of 1913. At Cherwell they met more of the University's dignitaries including Sir W Rayleigh, and Wilson dined in Hall at New College with John Haldane. By contrast a brief visit in November to Cambridge where they toured the Colleges and had tea at St Johns with W H R Rivers was perfunctory. Plans however 'gang aft agley'.[38]

The shadows of war were lengthening as the Wilson family set sail from the heart of empire for the Australian periphery in early

February 1914. Fighting in the Balkans had been going on since 1912 and in the Mediterranean they sighted transports of Italian troops. For Australians, however, 1914 was still to be 'the year of the British Ass.' Public interest was extraordinary. Membership enrolment was far greater than for any previous meeting of the British Association: a total of 4,930 of whom 4,630 were resident Australians.[39]

When Wilson arrived back on 12 March 1914 Sydney was in the midst of final arrangements. University and city buildings were having a clean-up, gardens being prepared for spectacular spring flowering and eyesores screened from view. Pamphlets and handbooks, some of permanent value, were coming off the press and elaborate plans for excursions, hospitality and entertainment were well in hand. Wilson threw himself into organizing, as local secretary, the Sydney meeting of the Anthropological Section. Anthropology was to be spotlighted: its representatives were mustering in strength for discussions on fundamentals because the focus was to be Australian Aborigines, 'the most primitive of existing human types'. In the anatomy department S A Smith, assisted by Raymond Dart, prepared a contribution on a series of Solomon Island skulls and another on the Aboriginal Australian humerus, while Wilson wrote one on the symmetrical exostoses (cartilage-capped protuberances) in the external ear passages of Australian Aborigines.[40]

The outbreak of war upstaged the British Ass. On 4 August when war was declared the Overseas Party was on the high seas approaching Adelaide. The seven German scientists among them were assailed by apprehensions about their reception and the organizers ashore by diplomatic headaches. There was doubt that the meeting should proceed. Professor Orme Masson met the situation by obtaining assurances from the Governor-General and the Prime Minister that, since the German scientists had been invited to Australia, the obligations of courtesy and hospitality would be honoured as if nothing untoward had occurred. The military status and behaviour of two of the Germans did give rise to official concern later on and national exigency did affect the concluding phase of the congress: the return passage of the Overseas Party had to be completely reorganized as a consequence of the Government requisitioning three ships, forcing some visitors to depart prematurely; arrangements in Sydney and Brisbane were affected, social functions were modified and the official New Zealand meetings cancelled. The gravity of the times and war hysteria robbed the occasion of much of its sparkle and some of its scientific impact, but the Association's imperial mission was fulfilled and Australian science internationally commended. The further investigation of marsupial reproduction was among the Congress's special recommendations.[41]

There were many celebrated scientists among the visitors but for Australians the most important of them was Grafton Elliot Smith. Sydney University preened itself in reflected glory. An FRS since 1907, royal medallist and recently Vice-President of the Royal Society, at 43 Elliot Smith was the world's leading comparative neurologist, an authority on mammalian and primate cerebral evolution and an eminent anthropologist. On Friday 21 August from the platform of a crowded Town Hall, in the red robes of the Sydney MD, he delivered an address on 'Primitive Man': 'Smooth serene and thoughtful of countenance, with all too early whitening hair, he looks the picture of benevolent abstraction', wrote *Hermes* which went on to give an account of the Piltdown skull, 'the nearest ever found to a relic of the "missing link".' Raymond Dart, then a second-year medical student in whom the passion for neurology had already been aroused, was dazzled. 'I fell under his spell ... and prayed that at some time I would be allowed to work under him.'[42]

Fate had supplied the occasion with a dramatic revelation of the great antiquity of human settlement in Australia. On the morning of this public lecture, in a communication to the anthropological section, Edgeworth David had announced the discovery of a highly fossilized Aboriginal skull found 30 years previously at 'Talgai', a property on the Darling Downs in Queensland whose owner, noting the flurry of interest in anthropology, had brought it out into the light of scientific inquiry. It was, said David, about 25,000 years old. 'Now', he concluded, 'if we are asked, "Is man a geological antiquity in Australia?" we can reply, "Yes, he is."' Wilson had then described it briefly. The strong tusk-like canine teeth, the small, elongated prognathous skull and its small cranial capacity, together with a distortion to the skull due to the steady weight of a thick overburden of clay, indicated great antiquity: it was probably of Pleistocene, perhaps early Pleistocene age. Congratulatory comments from Professor W J Sollas of Oxford, Professor Klaatsch of Germany and Elliot Smith followed and another 'Jummy' anecdote was born, as related by Raymond Dart

> Only those intimately acquainted with J T Wilson's tutelary guardianship of each and every delicate anatomical specimen from

his museum could possibly appreciate fully the apprehension in his restless eyes, following each movement of Sollas's gesticulating right hand while holding aloft in his left hand this pre-eminent skull. Momentarily, as the speaker became lost in congratulating its discoverers, a burst of applause and relief greeted Wilson's sudden rising and rescuing it from orator's rear overhead.

So that evening Elliot Smith adjusted his lecture on the remains of primitive man of Pleistocene and later periods around a discussion of the Talgai cranium, for which he claimed international evolutionary significance.[43]

The Talgai skull led Elliot Smith to a further interesting discovery. With the vertebrate palaeontologist D M S Watson who accompanied him to Australia he sought to establish the age of the skull by examining similar fossils of assumed similar age in the MacLeay Museum in Sydney and the Queensland Museum in Brisbane. They came across mummies from the Torres Straits which for Elliot Smith afforded remarkable confirmation of his recently expounded theory of the 'diffusion of culture'. This had grown from reflections during his anthropological labours in Egypt on the spread of certain Egyptian beliefs and practices – especially those involved in mummification – to areas far distant and in quite different climates and cultures. The Torres Straits mummifiers he discovered had followed precisely the practice of Egyptian mummifiers, without the cultural pressure of their beliefs. The Egyptians, seeking to restore a semblance of life, had followed the practice of filling the mummy with mud, after removing the viscera through short slits in definite positions in the body; the Torres Straits mummies had slits in the appropriate positions but no padding; they served no purpose. Watson, impressed by Elliot Smith's appreciation of the significance of these new facts and his capacity to coordinate them into a logical scheme, found both the evidence and the argument convincing. Twenty-four years later he had not changed his opinion.[44]

The Australian meeting of the British Association severely taxed Wilson's time and energy. Besides organizing and overseeing the Sydney meetings of the Anthropological Section and preparing his own contribution, which in the event he was unable to deliver personally, he was involved with Edgeworth David from late July till late October in negotiating the purchase of the Talgai skull for the University from its capricious owner, E H K Crawford of Greenethorpe, NSW. Also, as one of the university's scientific

233

leaders, he was committed to the formalities and festivities of the meeting. Specially welcomed were many personal friends among the overseas scientists, including Annie Lorrain Smith who was a family guest till the end of September. Yet he found the time to show D M S Watson his notes, sketches, sections and models of foetal monotreme skulls, and 'with extreme generosity', Watson recorded, 'suggested that I should publish an account of them'. Wilson's considerable work on them became incorporated in his major treatise, published in the *Philosophical Transactions of the Royal Society* in 1916. S A Smith was similarly favoured. Wilson handed him the Talgai skull for description: 'superb evidence of generosity in a scientist', observed Smith.[45]

At the conclusion of the Sydney meetings, as the British Association entrained for Brisbane, there was a Wilson family wedding. On Saturday 29 August in a quiet ceremony 'because of the war' Jeanie married Tom de Burgh following a romance that had survived the disapproval of both families and more than a year's separation while the Wilsons were in Europe. Jeanie and Tom began married life in a splendid tent lined with blue linen, at Nimmitabel in Southern NSW where Tom, a civil engineer, was supervising the construction of railways.

This was one of the busiest times of Wilson's busy life. He was of course generous in handing over prized anatomical specimens by which others might make reputations, but in late August 1914 there was another consideration. For the foreseeable future he was to be fully occupied with quite other affairs and what could be more appropriate than handing his work on foetal monotreme skulls to Watson, an eager researcher trained by Hill, or in giving the Talgai skull to the current occupant of his chair? At midnight on the day war was declared, 4 August 1914, Wilson had been called to Victoria Barracks to organize and command the Censor's Office in New South Wales. His appearances at the proceedings of the British Association meeting were interruptions to his new duties. He was on leave from the army.[46]

Notes

1. Sabbatical leave: papers by Allen Mawer, JTW and E H Alton on 'Interchange of Teachers and Students', Alex Hill (ed.) 1921. 'in vital' and 'Professors should...': JTW, *ibid.*, 394–5.
2. LH and KR, Notes.
3. JTW Diaries for 1913. Background on Fabricius: Nordenskiold, 105.
4. Report of Congress: JTW Diary; *Nature* Vol. 91, 17 April 1913,

162–5. There were 720 delegates, at least 80 British. Zoological Nomenclature: S J Gould 1991, 79–83. 'the fulcrum': *ibid.,* 83.

5. JTW Diary. BNA: Barclay Smith, 40–8.
6. JTW Diary.
7. GES' advice: GES to Broom, 10.5.1913, Abbie m/film.
8. Royal Society meetings: JTW Diary; *Nature* Vol. 92, 131.
9. John Haldane's work: JTW Diary 21.4.13.; C G Douglas on Haldane, *RSO* 1936, 130–1.
10. Curtis and imperial relations: Kendle, 160, 170, 176; Rowse, 342. Organic union: Kendle, 161, 172. Dinner with Curtis: JTW Diary 10.5.1913.
11. Dual loyalties: Foster, Ch. 5. Sole sovereignty: Kendle, 175. Curtis: Rowse, 338–40; Kendle, *ibid.* 'I do not': JTW to Jeanie, 23.9.38. Round Table 1913: Kendle, 157–8, 176.
12. Earls Court: JTW Diary, 13.6.13. Round Table & navy: Foster, 74–8.
13. JTW Diary. Admiralty control: Robert Hyslop in *ADB*, on Creswell.
14. JTW Diary.
15. 17th Int. Med. Congress: *Nature*, Vol. 91, 7 August 1913, 585; Bateson, *ibid.*, 608–9. Almroth Wright: *BMJ* 1913, Vol. 2, 412.
16. 17th Int. Med. Congress: 'Proceedings of Sections', in *BMJ* for Aug./Sept. 1913. 'beautifully fixed', 'sympathetic': *ibid.*, 380, 456.
17. 'there were no': *BMJ*, Aug./Sept. 1913, 458.
18. Cerebral location of brain function: Riese & Hoff, 439–70; Clarke & O'Malley. Attack with microscopes: Woollard 1937, 292–3. Campbell: Abbie, 114; Ford *ADB*, Vol. 7. Confining of British anatomists: Keith, *J of A* Vol. 62, 241. GES' work: Cave, Stopford, in Dawson 1938, 192–3 and 154 resp.
19. Piltdown Man: Le Gros Clark, *RSO* on Arthur Keith, 150–1. GES' opinion: *Nature* No. 92, 319, 729; 'the glaring errors', 'must have felt' and 'brawler': Keith 1950, 327.
20. Waterston letter: *Nature* 13 Nov. 1913, 319. GES' error: Keith 1950, 327.
21. JTW Diary.
22. 'The cry of course': JPH to JTW from Univ. Coll. London, 3.4.1908. Flexner report: *Nature* 21 Aug. 1913, 639–40. Commission's report: Haldane (chair) 1913; Ashby & Anderson, 103–12. The report recommended elective studies, less emphasis on exams, more freedom for students to pursue special interests (an echo of JSH's criticism of Edinburgh in 1883). Consequences: Newman, 265–96.
23. GES' work for anatomy: Stopford in Dawson, 151–65. 'the teaching': GES 1918, 10.

24. GES' expositions: Stopford in Dawson, 152–3. 'Looking back': GES 1918, 8. 'could expound' and 'his lectures': Stopford in Dawson, 153.

25. 'one can never': JTW to J, 20.3.35. GES' work: Stopford in Dawson, 151–2, 154.

26. 'the real basis': GES, 'The Teaching of Anatomy', *Edinburgh Medical Journal*, March 1918, 10.

27. 'whose energies', etc.: GES letter in *The Lancet* 25 Oct. 1913, 1227.

28. JTW draft to *The Lancet* dated 25 Nov., WP. Weekend in Manchester: JTW Diary.

29. 1912 Congress of Univs: Alex Hill (ed.) Intro and 319–23.

30. Plans for 84th British Ass.: BAAS 1915(1), 6–13. 'additional step': MacLeod 1988, 5–7.

31. M E David, 206; JTW Diary.

32. WEA in UK: Orwin, 'Mansbridge, Albert (1876–1952)', *DNB*.

33. WEA in Australia: Crew, 9–14.

34. Meredith Atkinson: JTW Diary. 'Long ago': J Clunies Ross, 'The Australian Highway', 1952.

35. 'to higher works': Mansbridge, quoted in Crew, 9. 'We think': quoted in Ashby & Anderson, 110.

36. JTW's support: letter to F A Russell, cited Turney *et al.*, 320. 'nothing less than': JTW, Address to WEA 1920, ms, 16–17. Idealists and education: Henry Jones 1919, 'The Education of the Citizen', *Round Table*, June 1919, 480–90.

37. JTW Diary. JTW 1915 (with JPH).

38. JTW Diary, esp. 7.4.13 and 5.11.13.

39. Enrolments for British Ass.: *Report,* BAAS (2).

40. 'the most primitive': *Nature* 22 Oct. 1914, 211. Items for presentation: Brit. Assn *Report*, 536; Dart 1973, 418.

41 War & British Ass.: Scott, 30–5; Brit. Assn *Report*, 16–35. Congress recommendations: MacLeod, 57.

42. 'Smooth serene': *Hermes*, August 1914, 56–8. 'I fell under': Dart 1972, 418.

43. Talgai skull: Edgeworth David in *SMH* 20.8.14; *MJA* 29.8.14, 205; British Assn *Report*, 531. 'Only those': Dart 1973, 418.

44. GES and Torres Strait mummies: DMS Watson, in Dawson.

45. Purchase of Talgai: Mackintosh, 189–91. Annie Lorrain Smith: JTW to J, 13.9. and 29.9.14. Wilson's generosity: Watson 1916, 312; S A Smith, 7

46. Appointment as censor: J Clunies Ross, Biographical Sketch of JTW, 24 WP; *Calendar* 1915, 580.

11

War

Despite the long build-up of international tension, or perhaps because of it, the declaration of war on 4 August 1914 caught Australia by surprise. A federal election campaign was in progress and government ministers were scattered across the country. The head of the Defence Department, Commander Pethebridge, and Colonel Legge the Chief of the General Staff were on the high seas, and the Inspector-General of the Commonwealth Military Forces, General Bridges, was on an extended tour of Australia's north. Nevertheless in the preceding two days the defence scheme for Australia had been put into operation in all military districts by the Acting Chief of the General Staff, Major C B Brudenell White: the manning of port defences, the examination of ships entering port, and the censorship of submarine telegraphs. The machinery for cable and wireless censorship was set in motion on 2 August by a cable from the Secretary of State for War in London to Sir Ronald Munro Ferguson the Governor-General, and the next day Australian newspapers became aware that incoming cable messages were being heavily censored. Control of international telegraph links by a Chief Censor in London and Deputy Chief Censors in the Dominions had been adopted as the Empire's primary barrier to enemy intelligence. Australia had taken the added precaution of planning as well for postal and press censorship.[1]

On 3 August the Federal Government appointed Colonel J W McCay Deputy Chief Censor at Defence headquarters in Melbourne. By 6 August district censors for the mainland States had taken up their offices in Brisbane, Sydney, Melbourne, Adelaide and Perth. For this quite new field of work the disbanded Australian Intelligence Corps supplied the cadre of early appointments: McCay and Monash briefly as Deputy Chief Censor before taking up commands in the army's expeditionary force; the district censors in Queensland (Lt Col. Pye), New South Wales (Lt Col. Wilson), and Western Australia (Capt Corbet). Many on their staffs were also former members. Wilson was given leave from the University for Michaelmas term to take up the appointment of 'Censor, Sydney' on 4 August, for the 2nd Military District. He thought the war, and the job of censor, would be over in six months and that he would be back at the University by March 1915.[2]

Australian nationalism, which had previously seemed at odds with British policies and sentiments, was now right behind the cause of Empire. 'Remember that when the Empire is at war, so is Australia at war', said the former Prime Minister Joseph Cook during the election campaign just before war was declared. On the same day Andrew Fisher, who became Prime Minister of the new Labor Government, promised that 'Australians will stand beside our own to help and defend her to our last man and our last shilling'. Prominent figures like Professor Wood who had been opposed to fighting the Boers actively promoted the imperial cause. Support for involvement in the war with Germany was almost unanimous. But in serving that cause Australian nationalism had to be recognized. Australian soldiers had shown at the Boer War that they were different from the British, and General Bridges had decided that they should fight as a coherent national force with a distinct national identity: 'I want a name that will sound well when they call us by our initials' he said, finally settling on the 'Australian Imperial Force', his own suggestion.[3]

Huge crowds cheered the newly formed battalions of the AIF as they marched through their State capitals for embarkation overseas. Censorship of all information relating to the AIF's subsequent movements was strictly enforced, and the convoy of Australian merchant vessels that assembled with the New Zealand contingent at Albany on the south coast of Western Australia in October 1914 took the further precaution of a delay to avoid German raiders known to be in the Indian Ocean. The troops' prevailing spirit of derring-do encouraged defiance of the censorship rules. As the convoy of vulnerable merchant ships steamed westward on 1 November, escorted by ships of the Royal Navy, one soldier slid down a rope to pass a letter for posting by a tug crewman. But the censor still got it. In this carnival atmosphere Australia's young manhood was going to war as if to an international picnic or sporting contest which, if they did not hurry they might miss. The censor was just a dry old kill-joy.[4]

The Australian censorship had to be constructed quickly from the barest of guidelines set down by Bridges' defence scheme. Not surprisingly the structure and *modus operandi* of each district office bore the stamp of its first chief's approach to this new and delicate task. Drawing on his background and contacts in the University and the Australian Intelligence Corps, Wilson took over rooms above the General Post Office where he recruited and trained staff to work with the press and to selectively censor postal articles. His initial full-time staff of 12 included two assistant censors, who were ex-Intelligence Corps colleagues, another was Mungo MacCallum's son Mungo (or 'Boy') and several were older men from the reserve of officers. His part-time squad of interpreters included University colleagues, Professors Holme and Todd and Assistant Professor Nicholson. By September five of his full-time staff had transferred to other work, two of their replacements being the Professor of Engineering, S H E Barraclough, and another Intelligence Corps colleague, R N Teece. Two more interpreters were taken on in October to cope with huge piles of foreign mail and by early 1915 the staff numbered 18. University colleagues continued to be a reservoir of talent which Wilson probably recruited personally. G V Portus for example, a recent Rhodes Scholar on the point of changing from preacher to historian, was summoned by Wilson to join the censorship at the end of 1915. 'I told him of my tentative plan of serving the RAMC' recalled Portus, 'but he overruled that and said he wanted me at once for a particular job. Glad to be told authoritatively what to do, I agreed. So it came about that I spent the next three years as an Assistant Military Censor in Sydney.'[5]

In the early months the censors had frequently to follow up with military intelligence on reports by nervous civilians of flashing lights, radio transmissions and suspicious behaviour of all sorts. 'I wonder if you get all our myriad scare stories up at Nimity' wrote Wilson to Jeanie on 29 September. 'We are getting callous down [here]. It takes a real scary one to get our hair erect.' But a few early frights did make the censors wary. In the first week firms with German connections were found to have set up a system to evade the censor by transmitting overseas telegrams from remote coastal towns. On 28 October the Melbourne *Argus* published a photograph of the embarkation of troops 'with the permission of military authorities', an indiscretion which, the Naval Board pointed out, put at risk a fleet of merchant ships carrying 30,000 men. This and two similar incidents served to smarten up coordination between the Australian censorship offices and between the Army

and the Navy. Independent Naval censorship under the control of
the Naval Board was established in December 1914, commanded by
another former colleague of Wilson's from the AIC, Arthur Jose.
Newspapers were stopped from leaving the country within a
fortnight of publication and all subsequent information about the
embarkation of troops was censored.[6]

Censorship command at military headquarters in Melbourne
passed rapidly from Colonel McCay to Lt Col. Tunbridge and then
to Colonel John Monash as each chief was assigned a command in
the AIF. When his turn came Monash sent a telegram to Wilson on
13 September, asking him to take over as Deputy Chief Censor.
Wilson's sense of duty forbade him refusing outright but it would
have meant a great personal upheaval and his reply the same day
dwelt on his poor state of health

> I would greatly prefer to be left to fill my small niche here than to
> take the more responsible position in Melbourne. For one thing I
> am subject to long continuous attacks of dyspepsia brought on by
> worry and lack of exercise. I am suffering in this way at the present
> time and have to diet myself rather carefully. I have hopes that I am
> improving but I am by no means anxious to increase my
> responsibilities. Whilst I will not go to the lengths of absolutely
> refusing if it were requisite in the interests of the service that I
> should accept, I hope I have sufficiently indicated my personal
> disinclination to assume the higher office and my reason for it.
> Nevertheless I am prepared to put personal inclinations aside if any
> really useful purpose will be served by my doing so.

Colonel Hall took over as Deputy Chief Censor ten days later, and
Monash left to command Australian troops in action at Gallipoli
and in France. Wilson settled down in his niche in Sydney for the
next 16 months at a job that Monash described as 'most worrying,
anxious and strenuous'. It had a high casualty rate.[7]

In October Wilson's staff opened an envelope addressed to
Columbia University in New York from a respected fellow scientist,
containing a letter dated 29 September for re-direction to his wife in
Germany, which dented Wilson's faith in the international
community of science. It was from Dr F Graebner, an
anthropologist who visited Australia to attend the 84th Meeting of
the British Association, one of the seven German scientists whom
Professor Masson had gone to great lengths to protect by obtaining
expressions of hospitality from the Commonwealth Government
and an undertaking that they be allowed, after the meeting, to travel

to a neutral country. Two of them, Dr Graebner and Dr Pringsheim
who were reserve officers of the German army, were first required to
take an oath of neutrality. They refused, so could not leave, but the
authorities decided to allow them to pursue their studies in Australia
with minimal supervision while the war lasted. Dr Graebner
changed his mind, taking the oath on 12 October, but then an
outraged Wilson read Graebner's letter to his wife via an American
address, repudiating that oath in no uncertain terms: the Allies were
'Entente-Bandits', England 'the laboratory of hypocrisy' and her
government indulging in 'utterly loathsome conduct', parading 'as
the virtuous defender of oppressed innocence'. 'England above all
must get the coup de grace.' And finally: 'Police called 7/10/14.
Had to take the so called oath of neutrality or go to camp.' Wilson
showed Graebner's letter to the Commandant, 2nd Military
District, and on 16 October the Minister for Defence revoked
permission for Graebner to leave Australia on parole. A good thing
too according to Major R S Sands, Commandant of the German
Concentration Camp at Liverpool on the outskirts of Sydney where
Graebner was interned. His opinion of Graebner was that 'to trust
this man would be to fondle a serpent'. Wilson agreed. For him,
henceforth, the German scientist was as tainted as any other with
the poison of 'The Hun'. Feelings on both sides by now were
vehement and violent, beyond all reason.[8]

As well as the mail and the press, censorship interfered with a
wide range of information media including books, pamphlets,
periodicals (even the Government gazette), cartoons, speeches and
films. Its purpose was twofold: to maintain secrecy on information
useful to the enemy; and to prevent the spread of demoralizing
alarm in the community by irresponsible rumour or enemy
propaganda. The latter called for systematic scrutiny of public and
private information at its point of outlet to the community, so
Wilson had to lay down a plethora of rules to guide his staff in
carrying out the growing list of regulations made by the Governor
General under the War Precautions Act. With characteristic
vehemence Wilson insisted on strict observance of them. Portus
tripped up more than once. 'I made several mistakes in interpreting
our voluminous instructions' he wrote many years later, 'which I was
told, by an irate senior who was the author of most of them, might
well have cost us the war. Fortunately they did not.' He did once
'have to eat a piece of paper on which was written a secret address,
lest it should fall into the hands of the uncircumcised.'[9]

The postal censors concentrated on external mail and the

241

correspondence of suspects and internees to prevent useful information from reaching the enemy, trace the lines of enemy trade (a complex matter which uncovered an alarming degree of German involvement in the metal industries), and detect disloyalty, enemy sympathizers and propaganda. How censorship should be applied to prisoners of war was a question Wilson dealt with in a report to his chief late in 1915. Wilson pointed out that the conventions of war allowed them to receive newspapers from their own country subject to censorship as to contents, but that that privilege meant nothing if pro-enemy matter was 'regarded as inadmissible to Prisoners' Camps'. On the other hand he saw no difficulty in prisoners receiving locally published material. The Commandant, 2nd Military District, thought enemy newspapers would only stir up discontent, citing the case of a 'disturbance at Liverpool [POW camp] which ended in the shooting of a prisoner [that] coincided with the reported capture of Warsaw'. Prisoners had to be content with the local newspapers. The censoring of prisoners' mail became a major task for Wilson's staff: 4,000 letters a week, requiring linguists in all the main European languages plus others including Persian, Chinese and Afghan.[10]

Mail handled by the navy and army censors showed that Australian servicemen took a long time, especially the officers among whom Monash was said to be a chronic offender, to appreciate that the clues in their letters could be valuable to the other side. The home-based censors had similarly to remove a lot of innocent-seeming news or gossip from civil mails, a habit Wilson found hard to shake off: 'it is difficult for a Censor to write letters' he wrote to Jeanie after only six weeks in the job. 'I feel inclined to blue pencil all I have written just from the Censor's natural perverse instincts. There are so few subjects too which are not censorable.'[11]

Press censorship was much more difficult and contentious. Bridges, who had a powerful distrust of the press, had drawn up orders for wartime controls which to his surprise in 1914 the press dutifully observed. Press relations with the censor were clarified by the issue of a set of instructions for newspapers on 28 September but this did not avoid frequent press complaint, sometimes about breaches by other papers. The Sydney *Mirror* was a frequent offender and as early as 30 October Wilson's office was authorized to seize any copies of the paper containing reference to torpedoed Australian Transport. In 1915 he placed a censor in the *Mirror* office which eventually had to submit copy on all naval and military matters before publication. The press deeply resented the censor's powers under the War Precautions Act to enforce his rulings and friction worsened as censorship mutilated the sense of cable messages and instructions forbade the publication of certain items. Critics included the editor of the *Sydney Morning Herald* T W Heney, who was 'heartily in accord with the Imperial policy and [a supporter] of the Australian Government'. Exasperated journalists found that 'when they had got beyond clerks and embryo reporters, and had reached to university lecturers or even professors, they had at last to take the word of command from a Deputy Chief Censor who had no personal knowledge of journalism, and who apparently never troubled to acquaint himself with the hours, routine, or system, of a morning or an evening newspaper'.[12]

The reading public was being kept largely ignorant of tragic and terrible action on the battlefields of Gallipoli and France, but uneasiness grew as long casualty lists began to be released. Journalists, parliamentarians and the general public found it hard to accept that news passed by the censor in Britain was prohibited from publication in Australia, but the Prime Minister defended the censors. The press was irked by a system which operated as a branch of military and naval administration (unlike Canadian censorship which was vested in a committee of the principal government departments). Organization and methods with the public were questioned, rather than the need for effective censorship: Australia's large commitments to remote theatres of war carried higher transport risks than crossing the English Channel, and remoteness was no barrier to the enemy obtaining useful intelligence from Australia. The censor had to stand firm, and his actions when tested by recalcitrant papers like the *Mirror* made him an easy target. Almost everyone, as Wilson later observed, 'indulged in jeers and jibes and often enough in bitter attacks upon those who were endeavouring to protect the national interest under the seal of official silence and secrecy'.[13]

Wartime controls over all aspects of trade with the enemy led to widespread surveillance of commerce. John Hattrick, a Scottish chemist and the Australian manager for a German supplier of potash, approached Wilson in December 1914 about cabling back to his employer so as to accept salary payments specially authorized by the German Chancellor for the previous three months and Wilson telegraphed his chief on 27 December for approval. The Attorney General's view was that Hattrick's relations with his employer did not break the law if he intended merely to keep the office open so as to resume business after the war. But suspicion fell on Hattrick in March 1915 when, after being told by MacCallum of Wilson's office he could have no further communication with Germany, he unwisely posted three letters intended for Berlin but addressed to intermediaries in the USA, Holland and Sweden so as to evade the censor. Hattrick's naivety in trying to keep in touch with his employer looked more serious after the Attorney General, William Morris Hughes, decided to break the hold of German firms on the market for Australian resources, in particular the lead, copper and zinc needed to produce munitions. For Hughes, and for most Australians including Wilson, the issue was now clear: total war was a new phenomenon requiring the efficient organization of all the Empire's men and resources in total national commitment. Hughes' proposition conflicted with international commercial law and ethics (which would have merely suspended trade contracts with the enemy during wartime) so the British government and Australian producers equivocated. But Hughes achieved his purpose by passing the Enemy Contracts Annulment Act in May 1915. This made any hint of a German connection suspicious. Hattrick's membership of the Woollahra Rifle Club, efforts to become the agent for 'an entirely British' firm, and technical advice to the Munitions Committee on the production of gun cotton and glycerine were not enough to prevent his arrest in March 1916 'on false information prompted by malice of a worthless son of a german in sydney', according to David Hall the NSW Attorney General in his telegram to the Minister for Defence on 14 April 1916. For a month Hall protested at the internment without trial of Hattrick, a British citizen, in the belief that the Australian people 'would rather endure the possible injury done to the Empire by its enemies by bringing men to trial, than the certain outrage that will overtake Australian citizens if their liberties are to be entrusted to any military body'. The Minister authorized an 'in camera' inquiry, held over four days in May/June, and Hattrick was finally released in December 1916. Early in 1917 he returned to Britain. The government used the censorship service to pursue its investigation of industry involved in the trade in metals, leading to some highly respected figures being accused of disloyalty by Hughes, who was now Prime Minister. In time the censorship itself would become the focus of contention on another issue in which Hughes passionately believed: conscription.[14]

As 'Censor, Sydney', Wilson was the first to learn of NSW casualties. Among them were friends, ex-students and the sons of colleagues and friends, and in many cases Wilson felt obliged to break the news to their families himself. Time and again he put himself through these ordeals and the Wilson family was plunged into grief for their friends. The first Australian killed in the war, on 11 September 1914, was a former medical student and a friend of Jeanie's, Brian Antill Pockley, a member of the Army Medical Corps in the Expeditionary Force sent to capture German New Guinea, in which Mabel's nephew Julian Simpson also served. On 27 April 1915 at Gallipoli, two days after the landing, Wilson's colleague from the Scottish Rifles and son of the late Chancellor of Sydney University, Col. H N MacLaurin, was killed in action. Others who were friends of the Wilsons included W R Aspinall, Egerton and Robert Clunies Ross, Edwin Hutchinson, Clement Rennie, Adrian Stephen, Lawrence Street, and the Dight Walker brothers from the Woollahra Presbyterian Church: 'we prayed for them for years', wrote Louise, 'in vain alas'.[15]

The wild enthusiasm with which Australians entered the war had subsided after a year. They now realized that the landing at Gallipoli was triumphant proof that Australian soldiers were superb fighters; and a tragedy. The accounts that filtered through the censor, and from the beginning of May the long casualty lists, were greeted with a confusion of pride and grief. Then on 24 May came the news that General Bridges, creator of the AIF and its first commander in the field, was dead. By August when his body was returned to Australia for a military funeral – the only soldier to be so honoured in that war – there were families in mourning all over the country. His funeral procession, in Melbourne on 2 September and the next day at the Duntroon Royal Military College in Canberra, was followed by large crowds. It stood for thousands who would not be brought home. The miracle of an evacuation in December that cost not one additional life to the 7,594 already lost in eight months of holding a tiny triangle of Turkish soil, gave Christmas 1915 some joy in the blur of sadness and disappointment for the survivors and their families, and for Mr Hughes who left Australia on 20 January 1916 'to say the things that need saying' to the British Government about the conduct of the war.[16]

In the early days of the war there had been talk of Sydney University closing down, so heavy was the response of staff, students and graduates. But its affairs were not seriously disrupted despite the many staff vacancies. Professor Barraclough left the University, and the censorship, in October 1915 to direct the work of 5,000 Australian munition workers in Britain and France. His secretary young Marnie Masson, the daughter of Melbourne's Professor Orme Masson and a close friend of the Wilson family, accompanied him.

Professor Edgeworth David ingeniously manoeuvred himself into active service at the age of 58: he initiated the formation of the Australian Mining Corps, then contrived his appointment to it and went to France, where his doctor son William was also serving.[17]

The war gave the stimulus of urgency to the University's medical faculty because it increased the demand for medical services. More students and fewer staff produced great pressures. Professor Sir Thomas Anderson Stuart (he was knighted in 1914) offered himself as Principal Medical Officer of the Forces of New south Wales but the Defence Department turned him down. He lectured to soldiers on fitness and to sailors on elementary anatomy and physiology; he accelerated the flow of medical graduates by virtually abolishing the vacations and facilitated the enlistment of medical students to war service as soon as they were allowed under government policy (after their third year); and he threw the resources of the Royal Prince Alfred Hospital behind the war effort. A E Mills, lecturer in medicine, enlisted in May 1915 but was fated to frustrating inactivity with the Australian Army Medical Corps in London. Sir Alexander MacCormick (he was knighted in 1913) joined up in September 1914 and served at Gallipoli and in France with the Australian and British armies. His old comrade-in-arms Robert Scot Skirving, who was in England at the outbreak of war, served with the British army. His son Archibald, a fully qualified surgeon and in England to do his FRCS, enlisted in the Royal Irish Fusiliers as a combatant and, following the landing at Suvla Bay, died on board the *Valdivia* in August 1915 of abdominal wounds that both he and his father knew could have been successfully treated.[18]

Because of a ruling that only Australian residents could join the AIF, those who happened to be in Britain at the outbreak of war could only serve with its forces. Mabel Wilson's nephew Brian Simpson, who was in London, joined the Royal Horse Artillery and died of wounds in France in July 1915. A future son-in-law, Lloyd Hutchinson, who had sailed for England on 1 August 1914 to enter Cambridge University, joined the East Yorkshire Regiment and was twice wounded while serving at Gallipoli and in France. Sir Alexander MacCormick's son Campbell, on completion of his English schooling, joined the Argyll and Sutherland Highlanders and was killed in October 1916 near Loos in France, aged 19.[19]

A distinguished exception to the rule forbidding enlistment to the AIF from outside Australia was Wilson's great friend Charles Martin, Director of the Lister Institute in London. In July 1915 he was recruited to the 3rd Australian General Hospital, then in

London *en route* to the Dardenelles, because of his special
knowledge of typhoid fever, a serious problem at Gallipoli.
Vaccinated men were getting typhoid and on-site laboratory
investigation was required. With equipment begged, borrowed or
improvised, and with the resources of the Lister Institute to fall back
on, he established a pathological laboratory at Lemnos for the 3rd
Australian General Hospital and investigated every case of the fever
unaffected by the typhoid vaccine. His team then made and
standardized a new vaccine which gave immunity to typhoid and to
two recently-discovered paratyphoid organisms researchers had
labelled 'A' and 'B'. The Lister Institute then quickly produced the
new TAB vaccine in considerable quantity, enabling Australian
troops to be promptly inoculated, six months before the British.
Martin's scientific authority, easy manner and administrative ability
drew him into the task of integrating laboratory services into the
Australian army in France near the front line, at base hospitals and
at headquarters in England. He was then lent to the British army to
do likewise. Based at Rouen and backed mainly by Australian staff,
from 1917 Martin controlled the laboratories of the Southern
British Sector till the end of the war.[20]

Martin's counterpart in the British army was another friend of
Wilson's, Sir Almroth Wright. He and Martin had both spent part of
their early careers in the same job at the Sydney Medical School, and
both had become leaders in laboratory medicine in Britain: Wright
after making his name in the fight against typhoid fever during the
Boer War, Martin with his work at the Lister Institute. Both knew
that the products of War – overcrowding, insanitary conditions, dirty
and ragged wounds – would sweep away the barriers erected by
civilized society to the spread of infection and disease. At the
outbreak of war Martin mobilized the mass production of tetanus
anti-toxin and Wright from his laboratory at St Mary's Hospital in
London produced anti-typhoid vaccine. Appointed in September
1914 as a Colonel in the Army Medical Service, Wright quickly set
up a laboratory on the roof of the Casino at Boulogne to combat the
horrors of septic infection. Every day he witnessed the pain and
anguish of hundreds of wounded men lying shoulder to shoulder in
the great hall of the Casino knowing 'these wounded boys lose their
limbs or their lives through infection, which could – if we had the
knowledge – be cured'. One of these boys was Mabel's nephew, Brian
Simpson, who was wounded in Flanders in July 1915 after climbing
a tree in full view of the German lines to shoot a sniper. Almroth
Wright could not save him, but he was able to arrange for his mother

Lilian to see him before he died. In the same year Lilian was bereaved of her husband John Ashburton Thomson, her father-in-law Sir George Simpson and her daughter Norah's fiancé who was killed in France. By the end of that year there were no longer any illusions about the war: it was a black iniquity which would not end soon.[21]

Wilson had lasted much longer than most of the early censors but at the end of 1915 he advised that he wished to retire from the job. He had begun the year abnormally fatigued though a week of rest at Bayview in early April had restored him enough to do some hard physical work without more than physical tiredness. By July he was again exhausted and by the year's end he had bankrupted his physical reserves. On 7 December the Deputy Chief Censor, Colonel Hall, arranged for him to be 'relieved from anything but necessary duty at once'. Promoted Honorary Colonel in recognition of his service, he ceased duty altogether as 'Censor, Sydney' on 1 January 1916. Two months later his replacement Laurens Armstrong resigned and Wilson's old friend Hubert Foster, who by then was Chief of the General Staff, sounded him out for a possible return or a successor. Wilson recommended Professor Nicholson who was thorough and systematic like himself. An alert journalist, perceiving Wilson's imminent departure, sent him an unsolicited testimonial:

> At first everyone was new to the work and there were mistakes on both sides and misunderstandings on the part of the press. This was soon righted, and for the greater of the term the censorship has been in operation it has, in my humble opinion, been conducted with consideration and judgement, under difficult conditions. Personally I desire to thank you for the willingness and promptitude wherewith all reasonable requests and suggestions made on behalf of our association have been received and acted upon, and for the way our business has been handled by the censors' department.[22]

For a year and a half the war had taken a 24-hour station in his household, with Wilson rarely getting home before midnight and then being on-call to the military and the police. He had fitted out a small dressing room as a bedroom with desk and phone so that Mabel would not be disturbed, but that put him close to the verandah and the beds of his young and early-rising children. They became as familiar as generations of medical students with his stentorian bellow for peace and quiet, but enjoyed his close presence nevertheless, as he did theirs. The children had thought at first that this exciting wartime regime must surely bring an end to school. But it was not to be and before long they discovered, through Mabel's war work with the local branch of the Red Cross, the additional challenge of learning to knit scarves, socks and balaclavas for soldiers.[23]

Wilson took up the full harness of his university offices again from the start of the academic year in March 1916 when he was re-elected Chairman of the Professorial Board, an office that now entitled him to a seat on the Senate. Despite the pressures of the censorship he had kept in touch with research through close association with the work of Dr Reg E Nowland (a prosector of 1911) on the treatment of acute epidemic cerebrospinal meningitis at Royal Prince Alfred Hospital, and by spending one night a week in the Anatomy Department with Raymond Dart trying to unravel the mysteries of Froriep's ganglion. 'In all seriousness' said Dart 'he would tell me, "This is the only way I can relax and gain a respite."' Dart had completed his BSc at the brand-new University of Queensland before enrolling for medicine in Sydney in 1914. For two and a half years, till he graduated in August 1917, Dart was Wilson's assistant. It was an association which Dart 40 years later recalled was 'intimate and treasured.... His influence on me was so great that even today, I find myself guided by the standards he implanted in my young mind ... his interests were automatically mine....' Dart saw this research project as part of Wilson's continuing fascination with the problems of evolution.

> With his Darwinian respect for all vestigial anatomical structures, the transitional area between the brain and the spinal cord had evoked from him an earlier paper on the area postrema of the *medulla oblongata*. He probably suspected that this vestigial sensory nucleus of the hypoglossal nerve, the last cranial nerves and one supplying the muscles of the tongue, should also throw light on the evolutionary history of the hinder part of the brain. No problem could have enthralled me more profoundly. How many body segments had been needed to make the human head?[24]

Wilson's work with Dart on Froriep's ganglion, like much of his research, did not appear in print. He put this disparity between work and publication down to laziness, which was manifestly untrue: it was more likely his passion for thoroughness and his aversion to writing, and because he did not feel proprietorial about his projects. As Dart observed,

> he loved collaboration but the giving would be all his, just as he helped unstintingly all his fellow scientists: to him that community of interest was reward enough.[25]

Like his venerated mentor, Raymond Dart stretched himself in university affairs, combining research and a crowded medical course with the positions of demonstrator of anatomy, tutor in biology at St Andrew's College and secretary of the Sydney University Medical Society. And it was he who drew to Wilson's attention a new rising star in the medical school: John Irvine Hunter, in his second year in 1916, was showing a versatile brilliance reminiscent of the young Grafton Elliot Smith who, during the Australian tour of the British Association in 1914, had reminded his Alma Mater and Australia at large of his great capacities. Like Elliot Smith, Hunter blossomed in the medical school, and both were attracted to neurology. According to Wilson it was in teaching that Hunter really found himself, first in the private coaching thrust upon him by economic necessity and later as a demonstrator and lecturer. For Hunter and Dart the glamour of Elliot Smith's career added to the attractions of medical research, but the most significant influence in the intellectual development of all three was their professor, Wilson.[26]

He always had a project on hand, the harvest thereof being delivered informally over tea or in more formal talks like the one he gave in July 1916 to the Sydney University Medical Society on 'some facts which have not yet become the current coin of textbook literature' concerning the neurones of the sensory ganglia. Essentially this paper was an updating of his 1908 address to the Australasian Medical Congress on developments in neurology, and focused on two questions of special interest. Firstly there was the method, as yet not explained, by which single nerve fibres transmit a variety of messages – pain, temperature, touch, pressure and muscle sense – from the periphery of the body to the central nervous system. Wilson thought this capacity might be explained by neuronal structural differentiation but researchers were as yet unable 'to pick out this or that group of ganglionic neurones as being dedicated to the conveyance of any particular subvariety of peripheral sensibility'. Secondly there was the question of the enlarged sensory nerve cells and how they acquire highly specialized functions as an individual grows to maturity. Wilson drew attention to the important work of Henry Head at the London Hospital, citing a paper he published in *Brain* in 1915, and to the proposition by S W Ranson of the Northwestern University Medical School in Illinois, also in *Brain* 1915, that the capacity of primitive nerve fibres could be due to the development of a myelin sheath. Wilson thought this interesting idea could be tested 'by education of the senses' to answer the question 'Could a protopathic [primitive] nerve fibre ever become epicritical [finely discriminatory, e.g. to touch, heat] in its functional capacity?' – an apparently simple suggestion typical of Wilson, produced by his long preoccupation with the neurology, embryology and phylogeny of mammals.[27]

The times did not favour research, for these were dark and anxious days. Throughout 1916, despite monstrous losses, the fighting in France hovered between stalemate and disaster. At Pozieres where the AIF fought a great battle in July, August and September, Australian casualties rose to nearly 23,000, all to no avail. Prime Minister Hughes returned to Australia on 31 July, just as the first news of those losses was beginning to arrive. Weary from his rousing tour of Britain and France, and jaundiced like the troops of British army leadership, he still held a passionate belief in the British cause. To execute the new strategy to win the war within a year – by relentless and sustained pressure on a narrow front to break the German lines – Hughes believed conscription was the only way to reverse declining recruitment and provide the AIF with the reinforcements essential for that effort. In May 1916 Britain had adopted this course and New Zealand did so in August, but during Hughes' absence the prospect of conscription had begun to stir up deep divisions in Australia.

The 1911 scheme of compulsory military service in Australia was not for expeditionary purposes; it was for the defence of the country against an invading enemy. Only the Navy was seen to be needed in an Empire war. The massive and urgent military needs of the Empire in Europe in 1916 were beyond all imaginings of 1911 and conscription seemed to Hughes and Australia's military leaders the only way of meeting Australia's imperial obligations. But by 1916 opposition to conscription by organized labour, both industrial and political, had solidified. The Labor movement opposed 'militarism' on principle, fearing contingent industrial conscription and the loss of hard-won working conditions, and it resented the censorship and the police as agencies hindering the anti-conscription cause. Campaigning for conscription were the Australian Natives Association, a friendly society with a strong patriotic flavour, the Universal Service League formed in Sydney in September 1915 (an updated National Defence League), and most of the press, leading academics and Protestant church leaders. Sectarianism, never far below the surface in Australian life, erupted again with Irish Catholic antagonism to British war purposes given fresh stimulus in April 1916 by the ruthless military suppression of the Easter Rising in Dublin. 'I wish Ireland was at the bottom of the

sea' exclaimed an exasperated Mabel Wilson, unfortunately in the
hearing of an Irish maid who forthwith announced 'I'm leaving!'
Mabel's calm and astute management of the Wilson household was
tested as she on the domestic front absorbed the stresses of these
contention-ridden days, while out in the community Wilson
campaigned for conscription.[28]

Lacking the full support of his party, and even his Cabinet,
Prime Minister Hughes appealed for popular approval of
conscription for overseas service by referendum, fixed for 28
October. He toured the nation in an all-out effort to secure a 'Yes'
vote, while governing the country in nomad fashion. Like most of
his generation, certainly his peers, Wilson supported Hughes'
mission and argued for it in his own areas of influence, primarily the
University. He represented Hughes as the responsible head of
government with 'full knowledge of the case', which few would have
disputed: it was a grievance of Australian citizens that the censorship
deprived them of full knowledge. But the urgency of that case many
did dispute, for the numbers of men sought by the British
Government as reinforcements for the AIF did seem suspiciously
high. In his public speeches Wilson challenged the views of the anti-
conscriptionists in a series of questions:

> Is the Allied cause just? Is the task accomplished? Should Great
> Britain be involved? Should Australia be involved? Are we or are we
> not part of the British people? Has Australia done enough? Should
> Mr Fisher's pledge to fight 'to the last shilling and the last man' be
> repudiated because the going was too tough? Should Australia's five
> divisions of volunteers not be reinforced? What of honour and duty?

A 'no' vote would be a 'war' vote he concluded, for it would
lengthen the war and cost more lives. Compulsory service lay at the
root of all citizenship:

> Govt. of the people for the people & by the people involves all sorts
> of compulsion in civic duty in personal behaviour & in defence of
> the common weal against aggression. Only in the deepest things of
> the individual soul may the individual claim immunity from
> compulsion.[29]

The Australian people rejected conscription by a narrow margin, less
than 4 per cent of the valid votes, after a campaign that exposed deep
antagonisms in the nation – political, social, economic and sectarian –
and led to bitter and enduring divisions. The Labor Government was
scuttled by the 1916 referendum result and in January 1917 Hughes

and the Labor ministers loyal to him formed a National Government with leaders of the Liberal Party which won convincingly at the general election in May. The United States entered the war in April employing a form of conscription called 'selective service', but it was temporarily off the Australian Government's agenda: Hughes had promised before the election that he would not introduce conscription without the consent of the people, and only 'if the tide of battle which flows strongly for the Allies turns against them'. The Canadians introduced conscription in August.[30]

The University did not need to be persuaded by Wilson's sophisticated and cogent advocacy for it was a stronghold for conscription, the only centre of resistance being the Catholic St John's College. From the beginning of the war voluntary enlistment by staff and students was strong, but a Defence Department ruling prevented medical students from doing so until they had completed their third year. Johnny Hunter formed the determination to enlist while in his second year of medicine, waiting till the Christmas long vacation to join the ranks down in Albury on the New South Wales-Victorian border where he had attended high school. He had paid farewell visits to relatives and friends by the time an official notice arrived ordering him to return to his studies. It was widely supposed that Anderson Stuart had intervened, but in fact it was Wilson and he had made the long journey to Albury to do so. Many years later he explained his reason: 'He had such a frail body and such a brilliant mind I couldn't let him do it.'[31]

Conscription was one national issue that engaged the University's ardent concern in late 1916. Another was the spread of venereal disease, an alarming health problem greatly exacerbated by the conditions of war. Under the stimulus of a British Royal Commission Report and State and Commonwealth Government inquiries a group of fifth-year medical students led by Raymond Dart organized a University Society for Combating Venereal Diseases. Its inaugural meeting of 300 staff, students and graduates at the Union on 12 October was presided over by Anderson Stuart and addressed by Wilson and D A Welsh the Professor of Pathology. Student zeal, as revealed by the published proceedings of this launch, exaggerated the University's scientific, educational and moral resources to meet the problem, and couched the Society's aims in a high-flown exegesis of the civic role of the University, redolent of Wilson's views on that subject:

> ...it is essentially from a University that there should pour those
> streams of beneficent social influence and enlightenment without

which no problem, with such deep roots and ramifications as that
of venereal disease, can be adequately solved. A University is not
merely a school of professional training ... its highest purpose ... is
to provide a source of light and leading to the whole community ...
a guide to all who seek knowledge that will fit them to play their
part in the uplifting of the race.

If this reflects Wilson's influence it also caricatures his argument. In
his address Wilson pulled attention from the 'comprehensive and
optimistic' down to the practical, the need to limit and concentrate
efforts in certain definite areas. Venereal disease should be treated as
far as possible like any other transmissible disease and the source of
the difficulty, moral stigma, combated by education, in particular
the sex education of the young: 'it is high time we gave up the
assiduous cultivation of ignorance in these matters'. On the
associated problem of prostitution Wilson could not agree with the
'realists' that it was an ineradicable vice, though he conceded that it
was 'more fundamental ... both physiologically and sociologically,
than easygoing optimists imagine'. As a 'convinced evolutionist' he
argued that there had been progress in sexual morality from
promiscuity through polygamy in some cases, and polyandry in
others, to a condition of monogamy; to legally recognize and
regulate prostitution as some advocated would be to return to a
system of slavery. Before the end of 1916 the WEA organized a
conference on 'Teaching of Sex Hygiene' in which Wilson
participated. He served the Society as chairman of its executive
committee during 1917–18 when it boasted a membership of over
600, and organized lectures, conferences and other meetings
'inspiring all who desire to do their share of social service'. Wilson
was high-minded but no prude.[32]

Wilson was in demand everywhere, partly because professorial
ranks were depleted, partly because of his growing influence in the
University. His military associations made him an appropriate figure
for war-related ceremonies or activities at the University. He was
continually being asked to address societies, contribute articles to
Hermes or read the lesson at church services. All this was in addition
to the usual administrative university affairs. In March 1918 he
complained that 'Meetings are the plague of my life – Senate, Prof
Bd & Committees & Boards of all sorts. One cant get one's proper
work done for them' and 'there are always either on hand or
looming ahead little duties outside of one's regular work which add
to one's burden a good deal'. But as Mabel observed, 'He always says

that he has far too many committees to attend to, but he wont hear of giving any of them up.'[33]

For the first two and a half years of the war the executive powers of the Empire for war purposes rested solely with the British Cabinet. Then 'it at last became clear to the rulers of Great Britain that a Cabinet representing all the self-governing States of the Empire was a necessity'. The new Lloyd George government invited the Dominions to an Imperial War Cabinet in the spring of 1917, on the eve of the planned Allied break-through in France. Hughes wanted to go in order to see that the problem of Home Rule for Ireland, which weakened the Empire morally and in the field, was settled as an *Imperial* question. But because of the May election Australia did not attend. At a War Conference held after the Cabinet meetings, which lasted from 20 March to 2 May, the Dominions made it clear that they wanted recognition as 'autonomous nations of an Imperial Commonwealth' after the war. In France the Allies did not burst through to victory as General Haig had predicted, and for Australia 1917 became the worst year of the war. The 'heroic, bloody and bungled' battles of Bullecourt produced 23,000 Australian casualties and a drastic drop in troops' morale; in the mud of Passchendale there were 38,000 more casualties in October and November. The collapse of the Russian army added to the deteriorating position in Europe and the revolutionary rhetoric of anti-war groups in Australia.[34]

The war weariness of all the belligerent countries was fostering social and industrial unrest. Eastern Australia, immobilized by a massive transport strike from August to October, seemed under threat of union action aimed at destruction of the state. Hughes, overstrained by the war and isolated after splitting from the Labor Party, thought he saw a traitorous alliance of Irish Sinn Feiners, the Catholic Church, members of the Industrial Workers of the World (IWW or 'Wobblies') – a small but active organization of American origin operating in Sydney since 1907 – and assorted anti-war groups. There was no alliance but all had their reasons for attacking the established order, with virulent advocacy of direct action in the case of the IWW. In September 1916 12 IWW members were charged with treason, later altered to arson and conspiracy after a series of fires in business premises in Sydney. There were acts of sabotage linked to dock workers: fires at Cockatoo Island Dockyard; the cruiser HMAS *Brisbane* deliberately disabled in October 1916 while docked in Sydney; in April the merchant ship SS *Cumberland* crippled by an explosion at sea, apparently in cargo loaded at a

Queensland port. The IWW was banned under the Unlawful Associations Act (1917), and early in that year special officers were appointed to military and naval intelligence to investigate security problems. In August demonstrations began to be held in favour of an immediate peace and the Stop the War movement gathered strength after the October Revolution in Russia.[35]

With enlistments down and reinforcements urgently needed in France, Hughes on 8 November announced a second referendum on conscription, set for Thursday 20 December. This campaign was even more bitter than the first, conducted in an atmosphere of violence: Hughes' life was threatened when a bomb exploded in his garden and he took to carrying a pistol as he once again stumped the country for a 'Yes' vote. Leadership on the 'No' side came from the oratory of the new Archbishop of Melbourne, Irish-born Daniel Mannix, and the political skill of the Premier of Queensland, T J Ryan, who managed to get a censored anti-conscription pamphlet published in *Hansard* a few days before Hughes was due to speak in Brisbane. This provoked Commonwealth seizure involving military action against Queensland police, and set the scene for confrontations on 27 and 28 November and a hysterical encounter next day at Warwick between Hughes and Irish Catholic supporters of Mannix. The violence of the campaign reached a climax among a crowd of 100,000 people in Melbourne on 10 December where hundreds of eggs, road metal and broken pieces of glass were hurled at the speakers.[36]

Hughes had already approved the augmenting of Military Intelligence and on 1 December Colonel Wilson – he had been transferred to the unattached list on 6 October – and Mr A G Ralston KC were recalled to duty as honorary advisers to NSW Military Intelligence, General Staff. Detailed orders were issued to Military Districts: 'In view of the possibility that there may be organised opposition, and possibly rioting and even an armed insurrection in the event of conscription being enforced', Intelligence Sections were to make 'inquiries as to the persons who might organise or lead any such opposition and as to their plans'. Wilson and Ralston were to advise the Commandant in New South Wales on the significance of the information collected and 'the scope of any further inquiries they think desirable'. The Australian people again rejected conscription, this time by a margin of 8 per cent, but civil unrest did not cease. Wilson's advisory role with the Intelligence Section brought him into regular contact with T R Bavin and J G Latham, of Naval Intelligence, and E E Longfield

Lloyd of NSW Military Intelligence. They met in the Section's offices which at first were located discreetly in the Commonwealth Bank Building in Martin Place, but after the presence of the Section became common knowledge it was moved to Victoria Barracks.[37]

In April 1918, with Europe suffering the final German offensive in France, Wilson once again delivered the annual address to the University Medical Society, entitled 'The "Social Inheritance" and the Undergraduates' Share in it'. He reappraised his personal philosophy against the exigencies of the times. The Hegelian parable of progress he stood by, and he reviewed the evolution and elaboration of civilized society with all its great achievements: a priceless 'social inheritance' which the University to a large extent embodied and had a duty to enrich and transmit from one generation to the next. The ideal of university life was to train its students in character, culture and craftsmanship to serve society as citizens. The present threat to civilization was unprecedented, but since the warring parties had a common heritage there was some hope for its survival. On the other hand, like a higher organism which is delicately adapted to its environment, Western civilization would be far less tolerant of gross disturbances than simpler societies of earlier times. His conclusion was chilling:

> As those sons of the University counted not their lives too dear, but freely offered them in the righteous cause of their country, so may you also be ready to spend and be spent in the service of the community, whether in peace or in war. So shall you realise the best that is in you. It is the only way. Nothing greater on this earth can you aspire to. Nothing less is justly claimed from you.[38]

This Idealist creed, drawn from the teaching of T H Green and fashioned in tranquil Victorian Oxford, when none could imagine that civilized Europe would be mired in the carnage of a terrible war that would make Idealism dated and inadequate, sustained Wilson throughout his life. The young men he now addressed, respectful though they were of this man 'whom no amount of stamping would ever frighten', were not so sure of any eternal truths, or eternal progress. As the desolating lessons of modern warfare were slowly absorbed they would look for explanations that accounted better for tragedy, capricious fate and the baser aspects of man's nature. But in 1918 the personal adventure promised by the war still appealed to young medical men. So when, in accordance with the custom of the day, the new recruits among them lined up to say goodbye to their teachers, some were moved but more were amused by Wilson's saying a prayer over them, a half-hour sermon according to one recruit. Either way, another 'Jummy' anecdote was added to University folklore. But Wilson knew that two out of every three would be casualties and one in five would be killed.[39]

Wilson's relations with Anderson Stuart had long been estranged. In response to an unctuous 'forget and forgive' letter from A E Mills, Wilson had stated the case plainly in March 1916: while the difference between them was 'too radical and too essential' to permit genuine friendship, he was ready to restore friendly and collegiate relations. But he could not approach 'one who has deliberately chosen to cut me dead when he passes within a yard on the road or in the precincts of the University ... I cannot undertake to penetrate armour of this degree of resistance.' He could only hope that an opportunity would arise 'towards the amelioration of our present relations'. This did not happen, and in the middle of 1918 they clashed publicly about whether medical students should continue to be prevented from serving in the war until after they had completed the third year of their studies.[40]

Following German successes in the spring of 1918 and General Haig's 'Backs to the Wall' rallying cry in May, the Australian Defence Department allowed minors to enlist without parental consent and removed the embargo on second and third year medical students. The latter issue ignited controversy. In the *Sydney Morning Herald* on 30 May, and again on 20 June, Anderson Stuart as Dean of Medicine pushed the view of an editorialist in the *Medical Journal of Australia*, who in turn relied on British practice imperfectly understood, that to use precious medical material as combatants was 'the acme of extravagant waste'. Since the war might well last five years it was in the interests both of the nation and the Empire to conserve medical expertise for future needs by sending medical students back to their books. To prevent the abuse of medical studies to avoid enlistment he recommended the British practice by which students were obliged to enlist when they entered medical school and be given leave to complete their courses, whereupon they received commissions and went to war. Failure in examinations meant a call to the colours forthwith.[41]

Wilson's rejoinders were immediate on both occasions. The *Medical Journal of Australia* was not speaking for the Australian medical profession, whose views had not been ascertained; nor was Anderson Stuart speaking on behalf of the medical faculty at the University. He held opposing views. Wilson believed that achieving the maximum manpower to meet 'the immediate, highly critical and probably decisive' situation in France was incomparably more important than making prudent medical provision for the future, which could be met perhaps by an early increase in the numbers of women medical students. He objected to a policy of compulsion whereby a medical student was forbidden to serve regardless of how he felt about the obligations of conscience, honour and tradition. Medical students should be applauded for accepting 'in common with their less favoured brethren all the risks of a soldier's life'. Anyway, the idea of obliging a student to enlist on medical enrolment was beside the point. '"Obliged to enlist!" By whom? Has Sir Thomas forgotten that the conscription campaign was lost? Nor has the University any right or power to reject otherwise qualified candidates who are of ordinary "good fame and character". The suggestion is perfectly futile.' Removal of the embargo simply meant that personal decisions for or against enlistment must now be made on independent grounds.[42]

This public argument mirrored the anxiety and division in the general community about the war and in particular recruitment. Public criticism focused on privileged university students who had not enlisted. In May 1918, as the 'only one unanswerable way of vindicating our honour', Assistant Professor Holme on behalf of the Undergraduates Association, launched the proposal of forming the Sydney University Company as a fighting unit to reinforce the AIF in France. The Senate approved the initiative and in support set up a Committee of Advice of its five leading Fellows which students and their parents could 'consult frankly and confidentially' before making the enlistment decision. Wilson was one of those counsellors, and among the 118 medical students who enlisted was Johnny Hunter. A total of 493 university recruits were in camp at Liverpool by the end of October.[43]

Sooner than anyone had imagined the war ended and the Armistice of 11 November was greeted with the relief of exhaustion. The University held a simple and dignified celebration in the Great Hall on 14 November, attended by 400 students. After a formal address to the King by Chancellor Cullen, Wilson made a speech condemning German repudiation of the ethical ideal of civilized humanity for the doctrine of force and the right of the strong, grounded they believed on evolutionary principles: a 'crude and shallow and doctrinaire interpretation of the Darwinian idea of "survival of the fittest" through natural selection'. From this perversion of Darwin's theory arose a mission in which the 'State-fettered universities of Germany showed themselves from the outset to be eager and willing instruments'. Justice and righteousness had prevailed because 'millions of free men of all the continents of the world' had sacrificed their lives.[44]

Great ideals were defended in this war by the British Empire and her allies. Western civilization had faced Armageddon and won through. But the war had been fought as if the side which suffered the most casualties would win. Australia's fallen – 60,000 dead and 120,000 wounded – and their reputation for valour, expanded the national self-consciousness of Australians and earned them an independent seat at the Peace Conference of Versailles and in the League of Nations. Australia won full nationhood by being blooded in a terrible Imperial war. There was irony in the fact that the nation which entered the conflict last and suffered the least casualties and the least disruption to its domestic affairs came out the victor in terms of power and influence. The United States of America, which commanded the Peace negotiations and weakened the peace by not joining the League of Nations, became the centre of the world's attention. The British Empire never recovered from the war. The Imperial idea was broadened to embrace the United States in a loose association of the English-speaking peoples, and its representation as an 'organism' with a centre and a periphery became an anachronism. The new image was of 'a chain of States round the world, each of which regarded itself as a centre of the whole'.[45]

Notes

1. Scott, 8, 14, 59, 200–2.
2. Establishing censorship: Scott 59–62, Coulthard-Clark 1976. Leave arrangements: JTW to JCR 13.9.14.
3. Cook's pledge at Colac in Victoria, and Fisher's at Horsham in Victoria, on 31.7.1914: quoted Scott, 22. Wood's pro-war reasoning: *Hermes*, Aug. 1915, 48–56. The AIF: Coulthard-Clark 1979, 118; Bean Vol. I, 36.
4. Incident at Albany: Scott, 83. War a picnic: Bean Vol. I, 43.
5. Sydney Censor's staff during Wilson's time also included: R S Murray-Prior, A R Wheeler, H Wilshire, E Brennan, Capt. C S Cape, Lt J W Cornforth, H A Rorke, J T C Richmond, Capt. S N Stokes, L F Vasok, A J K Taylor, A Archey, C M Smith, L F Smith, W E Vincent. AA, B543, file W363/4/700. See also, Military Orders for 1914 Nos 469, 510, 569, 654; for 1915 Nos 20, 69, 109, 143, 155, 590, 698, 735, 809; for 1916 No. 23. 'I told him': Portus, 163.
6. Early censorship frights: Scott, 67, 90, 106; Jose, 444. 'I wonder if':

JTW to J, 29.9.14.

7. Censorship headquarters: Scott 60–1. 'I would greatly': JTW to Monash, 13.9.1914. 'most worrying': Monash quoted in G Serle, 202.

8. German scientists: Scott, 32–5. Some authorities say there were seven German scientists, others say eight. Graebner and Pringsheim say seven in letter of 28.11.1918. 'Entente Bandits': Graebner, quoted Col. Wallack, Cdt of 2MD memo 20.10.1914 to Sec. Defence. 'to trust this man': R S Sands to AAG 2MD, 5.11.1914. All from AA, MP 367, file 567/8/403.

9. Censorship: Jose, 445. 'I made several' and 'have to eat': Portus, 164.

10. 'regarded as': JTW memo to Deputy Chief Censor, 3.12.1915, AA, MP 367, file 512/1/864. Postal censorship: Scott, 62, 82–3, 88–9.

11. Army and navy censors: Serle, 303; Jose, 55. 'it is difficult': JTW to J, 29.9.14.

12. 'heartily in accord' and 'when they had': Heney, quoted in Scott, 80–1. Sydney *Mirror.* Dep. Chief Censor's Diary, Sat. 30 Oct. 1914 and 4 Nov. 1915, AA, B543, file W363/4/700 and MP 390/8, Vol. 1.

13. Discrepancies with British censorship: Scott, 58–9. 'indulged in jeers': JTW, ms of speech to Censorship Reunion Dinner 16.8.1919.

14. Hattrick case: AA, MP367/1/0, file 512/1/1149. Hughes' and German firms: Fitzhardinge, 16–26.

15. Brian Pockley's death (shot after removing Red Cross coat to cover a casualty): *Hermes*, Nov. 1914, 98. Pockley: JTW to J, 13.9.1914. MacLaurin's death: Bean Vol. I, 521. Friends of the Wilsons: LH to author. 'we prayed': *ibid.*

16. Bridges death and funeral: Coulthard-Clark, 179–81. Evacuation of Gallipoli: Bean Vol. II. 'to say the things': R Munro-Ferguson, Novar Papers, ANL Archive, MS 696/10595 S21–22.

17. Edgeworth David's service: M E David, 211–14, 215–39. Barraclough's service: MO 698 of 1915; *Institution of Engineers Australia, Journal,* Dec. 1958, 381.

18. Anderson Stuart's work: Epps, 105. Active Service by medical school people: University of Sydney 1929. There were reports that some 'great swells' among the medicos 'demurred at being detailed to do work' they were too good for: Munro-Ferguson, 29.6.1915, Novar Papers, ANL Archive, MS 696/10594. Archibald Scot-Skirving: *RSS* Vol. III, 117, and University of Sydney 1929.

19. Brian Simpson: *Hermes*, Nov. 1915, 139. Campbell MacCormick: *MJA* 24.1.1948, 119.

20. C J Martin: Morison, *ADB* 10; Chick; Chick, *et al.*, 122–6; Butler Papers, AWM.

21. Wright's work: Colebrook, 70, 256. 'these wounded boys': *ibid.*, 268. Brian Simpson: University of Sydney *Calendar* 1916, 457.

22. fatigued: JTW to J, 15.4.1915 and 8.7.1915. 'relieved from anything': W H Hall to JTW, 7.12.1915, WP. Hubert Foster to JTW, 3.3.1916. 'At first everyone': J W Bradley of NZ Press Association to JTW, 30.12.1915.

23. JTW's sleeping arrangements and family activities: LH and KR to author.

24. Suppers: Dart to JTW, 1.11.1938. 'In all seriousness' and 'intimate and treasured': Dart 1959, 27 and 28. 'With his Darwinian': Dart 1973, 419.

25. 'he loved collaboration': Dart to author 15.3.1980.

26. Dart 1973, 418 and letter to author, 15.3.1980. On Hunter: JTW in *J of A* 1925, 59, 340–4.

27. 'some facts': JTW 1916, 102. 'to pick out this or that': *ibid.*, 105. 'Could a protopathic': *ibid.*, 105–8.

28. Conscription: Forward & Reece, 32–3. 'I wish Ireland': KR to author.

29. 'full knowledge of', and 'Is the Allied': JTW, MS notes, address to Women students, 1916. Reinforcements: F B Smith, 15.

30. Fitzhardinge, 216–36. 'if the tide': *ibid.*, 263. Canada: Forward & Reece, 42.

31. University of Sydney and conscription: *Australia's First*, 421–4. Hunter's enlistment: Blunt, 18–19.

32. University of Sydney Society for Combating Venereal Diseases, *Proceedings* Dec. 1916. Wilson's views: JTW, 1916a. WEA and later work: *Australia's First*, 423.

33. 'Meetings are the plague': JTW to J, 31.3.17. 'He always says': MMW quoted by J, Biog. Sketch of JTW.

34. Imperial War Cabinet: *The Times History of the War*, Vol. XII, 269–304. 'it at last' and 'autonomous nations': *ibid.*, 269, 303. Hughes and the Irish question: Fitzhardinge, 260–1. 'heroic, bloody': *ibid.*, 268. Passchendale: F B Smith, 26.

35. Transport strike, Hughes' state of mind, enemies: Fitzhardinge, 266–78. IWW: Kain, 1993. HMAS *Brisbane, SS Cumberland:* Scott, 688–95; AA, MP 1049/1/0, files 16/0258, 17/0153, and MP B197/0, file 1997/1/144. Special intelligence officers: AA, MP 1049/1/0, file 18/0155. Peace movements: AA, B197, file 2021/1/270.

36. Second conscription campaign: Fitzhardinge, 283–96. Hansard conspiracy: AA, B197, file 2021/1/270.

37. JTW, Honorary Col. on unattached list: MO 447, 770. 'In view of',

etc.: Maj. Piesse memo 1.12.17 to Intelligence Section 2MD, 'Expansion of Duties in Connection with Conscription'. On Bavin and Latham: J McCarthy, *ADB*, 7 and S Macintyre, *ADB*, 10; also AA, MP 1049/1 file 18/0155. Location of Section: Comdt to JTW, 22.3.18.

38. 'As those sons': JTW 1918, 37.

39. 'whom no amount': Dr Wallace Freeborn, quoted by J, Biog. Sketch of JTW, 16. 'Jummy' anecdote: Sir Douglas Miller to author.

40. Relations with TPAS: AEM to JTW, 28.12.1915. JTW to AEM, 20.3.1916.

41. TPAS proposals for medical students: *SMH*, 30.5.1918, 20.6.1918.

42. 'in common with': JTW in *SMH*, 30.5 1918. Other quotes: JTW in *SMH*, 22.6.1918.

43. 'only one unanswerable': Holme quoted in *Australia's First*, 424. 'consult frankly': *ibid.*, 425.

44. JTW Address, 14.11.18: JTW MS Notes; *SMH* 15.11.1918.

45. 'a chain of': Lt Col. Amery, Parl U/Sec for the Colonies, *The Times* 16.8.1919, quoted by E R Holme in Report 9 of Admin. Cttee of the Aust. Univs, 20.8.1919, 5. Senate Minutes, 1919, 324.

12

Expansion

Wilson's military sevice did not end with the Armistice in Europe. Threats to Australia's inner security kept him at his post as honorary adviser to New South Wales Military Intelligence, General Staff. By 1918 expressions of dissaffection had shifted from the issue of conscription – a focus for indigenous political, industrial and sectarian tensions, exacerbated by war – to the imported manifesto of Bolshevism, for which the American syndicalist movement, the Industrial Workers of the World (IWW or 'wobblies') established in Sydney in 1907, was an advance guard. A communist revolution, mounted behind the prevalent industrial unrest, seemed a distinct possibility and Sydney and Brisbane were regarded as the most likely centres for a coup. Sydney was the headquarters of the IWW in Australia, while Brisbane with its high Irish-Australian and even higher German-Australian populations had aroused the most determined opposition to Prime Minister Hughes and conscription, opposition supported by the Queensland Labor Government. Both cities had strong waterside workers unions.

Early in 1918 the Bolshevik Government in Russia appointed Peter Simonoff, a Russian-born, naturalized Australian (1916) and seasoned 'wobbly' in his mid-thirties, as its consul-general to Australia, an appointment the Commonwealth Government ignored. Supported by left-wing groups and generous funds of unknown origin Simonoff toured the eastern states publicizing the causes and aims of proletarian revolution, fanning the flames of disaffection as he did so. In the work-place others like the Russian-born Peter Timms spread transplanted images such as the 'serfdom of the workers' which drew susceptible audiences. Dodgers exhorted fellow workers to form secret groups 'for so permeating the minds of the people with the principles of Revolutionary Socialism that when the time arrives the change from capitalism to a system of Communism can be brought about peacefully, yet swiftly'. In Brisbane in September Simonoff was prohibited, under an Aliens Restriction Order, from taking part in propaganda connected with the war. In defiance he did so at meetings in Sydney around the first anniversary of the Russian Revolution and was arrested in Melbourne by military police on 30 October, charged with breaching the War Precautions Act. On 19 November the court put Simonoff on a bond to refrain from engaging in propaganda or addressing meetings. He broke the bond, was jailed and Bolshevik-inspired demonstrations began for his release.[1]

The surveillance authorities cast a wide net, keeping known dissidents, radical unionists, leaders of Irish-Australians and Russian-Australians as well as pacifists under regular surveillance. In New South Wales suspected dissidents living along the coast were periodically checked out. Occasionally innocent people were caught in the net, and they became subjects of public interest and political debate. One such was L H S Brodney. Spencer Brodney was born in Melbourne in 1883 of an Australian mother and a father of Russian parentage born in Prussian Poland (name of Brodsky changed to Brodney in 1914), who owned and published *Table Talk*, a political and literary journal in Melbourne, until he was bankrupted by a libel suit. The family moved to the United States. Spencer Brodney was a journalist of some standing in New York when, early in 1918, he came to the notice of Australian Military Intelligence by writing a letter to his friend Maurice Blackburn, a prominent Melbourne socialist and pacifist lawyer, requesting an article on the Australian political experience of war, conscription and industrial unrest. Brodney was a well-educated and well-read socialist with a student's interest in Russian affairs, a rare bird 'likely to create interesting developments' commented Longfield Lloyd. As luck would have it Brodney himself arrived in Sydney with his bride in the tension-ridden days of early November 1918 with news of Russia which insouciantly he claimed 'does not find its way into our capitalistic press'. The Sydney censor considered that the 'chief immediate aim' of such news was 'to goad workers into a state of frenzied hostility against employers'. The Brodneys moved to Brisbane where Spencer found work as a journalist with the anti-Labor *Daily Mail*. They rented a comfortable house and entertained a number of people of interest to military intelligence, like the Russian Zuzenko whom no one, according to their watcher, would invite home for pleasure.

Brodney's home was raided in January 1919 and again in March after a demonstration in Brisbane. Nothing incriminating was found but probably as a result of the raids Brodney lost his job with the *Daily Mail.* There was not 'any suspicion that he was dangerous', the army later admitted, nor did the raids disclose anything 'in any way detrimental to Brodney's character'. The justified indignation of such victims aroused the sympathy of fair-minded people who had no truck with Bolshevism, and threw a shadow over the justified concerns of surveillance authorities.[2]

Forgivable young firebrands like Sydney University's *enfant terrible* V Gordon Childe were also caught in the net. A brilliant student (BA, Sydney, 1914 with first class honours in classics; B Litt, Oxon, 1917 with first class honours), Childe returned from Oxford in 1917 and in November was appointed senior resident tutor at St Andrew's College. A confirmed pacifist and socialist, he joined the Australian Union of Democrats, criticized the Prime Minister for what he regarded as attacks on civil liberties, and joined the fray against conscription. Like all pacifists he came under the surveillance of Military Intelligence and had his mail censored. Over Easter 1918 Childe addressed a peace conference which led in May to his resignation at the request of the College principal. In July the University Senate refused to confirm his appointment as a tutor in ancient history for the Workers' Educational Association (WEA). The Sydney Censor remarked that 'it is good that the Senate have been strong enough to take action on their own initiative', but it is possible that the Senate was in receipt of advice on Childe from the Defence department. It is also possible that the initiative was taken by Wilson. Childe complained to the Chancellor and questions were asked in the NSW Parliament which helped Childe – in August 1919 he became private secretary to John Storey the Parliamentary Labor leader – but he was kept under surveillance till the end of the year.[3]

In December 1918, over 13,000 Australian soldiers, nearly all of them able-bodied, were on their way home from Europe and there were fears that they would engage the demonstrators in street-fighting. In mid-January the Chief of the General Staff, Lieutenant-General J G Legge, conferred with senior police officers from New South Wales and Victoria to discuss cooperative action to maintain civil order. It was agreed that the army would provide the police with military materiel, small groups of picked men with machine guns, and a few aeroplanes with improvised bombs, while the police would hold in readiness special reinforcements of mounted constables. When Military Intelligence in Sydney met early in February 1919, Wilson and Ralston in an effort to defuse the situation strongly recommend 'that Peter Simonoff be afforded the earliest facilities to leave the Commonwealth', indeed that 'all the Russians who desire to do so, be permitted to leave'. The British Foreign Office, however, had directed the Australian Government that all Russians returning to Russia should go via Vladivostock; they were on no account to travel via Britain, for the British Government was having similar trials with Bolsheviks. Peter Simonoff preferred jail in Australia because he feared arrest by Japanese police if he attempted to go to Vladivostock. He was released in July 1919, when the troubles had to a large extent subsided. After helping to found the central executive of the Communist Party of Australia he returned in 1921 to Russia, where he disappeared.[4]

The expected clashes between demonstrators and returned servicemen did occur, the most serious of them in Brisbane in the last week of March 1919. On Sunday 23 March 400 demonstrators protesting against continued enforcement of the War Precautions Act and carrying Red Flags – banned by a Commonwealth wartime regulation that was ignored by the Queensland Government – provoked an angry response from ex-servicemen, who aroused crowds of several thousand 'intent on teaching the Bolsheviks a lesson'. Violence mounted. The police were armed with rifles and bayonets. Property damage was substantial and 19 people were taken off in ambulances, while more than a hundred suffered bayonet wounds. The Commissioner of Police was injured and two constables and three police horses wounded by gunshots. Four days later at a public meeting in Sydney Peter Timms urged violent retaliation against the police: 'At all times the Master class has used the tools at their disposal,- the Armed Forces ! We must adopt the same method, which means force ! I am out for Revolution by any means!' Rumour had it that the Brisbane left was enrolling a Labour Volunteer Army. In Melbourne Major-General Legge was on alert, receiving telegraphed reports twice daily; he requested a list of the names of Russian 'undesirables'. The Brisbane Censor called on the Commonwealth Government to announce a policy on Bolsheviki. The *Sydney Morning Herald* reported the 'disgraceful scenes' in Brisbane and criticized political inaction. Wilson and Ralston advised 'deportation of Russians shown to belong to the Soviet and Russian Association, without requiring further evidence, as association with Timms should be sufficient proof of dangerous activity'. Cabinet felt that more evidence was needed, but Timms was deported. The disturbances fizzled out, a prohibition on public meetings to counter the influenza epidemic assisting the cause of peace.[5]

With the signing of the peace in Europe in July 1919 Wilson resigned from the New South Wales Military Intelligence Section General Staff, one of his last recommendations being the destruction of the Section's secret records. Back in October 1917, just prior to his appointment to this honorary post, Wilson had been mentioned in Military Orders for 'specially meritorious services'. Now in July 1919 he was thanked by the Secretary of the Defence Department and more fulsomely by the Minister for Defence for establishing the Censor's Office in NSW:

> The work on which you were engaged was of the highest importance to the Commonwealth and the Allies, and the valuable results attained by the Censorship in the 2nd Military District are a high testimonial to your organising ability and capacity for the solution of difficult problems.

A year later he was offered an Order of the British Empire. He declined it. 'It was worth more than that', was his opinion of his war services. On 21 September he was transferred to the Retired List with the honorary rank of Colonel.[6]

The repatriation of 160,000 Australian troops, and in many cases their wives and children, almost entirely within eight months, was an extraordinary achievement, masterminded by Lieutenant-General Monash. He considered it his finest achievement. Monash also presided over an excellent AIF education scheme directed from June 1918 by an army chaplain who in civil life was an Anglican bishop and educationist, Bishop Long, assisted from February 1919 by E R Holme, Associate Professor of English at Sydney University. They superintended the admission into British and French universities of Australian servicemen awaiting repatriation. By means of this programme Raymond Dart and Joseph Shellshear, both graduates of the Sydney Medical School, and H H Woollard a graduate of the Melbourne Medical School, were delivered to careers in anatomy under the auspices of Grafton Elliot Smith who in October 1919 became Professor of Anatomy at University College London. For Raymond Dart this was a dream come true.[7]

Prospective students in Australian universities were given preferentially prompt repatriation, so that many of them were able to enrol at the beginning of the academic year 1919. Student numbers increased by 40 per cent at the University of Sydney, placing great strains on accommodation and staff. The Medical School, already overloaded with 637 students in 1918, had to take on another 220 in 1919. In August Wilson had 500 students dissecting every day and simply did not know how he could accommodate the 250 first-year students programmed to start anatomy in October. He drew up plans for a new anatomical institute to better accommodate and equip his department, and to release space for the expansion of other departments. That, however, was a long-term solution: in the meantime he had to organize a way to avoid chaos. On 8 September 1919 he sought the approval of the Senate for the erection of a gallery in the Hunterian Theatre, which was referred to the Buildings and Grounds Committee. Complaining of an 'almost impossible position in regard to accommodation' the Senate's appeal for urgent government assistance was met with a generous grant of 5,000 pounds per annum over six years for new buildings.[8]

The returning troops brought with them from Europe quite literally the germs of another calamity: epidemic pneumonic influenza. The first cases of this virulent disease occurred in January and a vigorous government prophylactic campaign could not contain it. In New South Wales 6,000 were to die of it. At the university the Professorial Board under Wilson's chairmanship introduced emergency measures including the wearing of masks in classrooms, a bar on class attendance of anyone with a mouth temperature of 99 degrees or more, and three-monthly inoculations, together with strong exhortations to go to bed immediately on the manifestations of the first symptoms. In late March, because of overcrowded classrooms, the government closed the University for five weeks, which became six weeks. Wilson, Barff and the four deans adjusted the academic programme, mainly by curtailing vacations, to cope with the effect of the closure. In addition they enforced the wearing of masks for another two months after classes resumed on 12 May.[9]

Wilson also coordinated and superintended the University medical service which drafted medical students – some of them still in their 'teens and with no clinical experience at all – to assist the seriously depleted numbers of local doctors in the very hazardous work of attending the sick and the dying. Teenage Louise and Dorette Wilson assisted as nurses until they caught the 'flu themselves. Five of Wilson's children went down with it. There were emergency hospitals everywhere: at the Deaf and Dumb Institute, at

269

the Showground, in churches and in brothels. In some houses everyone was in bed with it and there was no food. Volunteers could not keep up with the needs and the medical profession suffered heavy losses. By June 1919 six of Sydney's recent medical graduates had died of pneumonia. It was a terrible time.[10]

In the midst of all this travail, in late July 1919, came a great windfall by which, in Wilson's words, all were 'set agog'. A wealthy pastoralist of Protestant Irish origin, Sir Samuel McCaughey, died leaving two-thirds of his wealth in trust to the University of Sydney and one-third to the University of Queensland. There were no strings attached: income from the monies was to be used as the senates of the two universities determined. The Sydney Senate estimated the income to its university as 15,000 pounds per annum, a munificent bequest which could not have come at a better time, for the University had reached a critical point of development which the aftermath of war had merely exacerbated. The time had come for a considerable expansion of its educational purpose, as had occurred in 1890 with the Challis bequest, and a radical restructuring of its organization. Wilson greeted the news as a deliverance for the University, but with some apprehension, as he informed Elliot Smith on 4 August 1919:

> It is tolerably certain that a somewhat strenuous period of organization and administration is in front of us. Already one's time is seriously taken up with this side of University work. I have been Chairman of the Professorial Board for the last four years or so and there are endless meetings so that I cannot get at my proper work. If only one could be a Professor and nothing else! I know the difficulty is the same everywhere, at least under the British system.

To Almroth Wright he confided 'I simply dread the worry of new organization at my time of life.' In fact he had been grappling with a radical restructuring of Sydney University's academic organization for almost three years.[11]

War had given science a stimulus for expansion. Thousands of doctors had served the cause, hundreds of Australian chemists had been recruited for the British munitions scheme run by Henry Barraclough and scores of mining engineers and geologists had joined Edgeworth David and the physicist Arthur Pollock in the mining battalion; the veterinarian J Douglas Stewart had commanded the Australian Veterinary Service; Douglas Mawson had distinguished himself in intelligence technology; Archibald Liversidge had come out

270

of retirement in England to assist the Admiralty; John Haldane had advised the War Office on gas while Jim Lorrain Smith had investigated gas, trench-foot and antisepsis (with his Edinburgh assistants he produced 'eusol'); Grafton Elliot Smith had researched the new phenomenon of shell-shock; Martin and Almroth Wright had taken their equipment and expertise to the battlefields. There were many others. In December 1915, as the Anzacs were being evacuated from Gallipoli, Prime Minister Hughes had wound himself up into a steel spring of national fervour to challenge the Teutonic prowess in science, announcing 'the idea of the national laboratory'. This resulted in the Institute of Science and Industry in 1916 which had a protracted birth and an early death, but did prompt the universities to review their science departments through its requests for reports on the 'future prospects of a regular supply of trained scientific investigators available for research work in connection with Australian industries'. The Professorial Board's response to this external request, in a report over Wilson's signature and dated 28 June 1916, gave the Senate a review of the Science Faculty's seven science and three engineering departments. The breadth of the science constituency in Sydney's academic structure was remarkable. Recent University developments, the Board found, had been almost entirely in the direction of science and applied science but congested accommodation and inadequate laboratory equipment (which for some departments like engineering was very expensive), specialized staff, library resources and research scholarships were major obstacles to teaching and research. There needed also to be a 'fuller acceptance of degrees and diplomas' by government and industry.[12]

A more comprehensive review of the University's resources and circumstances, initiated by the Senate in July 1917, resulted in similar findings. Reports by the Professorial Board and the various Faculties on 'each year's work: teaching done, original work, books and papers published and any pressing needs' revealed a somewhat alarming situation. Many departments were in serious difficulties due to increased student numbers without a corresponding increase in staff. While the reports indicated future policy developments with regard to subjects and curricula, it was clear that bringing staff, accommodation and equipment of the various departments up to full establishment must be the main priority. In late October the Senate postponed any comprehensive consideration of future developments for another year.[13]

Architecture and Medicine, however, had some success in lifting their status and expanding their teaching scope. Under pressure from the Institute of Architects and with an assurance of

Government funds, a Chair of Architecture was created in 1917 within the School of Engineering in the Science Faculty and in early 1918 Leslie Wilkinson was appointed to it. In December 1917, with an expedition suggesting the hand of Anderson Stuart, a Chair of Pharmacology was established by the Senate and in February 1918, without advertizement, Stuart's former assistant professor in physiology H G Chapman was appointed to the new chair. Wilson must have agreed with both of these decisions, for he was a member of both Senate committees which considered the two matters and he later refuted the charge that the position was created especially to make room for Chapman: there was great scope for pharmacological research in Australia and Chapman was well-qualified, he argued. It is probable that Wilson was not privy to all the facts, given the distance between himself and Anderson Stuart, and his distain for gossip. Wilson's support for Chapman against 'the intense objection and opposition to the man', of A N Burkitt and others, was most unfortunate on both professional and personal grounds. By the mid-twenties it was clear that Chapman was not abreast of his subject. His descent into fraud and promiscuity began about 1916 when he separated from his wife and ended in suicide in 1934 when, as Director of Cancer Research, he was faced with exposure for embezzling 20,000 pounds from the Royal Society of New South Wales and the Australian National Research Council.[14]

On 14 October 1918 when the University's circumstances, resources and future development again came up for review by the Senate, Professor Warren of the Engineering School proposed the creation of a Faculty of Engineering and Architecture. Under the superintendence of the Science Faculty he had begun teaching engineering in 1883 and architecture as an elective in 1884, in which year he was appointed to a new Chair in Engineering. Distinctive degrees in engineering (BE; ME) were introduced in 1884 but provision for a full course in architecture and a distinctive degree (B Arch) did not occur until a Chair in Architecture was created in 1917. By 1918 Engineering was a well-established professional school with about 100 students, issuing degrees in civil, mining/metallurgy and mechanical/electrical engineering. 'The Engineering School', said Warren

is now recognized as one of the best in the British Empire. It stands higher than any one of the schools in Great Britain in regard to investigation and research work on the materials used in Engineering and Building construction. The termination of this great war will stimulate enormously the production of all those things which are necessary for our development industrially, and will open up new avenues for the work of the engineer in all the various branches of the profession....The time has arrived, I consider, when it is desirable to establish a Faculty of Engineering.

Wilson gave wholehearted support to Warren's claim.[15]

On 4 November 1918 the Senate referred the matter to the Professorial Board. For Wilson, Warren's proposal raised a major issue: 'the organisation in faculty groups, of the various teaching departments of the University'. This was referred to a committee headed by Wilson which reported back on 9 December with a short paper entitled 'Committee Re Faculties'. It was Wilson's work. Academic organization is not unchangeable, he began; it must evolve. There was no need to restrict the university faculties to four and the engineering department's claim to faculty status was very strong indeed. Engineering was not appropriately governed by the Science Faculty which was 'comprehensive and heterogenous', embracing 'such extraordinarily diverse curricula' as chemistry, biology, physics, engineering, veterinary science, agriculture and metallurgy, most leading to distinctive degrees of BSc, BE, BVetSc, BSc Agric. The Science Faculty was bearing the brunt of this faculty problem which had arisen through the creation of new and distinctive degrees without a correlative differentiation of faculties. The other faculties had only minor difficulties in this respect, for instance in the relation of dentistry to the Medical Faculty, or the relation of economics to the Arts Faculty. For the solution of the problem Wilson put forward basic criteria for the constitution of faculties

The necessary unity of aim and interest which is surely the raison d'etre of a faculty would seem to be logically attainable only by a definite relationship between the personnel of the Faculty and a given curricula or curriculum embracing studies of cognate character, and leading to a distinctive degree.

The Dean of the Faculty who ought to be in the position of an expert administrative officer in connection with all the business of the Faculty [but he] cannot possibly be in such a position where the subjects and curricula included are so utterly diverse from one another.

He proposed an administrative system of ten distinct faculties comprised of the existing four plus Engineering, Agriculture,

Veterinary Science, Dentistry, Economics and Architecture, each with its distinctive degree. The objection that ten Deans sitting on the Senate (as according to law Deans were entitled to do) would throw out the balance of representation, could be met by the Senate deciding from time to time which should be the four faculties whose Deans were ex-officio members of the Senate. 'The adoption of the principle of correlation of Faculty and distinctive degrees would provide a useful regulative idea for guidance in future development', and it would, Wilson concluded, 'confer greater freedom and independence on groups whose real individuality is merged and lost in association with other groups with which they have little or nothing in common except the general University spirit'.[16]

Professor Warren endorsed Wilson's scheme except in one particular: he thought the criterion of correlating faculty with a distinctive degree was sound in principle but not the only one; the size of a department also mattered. Architecture for the time being should, he argued, be part of the new engineering faculty. This proposal was not upheld. The Board, on the motion of Barff seconded by MacCallum, adopted the report and recommended it to the Senate on 9 December 1918. The Board had now developed a framework for the Senate to handle faculty development. The Senate referred it to the faculties where it gathered dust for more than six months, partly due to the influenza epidemic. The Professorial Board sought on 28 July 1919 to prompt the Senate into action when it carried Wilson's motion as chairman, seconded by Barff, that the Board's reports be retransmitted to the Senate with a recommendation that the Senate from time to time decide which four Faculties be represented, the other Deans having the right to be present and to speak on matters relating to their Faculties.[17]

A week later came news of the McCaughey Bequest which cast a new and optimistic light on university affairs. The Senate immediately requested the various faculties to report through the Professorial Board on the 'best methods of applying the Bequest'. And on 8 September the Senate decided, on Wilson's motion as Chairman of the Professorial Board, to receive the Board's report on the creation of additional faculties and to refer the question of the legality of the suggested changes to a committee of the Senate's legal members. Re-elected Chairman of the Professorial Board on 11 November, Wilson set up a committee to draft the principles of new faculty constitution and on 16 December presented a paper which the Professorial Board adopted. Four months later it laid out proposals to the Senate on faculty developments in the light of the

McCaughey Bequest, and on 19 July 1920 the Senate recorded the names of the Deans elected by the six new Faculties. It was now obvious to all concerned that the Professorial Board had established itself as the key authority on the University's academic organization and management, and that Wilson with his fundamental principles and systematic approach to these matters was the driving force.[18]

The McCaughey Bequest was a handsome gift but it would have needed to yield 100,000 pounds, rather than the estimated 15,000 in yearly income, were it to fund all of the claims submitted for its application. The Professorial Board had the difficult task of selecting the most pressing needs and bringing them within the University's means, as well as coordinating them in the general purview of the University. There was a long list of unapproved items. The first claim on the Bequest went to strengthening the existing departments with considerably increased salaries to full-time permanent staff, increased annual grants to services common to all departments: the administration, the Fisher Library and a Research Fund to be administered by the Senate on advice from the Professorial Board, a new provision of primary importance to Wilson. A large commitment went to an unprecedented increase in academic staff: six new chairs, three associate professorships, six lectureships and two tutorships. Finally a list of good causes for any remaining funds was appended.[19]

The Bequest signalled a new era in the history of the University, in enabling a dramatic expansion of academic positions which the Senate expeditiously established and filled during 1920 and 1921, some by promotion or invitation, most by advertisement. Wilson was involved in nearly all of them. Coincidentally, senior posts were becoming vacant by retirements, primarily of the occupants of Challis chairs after 30 years' service. Haswell the Challis Professor of Biology (restyled zoology in 1915) had already retired in 1917, his position having been offered to J P Hill who declined it. MacCallum's Challis Chair of Modern Literature was discontinued and replaced by two chairs, two associate professorships, a lectureship and a tutorship. There was a ferment of excitement in the staff. For the first time at Sydney University senior appointments, as well as many down the line, went to the locally trained. Sydney graduates were coming into their own.[20]

Early in 1920 Wilson's attention was trained on a proposal referred to the Professorial Board by the Senate to establish the position of Associate Professor in Sydney's academic ranks. Wilson, the systematist, reviewed the whole academic staff structure, concluding that it should be five-tiered: Assistant Lecturer or Demonstrator; Lecturer and Lecturer/Demonstrator; Assistant Professor; Associate Professor; and Professor. In Wilson's view the third grade, Assistant Professor, would be filled mainly by promotion from the second grade, usually experienced teachers not fitted for the leader's role. The proposed new grade of Associate Professor would have no prescribed conditions; it could be a temporary substitute for a full chair, a means of retaining an exceptionally good teacher (as might have been the case of J P Hill in 1906), a consolation prize for a gifted assistant professor who had just missed out on a full chair; or an appointment to head a division of a large subject beyond the management capacity of one professor. This position might be filled by promotion 'possibly in a few cases overleaping the intermediate stage', or by advertisement from within or outside the Sydney staff, but it should be as jealously guarded as is the highest grade of full Professor to which it would be little, if at all, inferior except in title and emoluments. Wilson argued that the institution of this fourth grade would remove the objection to the appointment of assistant professors that, despite precautions, they were determined by seniority; and it would enable Sydney University to be strengthened by the appointment of teachers of the ablest kind from outside.[21]

The Professorial Board's meetings were lively, as was to be expected with a quarter of them naturally disputatious Scots. MacCallum, Anderson Stuart, Wilson and Carslaw certainly were, Francis Anderson and Alexander Mackie too, if episodically, though Haswell was conspicuously not so. Wilson was a confrontationist, a 'swords before breakfast' man, who according to university lore habitually slew a dozen men at a session. Fights were frequent between Wilson and Carslaw the Professor of Mathematics, the cause according to Carslaw being opposition from chairman Wilson and 'Barff & Co.' to his endeavours 'to get some very necessary reform through'. When Wilson 'took to jumping on Carslaw in the P. B. he could be heard in the Quadrangle', said Carslaw, who was nevertheless a Wilson admirer: 'A splendid type is and was J. T. W.', he wrote in 1942. Wilson liked Carslaw too 'in spite of his fuss & peculiarities'. Carslaw's background was very similar to Wilson's – a lowland Scot of Free Church convictions – but Carslaw had capped his Glasgow MA degree with three degrees from Cambridge and had become a devotee of English academic traditions. Carslaw was strongly opposed to the titles and grades of Assistant Professor and Associate Professor; he preferred the title Reader for a single grade between those of Lecturer and Professor. Wilson won that battle in 1920 but Carslaw was delighted when, in 1936, Vice-Chancellor Wallace turned the tables by abolishing Assistant and Associate Professorships, replacing them with the grade of Reader.[22]

In Senate meetings A B Piddington was Carslaw's counterpart, but much worse in Wilson's opinion. Elected to the Senate in 1910, Piddington was a distinguished Sydney graduate and former lecturer in English Literature, before embarking on a career in the law and politics, most recently as a Royal Commissioner on a number of issues concerned with social justice. He was a professional self-conscious do-gooder. His influence on Senate meetings was primarily delay, which under the pressure of business relating to the McCaughey Bequest was very frustrating. Taking a high moral stance he denounced alleged abuses and promoted at length laudable ideas like sending sympathy letters to the relatives of fallen soldiers of Sydney University, the entry of academic staff to either house of State Parliament, the appointment of staff only after advertisement and the admission of the Press to Senate meetings. 'After long consideration' his motions were usually postponed or, if he were absent from a meeting, deemed to have lapsed. He was tireless, however, skilled in debate and he commanded sufficient support to negative the Professorial Board's recommendation that a lectureship in entomology be not established. Having got the lectureship, Piddington immediately pressed for its conversion into a chair. MacCallum in exasperation moved that a time limit be imposed on speeches at Senate meetings. That, however, suffered the fate of many of Piddington's motions: postponed and finally withdrawn. Piddington was a persistent nuisance, always associated in Wilson's mind with the lines: 'I have seen five and forty leaders of revolt' who 'think the world will go right if they holler out "Gee"'. It was doubtful that such men would do any harm, he observed, but still more doubtful that they would do any good.[23]

Wilson's long service as Chairman of the Professorial Board formalized his differences with Anderson Stuart. Wilson's influence strengthened as the Professorial Board grew in size and authority, and as his grasp of the full spectrum of faculties and curricula firmed. With his faculty system of December 1918 he established a coherent basis for the University's academic organization and future development. At important university ceremonies like the official welcome-home to Professors David and Pollock and the unveiling of the Roll of Honour for the 197 university men who died in the war, Wilson delivered the address. Anderson Stuart on the other hand always stood for the special interests of the Medical School, extending his constituency by promoting dentistry, pharmacy and massage (physiotherapy) as ancillaries to medicine; pharmacy in his design for instance was a sub-department of a medical discipline, pharmacology, for which a chair had been created in 1917. The Medical Faculty then persistently lobbied for two clinical chairs, in medicine and surgery, to which on 8 October 1918 the Professorial Board's response (adopted by the Senate on 14 October) was that though desirable 'any proposal to establish these Chairs should be considered in conjunction with the claims of other faculties'. Professor Warren's claim for faculty status for engineering and architecture was tabled in the Senate and referred to the Professorial Board on the same day, 14 October. Warren's case was strong, as also was the Arts Faculty's bid for new chairs. New chairs for medicine were not approved. On 27 October the Medical Faculty expressed its regret 'that the Senate could not give preference to the Medical Faculty'. The need was urgent. It applied again for the two clinical chairs but, if only one could be afforded, preference for a chair of medicine was recommended. The Professorial Board was unmoved.[24]

Anderson Stuart's influence in the Senate had waned significantly since the inception of a reformed Senate in 1913 and the death of Chancellor MacLaurin in 1914. But his will did induce the Senate to create a Chair of Medicine. It was his final major achievement for the Medical School. By April 1919 it was known that Stuart was terminally ill and 'an anxious gloom fell over the school'. On 2 June at Senate the Chancellor, Sir William Cullen, proposed the establishment of a chair in clinical medicine and his motion was carried. On 1 December A E Mills, one of the University's earliest medical graduates and a close friend of both Stuart and Wilson, was appointed.[25]

Fate was cruel to Anderson Stuart. At the age of 63 while still straight, vigorous and fresh-faced, he was found early in 1919 to have a colloidal cancer of the abdomen. MacCormick assisted by Scot Skirving explored but would not operate since complete removal was impossible. Stuart rose to the occasion. Though this sentence angered him at first and he occasionally thought it was all a mistake, the next 11 months of pain and decline he traversed with great fortitude and consideration for others. He relinquished none of his offices and transacted business in his usual style. He destroyed documents that gave evidence of former antipathies and went to unusual lengths to make peace with colleagues he had fought with or offended. Wilson paid a special call for that reason. His last lecture, at the end of 1919, was an impressive farewell performance. His face gaunt, body swollen and gait shuffling, Stuart followed normal procedure with absolute precision until overwhelmed by a student demonstration of honour and affection. It began with the squeal of the bagpipes followed by song, revelry and champagne and ended with the students harnessing themselves to Stuart's car and pulling it like a Roman chariot out of the University precincts. On that day this brash and brassy man was a noble figure. All those present in the crowded lecture room took away with them an unforgettable impression of their leader's heroism. Anderson Stuart at the end won the applause he had craved all his life. He was cheered to the echo.[26]

Anderson Stuart died on 29 February and was interred in the cemetery on North Head on 1 March in the presence of a huge crowd of people. Wilson's tribute to his 'senior colleague' at the Medical School reviewed their association from around 1880 in Edinburgh. Most appropriately he concluded with the epitaph to Sir Christopher Wren in London's St Paul's Cathedral: '*Si monumentum requiris, circumspice*' [If you would see his monument, look around]. Against heavy odds and in remarkably short time Stuart had created a magnificent building which he believed had contributed much to the success of medicine as an institution in Australia. It had provided a place of honour for medicine in Australia and a link with medicine's European traditions. Raymond Dart, writing in 1923, believed there was a larger Stuart legacy:

Stuart's achievement

> For Australia, his work had a distinctive result in society-moulding,
> in that it was the initial step towards the quasi-aristocratic rank
> which the medical profession now enjoys in that country.[27]

On 22 March 1920 Wilson became Dean of the Faculty. Predictably he moved to arrange the affairs of the Faculty more to his liking. The vacant chair offered an opportunity for the redistribution of the work of physiology. In the first place 'it was of the utmost importance' that histology or microscopical anatomy be detached from physiology and put under the control and direction of the Professor of Anatomy if there were to be a proper co-ordination of the teaching of naked eye and microscopical structure. In Europe and America almost invariably histology was part of anatomy departments and before long, he predicted somewhat rashly, this would also be the case in British schools; Melbourne had already made that shift.[28]

JTW Dean

Physiology's proper study was function not structure, he continued. In recent years physiology had expanded considerably in

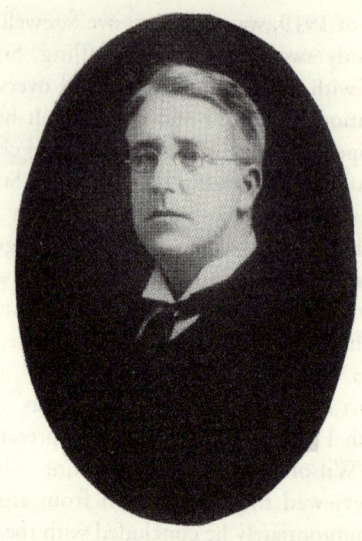

Professor Thomas Peter Anderson Stuart
SUMJ, March 1920. Courtesy University of Sydney.

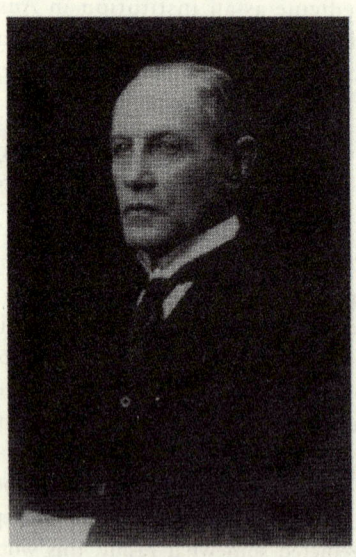

Professor James Thomas Wilson
Reproduced from Australia's First. *Courtesy SUA.*

theory of their subject, would coordinate the clinical teaching of all the related subjects in their divisions and bring order out of chaos.[30]

For the Medical School, as for the University in general, the McCaughey Bequest opened a new era in its history. The new professors, Mills, Sandes and Priestley were all Sydney graduates, the first to be appointed at their Alma Mater. Prejudice against the 'home-grown product' had been overcome and the 'Edinburgh clique' broken, it was said. Though probably overstated some such prejudice must have existed. There were also tensions inherent in the relationship between the academic and clinical sectors of medical training, some of which was generational and much wider than the school. Established eminent clinicians, mostly from Britain like Alexander MacCormick and Robert Scot Skirving (both Edinburgh men), showing a resilient disinclination for retirement, were an irritation to the aspiring younger Sydney-trained men. Both factions were clear about their adversaries. For MacCormick it was the 'Mills-Hinder push' of early Sydney graduates growing towards eminence. For the native-born it was the 'Edinburgh factor'. The prevailing post-war chauvinism found an outlet when A E Mills was elected Dean of the Medical Faculty on 16 September 1920. The natives were jubilant:

> That Dr Mills is our new Dean is not merely a tribute to his own high qualities: it is a tribute to the School that bred him. We were proud of that great man who guided the destinies of the School from its tender babyhood to its more mature years, and of his revered successor who hardly assumed the wand of office before he left us for more ambitious shores. But Sir Thomas Anderson Stuart and Professor Wilson were only our foster-fathers. Professor Mills is one of us, one of our own kith and kin, the first chief of our race. With his accession to the Deanship our School can truly be said to have come of age.

> ....The clinical side of the profession now has a very real representative at headquarters as distinct from the purely scientific side of Medicine, but even the physiologists and anatomists know that no better man could be appointed Dean.[31]

A by-product of this contention among medical men was the enshrinement of Anderson Stuart's materialist formula for success, which may have been as much Edinburgh-inspired as were Wilson's ideals in medical education. Edinburgh's eminent clinicians advertised their success in displays of material comfort: Wilson's respected surgeon 'chief' John Duncan drove around Edinburgh in a yellow dogcart drawn by two high-stepping horses. Aping their

282

eminent immigrant seniors in Sydney, the younger native-born generation mounted similar displays of success as a means to 'success': a Macquarie Street address, a car (if possible, chauffeur-driven), a good tailor, a cultivated interest in food, wine and cigars, membership of the Australian Club and the University Club, patronage of the arts, overseas travel. The archetype of this breed was Herbert (later Sir Herbert) Schlink, a disciple of Anderson Stuart, whose long career was so intimately woven with the fortunes of Royal Prince Alfred Hospital that it was to become known as 'Schlinktown'. The Sydney community cooperated in this abasement of medical practice to material success. A young doctor of pre-1914 Sydney instanced the case of a poor patient crippled with osteo-arthritis whom he treated for no fee – as an L.O.G. or Love of God case in medical parlance – who told him on one visit, 'I took a guinea from my savings and went over to Macquarie Street and saw *a really good doctor* ... and he says *just the same as you.*' The novice medico concluded that 'the doctor who treats for nothing has his services valued at the same price.'[32]

[margin handwritten note: Schlink – material success]

The Edinburgh ideals in medical education which Wilson championed – a strong scientific foundation, clear separation of academic from clinical training and the subservience of hospital to school – found little acceptance at Royal Prince Alfred Hospital, Sydney's principal clinical school. Practitioners adhered to a strictly utilitarian view. They wanted an abbreviated scientific foundation with more time and more emphasis given to clinical work throughout the curriculum so as to prepare students for practice, 'the destiny of seven-eighths of them'. But it seemed to some, who were in a position to know, that the medical staff at Royal Prince Alfred carried their teaching obligations too lightly. William Epps, the Hospital's lay secretary since 1902, wrote to Wilson in May 1920 of a serious situation there:

> I fear the Board [of Management of RPAH] appreciates very little the fact that this is almost firstly a clinical school, & is apt to look askance at the University side of its existence. Sir Thomas [Anderson Stuart] of course always had this in view & was able to get things done in the interests of the students & of teaching which but for his influence would not have been done.'

Epps wanted Wilson to take 'an active part in the management – ultimately a very active part – & be an influence which is greatly needed.' He was probably behind an item in the *Medical Journal of Australia* in April 1920, publicly inviting Wilson to become the

Chairman or Vice-Chairman of the Hospital's Board of Management. To Wilson in May he alluded delicately to the problem threatening the Board as:

> the rocks of medical sectionalism, which Sir Thomas avoided, but which I dread greatly now. Perhaps you will grasp my meaning without more detail. We know you would have a broadminded view of the various interests at stake & not be in any way a partisan.

All was not well with the Royal Prince Alfred Hospital and Wilson might have been able to straighten things out, but presiding over warring parties in this arena would not have been a congenial assignment. Whenever possible in public, in private and in committees Wilson gave emphatic voice to his conviction that the general scientific foundation of medical education was the most crucial part of it, especially for those who were to go into practice.[33]

In 1919 both Wilson and Elliot Smith had their futures under review and they exchanged confidences. Elliot Smith was not making ends meet in Manchester and would, he thought, be forced to write for money. He was no businessman and his was an improvident family. He enquired of his chances in Sydney if Wilson's chair became vacant, to which Wilson responded 'you would simply have to throw the handkerchief'. But by August 1919 Elliot Smith was 'booked to UCL'. Wilson was heartily delighted by this news for a number of reasons: London had got 'a really first grade anatomist who is really active', one who might 'rescue London anatomy from the strangle-hold of the College of Surgeons examinations'; London was more convenient since Elliot Smith had much business there; and he was glad for Hill's sake that Smith would be near him. And, Wilson continued

> If only we could reconstitute the Duckmaloi trio! U.C.L. has already a more or less homely association for me and if and when I am in London I shall claim citizenship there. You make some reference to my possibly taking a hand over there. Who knows what may happen?[34]

When he left London in early 1914 Wilson had had in mind the idea that in 1919 or 1920 he might be back in England, perhaps not to return to his Sydney chair or even to Australia. The war and its aftermath had precluded all such planning and now Stuart's illness and the McCaughey Bequest had complicated matters. Leadership of the Medical Faculty and indeed the guidance of the whole university at a time of prodigious expansion, were claiming all his attention and energy, and would continue to do so, 'at least for a time'. But after 33 years service he sometimes felt that both he and his department would benefit by a change. He would be due for leave at the end of 1920 and it was 'at least probable' that he would take it then, returning to his chair in 1922. Or he might retire at the end of his leave and remain in England for at least another year 'for purposes of education of the family'. By family he probably meant sons, for his daughters would by then be in the tertiary stage of their education. Douglas, the eldest son, would by 1921 be starting his secondary education, and for boys an English secondary schooling was generally thought desirable. But there was a firm proviso to his retirement:

> I shall not do so unless I find that the family resources are economically secure enough to allow me to be independent of an ordinary salaried appointment, which indeed at my age I should be little likely to obtain. And, again, if I have to sustain the burden of general routine anatomical teaching I should probably do so here with greater usefulness than elsewhere.[35]

There was indeed a possibility of reconstituting the Duckmaloi trio. Wilson's letter of 4 August reached Elliot Smith at 'a psychological moment' on 15 September, just as he was about to cable Wilson for permission to enter an application on his behalf for the Chair of Anatomy in Cambridge, made vacant by the death of Alexander Macalister a fortnight before. British anatomy had 'been harrowed ten times over' during the last three months by the death or retirement of senior men and there were no young men left of sufficient stature to take their place. As a result Elliot Smith had taken the 'bold course' of appointing Raymond Dart as his senior assistant at University College London. There was no one in Britain, declared Smith, capable of upholding the great reputation of the Cambridge school and it would be an ideal job for Wilson: salary about 1050 pounds per annum inclusive of a College Fellowship, i.e. 850 pounds from the University Chest and 250 pounds from a College with all a Fellow's rights; duties 'as much or as little formal work as you like, for in Cambridge a professor does his best for the place by means of social intercourse with students and dons'.[36]

This Cambridge opportunity, however, was complicated by local politics and 'things' moved slowly there. A 'Syndicate' – as Cambridge called its Senate committees – appointed in November to review the conditions of the chair reported in January 1920 recommending an increased salary and an expanded jurisdiction for its anatomy chair and the creation of a Readership to relieve the professor of the drudgery of human or topographical anatomy. Debate and 'pseudo-intriguing' continued and Smith and J P Hill – who was equally keen to reconstitute the Duckmaloi trio – observed diplomacy in building support for Wilson, to whom Smith reported periodically. Wilson made his position clear in a letter to Elliot Smith of 20 January [which has not survived], probably that he wanted a 'haven of refuge' – but he did not formally apply for the position until so prompted in a cable from Elliot Smith, J P Hill and W H R Rivers. On 15 May Wilson cabled the Cambridge Vice-Chancellor, Dr P Giles:

> I hereby apply for appointment Cambridge Anatomy Chair.
> J T Wilson.

On 31 May came the Vice-Chancellor's reply: 'Elected'.[37]

In confidence, but in rather matter-of-fact terms, the family had discussed the prospect of a move to Cambridge. The boys were eminently transferable – 'like a sack of potatoes', Jeanie remarked – and the others would adjust. The effect of the news on Mabel revealed a strength of feeling in favour of Cambridge that would have swept aside any reservations Wilson might have had. 'I am so excited that I must write though I shall see you tomorrow', she scribbled in a note from Bayview, 'It speaks much for my self control that I read your letter before the assembled family without them detecting any perturbation in me – since then I have made some pastry, but naturally can fix my thoughts on nothing – Naturally yours is the greater venture, but you know I feel sure of you & in your heart of hearts you know you can make good. I will not regard it as settled – but the chances are that we shall go.' Wilson was attracted by the thought of being among friends who called him 'Jim', but he evidently expected that the Cambridge appointment would be short, and a return to Sydney quite likely, for he replied to Professor J D Stewart's congratulations with

> Of course I am pleased at being chosen for Cambridge but pleasure is by no means uppermost in my mind. It is a painful thing to contemplate separation from so many friends & associations of an entire generation. Still I may see Sydney again when the few years of activity I can hope for in Cambridge are over.

Louise and Dorette, then staying in Melbourne with the Massons for the arrival in Australia of the Prince of Wales, treated the news with disbelief.[38]

Wilson's resignation was accepted by the Senate on 7 June, to take effect from 31 December. But a few weeks later came advice from Cambridge, that it was 'imperative' that he begin work there at the commencement of the academic year, on 8 October. From an abstract and slowly-unfolding proposition the Cambridge appointment suddenly became a concrete and somewhat daunting challenge, with an early deadline. On 5 July the Senate approved Wilson's request for leave of absence for the final term, and on his recommendation Dr F A Maguire was appointed Acting Professor and J I Hunter was charged with the delivery of lectures in introductory anatomy. Maguire, a graduate of 1911, had taught in the anatomy department since 1913 in positions from junior demonstrator to senior lecturer and had in addition a distinguished war record, rising to the status of General in the Medical Corps. Wilson's request, that his pension of 400 pounds per year be payable on his retirement from the Cambridge chair, had already been approved.[39]

The question of the succession at the Medical School took longer to determine. Wilson had in mind a far bolder step than Elliot Smith's in appointing Raymond Dart as his Senior Assistant. Wilson's chosen heir was the brilliant, popular, 22-year-old demonstrator, John Irvine Hunter, who had only graduated in April 1920 (with first class honours and the University Medal). The Senate Committee appointed on 5 July to consider the future of the Chair – it consisted of the Chancellor, the Vice-Chancellor, the medical members of the Senate, Judge Backhouse, Mr Leverrier and H E Barff – found a means of endorsing Wilson's wish, safeguarded within a long-term strategy. On 9 August the Committee recommended to the Senate that there should be an Associate Professor as well as the Challis Chair in Anatomy; that histology be incorporated within the Anatomy Department and a Special Lecturer and Demonstrator be appointed to conduct the histology course; that Professor F Wood Jones, then Professor of Anatomy in Adelaide, be offered the Challis Chair for five years; that John Irvine Hunter be offered the Associate Professorship, 'it being understood that Mr Hunter will be granted a year's leave of absence ... at as early a date as the exigencies of the Department permit'. Hunter was poised to overleap two intermediate steps in Wilson's five-tiered academic staffing structure: from Demonstrator to Associate Professor, with the view a few years later to taking the Challis Chair. By advancing Hunter, Wilson was furthering the chauvinist cause of the native-born, but strictly on grounds of merit. He had the highest opinion of Hunter's abilities, comparable to those of his famous namesake. As he said to Maguire, 'he is worthy to bear the name of John Hunter'.[40]

One factor in this strategy gave Wilson some misgivings: the offer of a five-year appointment to Frederic Wood Jones. Wilson admired Wood Jones' talents and attainments: at 41 he was a charismatic teacher and public lecturer, an experienced researcher who wrote well; much interested in anthropology – he had been Elliot Smith's assistant in the archaeological survey of Nubia in 1907–8 – he was a Lamarckian evolutionist and a Vitalist. London-born and trained, Wood Jones had 'something nearly approaching genius', Wilson wrote many years later, 'though perhaps a bit erratic ... [and] I feel that it might not be all smooth water in his vicinity'. But 'the same old aggressive Freddy', as Hill referred to him, might have been equal to the clinical 'push' which was about to test severely the authority of the teaching medical scientists at the Medical School. Wood Jones was inclined to accept the offer of the Challis Chair but Adelaide University would not release him from his contract. So Dr F A Maguire succeeded to it, as Wilson had hoped.[41]

Shock and dismay muffled the congratulations that poured in when Wilson's translation to Cambridge was announced. They came from the medical fraternity, scientists, churchmen and colleagues associated with all the various offices he had held. Old students paid tribute to his inspiring energy, enthusiasm and passion for accuracy; 'and we grudge losing a teacher like yourself from our midst', wrote Earle Page, now a politician in the Commonwealth Parliament. Dr A E Finckh deplored the loss of 'A very firm mind' to contend with 'that so-called democratic element, and, above all, that spirit of materialism, and of purely commercial aims which are becoming more and more evident in our scientific circles.' The messages of keenest regret came from the clinicians at Royal Prince Alfred Hospital. There must have been some in this fraternity who were pleased at the prospect of Wilson's departure but 'most of us', wrote Sinclair Gillies, regarded it as 'nothing less than a disaster', and he asked Wilson to reconsider; it was unfortunate wrote R Gordon Craig to 'lose the Dean whom we have wanted for so long'; Cecil Purser wrote of 'hopes dashed to the ground' after having been 'so buoyed up with pleasure & gratification' when Wilson took the helm at the Medical School; Charles Bickerton Blackburn was 'acutely conscious' of the 'almost irreparable loss'.[42]

The University as a whole was scarcely less affected than the Medical School, in two ways: Wilson's leadership of the University and his moral influence within it. Professor Carslaw's message typified the first of these:

> I had hoped to see you our Sir William Turner and that, as Principal, or Vice-Chancellor of the University of Sydney, you would set a standard for the Australian University. Often in these last years when you were Chairman of the [Professorial] Board this remark has fallen from several of its members.

From Brisbane Elton Mayo, who was striving to establish a chair in medical psychology, wrote, 'your departure is sheer disaster for Australia. We have too few real leaders of men and Universities in our Southern academic ranks; we can ill spare you'. On Wilson's moral influence Professor Edgeworth David spoke for many when he wrote

> I weigh my words well when I say that the grandeur of your character has greatly uplifted the whole of the University ... your whole life among us has been an inspiration.

G V Portus, the Director of Tutorial Classes, managed to 'chuckle at the thought of your championship of attacked causes in some Cambridge Senior Common Room after the fashion in which you tackle us at lunch!' Professor E R Holme complained that Cambridge had taken 'our best man', but consoled himself with the thought that Providence had placed him exactly where he would be of most value to Sydney University in choosing the right men for the major expansion in academic staff.[43]

An editorial in the *Sydney Morning Herald* put the matter in perspective. News of Wilson's appointment was received with 'positive consternation, on personal grounds no less than on academic grounds' and in the Medical School, bereft of two deans in a single year, by 'a feeling akin to despair'. But it would be wrong to pressure Wilson to stay, for his decision was not lightly made. The appeal of the wider sphere and greater opportunity for research in better-equipped laboratories which Cambridge offered, outweighed Sydney's claims. Despite heavy disabilities Wilson had demonstrated his capacity for research and it would be unfair to him and to science to grudge him the chance of fulfilling all that is in him. For Sydney there was consolation in the thought that Sydney University was also honoured by Wilson's translation to Cambridge:

> It speaks well for the standing of Australasian seats of learning that universities of the old world should covet our Wilsons and Rutherfords, Braggs and Gregorys.[44]

The magnitude of Sydney University's impending loss was well appreciated by MacCallum who had witnessed Wilson's influence on the proceedings on the Conference of Australian Universities, hosted by Sydney University in the last week of May. Its aim was to promote the coordination of university policies and practices throughout the Commonwealth as a lead-up to the first post-war Congress of the Universities of the British Empire, planned for July 1921 in Oxford. Wilson's interest was fully engaged and he took a leading part in the wide-ranging discussions: the interchange of examiners, teachers, students and material; the representation of Australian universities in British, American and other universities; the establishment of executive heads in Australia analogous to those in British and American universities; the relationship of the university to the state and to industry; the proposed extension of the medical course to six years. On this last matter Wilson took the opportunity of a national forum to give trenchant expression to his opinions on medical education, and they were given generous space in the Conference report.

> The majority of the medical faculty would cry out for the devotion of the extra time to practical clinical work among the senior students. [Wilson] would not be prepared to devote a whole extra year to this. He believed that a thorough grounding in the fundamental sciences was the most important part of the medical curriculum. A relative deficiency in medical training could be made up in the subsequent years of professional life, but a man would never go back to study physics, chemistry and biology. Yet more and more the practice of medicine was coming to depend on these sciences. The physician had more and more to think in terms of physical chemistry and biology. [Wilson] had, therefore, the utmost repugnance to the idea of shoving the study of such sciences back into the school curriculum.... more was required than a mere schoolboy understanding of these subjects;... The man who was to practice medicine or science all his life was the very man who could afford to put off his practical medical or scientific training for a little.

The Conference's most important decision was to establish in Melbourne (geographically the most central of the Australian universities) a Standing Advisory Committee charged with collecting information, framing recommendations, compiling a Year Book, and generally promoting common action by the constituent universities. In December 1920 the Senate of Sydney University appointed Wilson one of its four delegates to the forthcoming Oxford Congress. In March 1921, after nomination by the various

Australian universities in place of the ailing Sir William Bragg, he was elected Australian representative on the Universities Bureau of the British Empire and its Executive Committee; he also became a member of its Committee of Vice-Chancellors and Principals.[45]

The final few months of Wilson's time in Australia were as concentrated in activity as any in his busy life. To the management of a teaching programme almost overwhelmed with students was added a multitude of meetings through which he steered his plans for an expanded and radically reorganized school and his special arrangements for its leadership. The Senate did not approve his strategy for the succession to his chair until 9 August, 11 days before he left Sydney. He also became involved in plans for extensions to the Medical School, which included a large dissecting room. And there were ceremonial duties associated with university receptions for the Prince of Wales, and for General Sir William Birdwood who had commanded Australian troops during the war. J J Fletcher of the Linnean Society prevailed on him to unveil a Roll of Honour, as part of the celebrations marking the centenary of the birth of Sir William MacLeay; this occasion concluded with an expression of appreciation and farewell to Wilson by Fletcher on behalf of the Society. Wilson was under pressure from the many clubs and societies to which he belonged, to attend farewell meetings. He was able to accommodate most of them, but not General Legge's request to deliver a lecture to his military cadets at Duntroon.[46]

There were three large farewell functions at the end of July, reported at length in the newspapers. The Senate and staff of the University said their parting words at an evening gathering of distinguished guests, including the Governor of New South Wales, in the Great Hall. Wilson's final message to this company was directed at the politicians: Australian governments must give the universities the necessary means to do what was expected of them for the intellectual growth and development of Australia. To the Millions Club he took issue with the prevalent utilitarian view of universities, especially in scientific education. In the long run the most theoretical researches must lead to practical benefits, but even if this were not the case 'wisdom is yet justified of her children'. Private industrial enterprise could not be expected to fund disinterested ends, but nations might well be expected to rise to that mission. 'It will be an evil day when the burning desire to know and to understand is either eradicated or is swamped by interest in the merely utilitarian application of scientific knowledge'.[47]

The third occasion was no less grand, but more intimate. A

dinner at the Wentworth Hotel on Friday 23 July, organized by the University Medical Society, was attended by about 220 graduates and students. A E Mills, now Dean-elect of the medical faculty, delivered the main address. As a friend and privileged witness of Wilson and his works for over 30 years Mills gave a fresh and lively review of his contributions to the Royal Prince Alfred Hospital, the Medical School, the University, Australian science and Australian defence. These services had earned their honour. For other reasons, and Mills considered them the greater, Wilson had won their esteem and their love: for his 'heart and soul' dedication, his high ideals, and 'because he inspired in us the desire to seek knowledge, to love truth and to gain understanding'. Johnny Hunter then spoke for the students and the Chairman, John Paling, presented a handsome illuminated address in appreciation of Wilson's 'powerful individuality' and his international scientific reputation for original work in comparative anatomy and neurology. 'Visibly affected' Wilson rose to reply, to sustained applause. Like Mills he too cast his eyes backward to the early days, appalled now at the colossal extent of his ignorance and inexperience and, he insisted, this was not a pose but naked truth. He was still floundering. His redeeming grace was that he had always been 'gladly learning as well as gladly teaching'. He had accomplished something but, he concluded,

> my predominant feeling is of failure. I did wish to do so much more and I have accomplished so little! But it is better to have tried, even if one fails, than not to have tried. And I do claim to have been a trier! As Rabbi Ben Ezra says,

> 'What I aspired to be,
> And was not, comforts me.'
> I am not lacking in that sort of comfort.[48]

His final lecture in the anatomy theatre on 29 July was transformed into another farewell occasion with a lantern slide of his own image displayed on the screen that had thrown up thousands of anatomical illustrations. Students and staff presented him with a gold carriage clock and once again Wilson used the occasion to stress the importance of a broad scientific training. Another tribute behind the scenes had greater significance: Johnny Hunter presented Wilson with a carbon copy of the notes he had taken of Wilson's neurology lectures. In them lay an assurance that Wilson's distinctive legacy in neurology would, through Hunter, reach new generations of medical students.[49]

The Wilsons left Sydney on 20 August, on the SS *Miltiades*. On board for final goodbyes were Jeanie and her four-year-old son Patrick among many personal friends; A E Mills, F P Sandes, Edgeworth David, H E Barff, Francis Anderson, Arthur Pollock, H G Chapman, F A Maguire, Johnny Hunter, Henry Barraclough and many others, but not MacCallum who 'could not trust himself to come'. On the wharf was a larger crowd, many of them students, witnessing the end of an era. One was heard to say 'I feel as though the light of my life has gone out'.[50]

Notes

1. Simonoff: E Fried in *ADB;* Cain, 231–5. Prohibition, arrest and later reports: AA, MP 367, file 479/3/234. 'for so permeating': dodger 'Organise: Watch: Prepare:', AA, MP 367, file 479/25/190. Peter Timms: Censor's Intelligence Report for 12.2.19; Chief of General Staff to 2MD, 8.4.19 re arrest; all from AA' MP 367, file 479/25/190.

2. Brodney: Cain, 133–7. 'likely to create': Cain, 134. 'any suspicion' and 'in any way': Cain, 136. 'does not find' and 'chief immediate aim': 2MD Censor to Chief Censor, 14.11.18. AA, MP 367, file 512/1/989.

3. Childe: J Allen, *ADB*; Cain 129–33. Senate decision: Minutes Book for 1918, 77. SUA. 'it is good'; AA, MP 1049/1, file MB 51.

4. Returning soldiers: Scott, 826. Legge: Coulthard-Clark 1988, 177. 'that Peter...': 2MD to DMI, 12.2.19, AA, MP 367, file 479/3/234. On British Foreign Office: Cain, 231.

5. Brisbane disturbance: Cain, 161–7. 'intent on': Cain, 163. 'At all times': AA, MP, file 479/25/190. 'deportation of Russians': *ibid.*

6. JTW resignation: Commandant to JTW, 8.7.19 and Trumble (Sec. D of D) to JTW, 15.7.19. WP. 'specially meritorious': W J Sherbon to JTW, 16.10.17. Sec. Defence to JTW, 15.7.19. 'The work': A/Min for Defence to JTW, 18.11.19. Gov. Gen's Mil. Sec. to JTW, 5.7.20.

7. Repatriation: Serle, Ch. 14. Education scheme: *ADB* on Long and Holme.

8. Student numbers and Govt assistance: *Calendars* and *Australia's First,* 431–2. Anatomy classes and JTW's plans: JTW to A E Wright, 4.8.19.; Senate Minutes, 8.9.19. 'almost impossible'; *Australia's First,* 432.

9. Influenza epidemic: *Australia's First,* 432–3; Professorial Board Minutes, March to July 1919.

10. Nursing: LH and DC, to author. Wilson children: JTW to A E Wright, 4.8.19. Emergency hospitals: Dr Cawley Madden, quoted *Australia's First,* 433. Deaths: *SUMJ,* 1, 2, 7–12.

11. 'set agog' and 'It is tolerably': JTW to GES, 4.8.19. McCaughey bequest: *Australia's First,* 431–5; *Calendar* (1920) 'Senate Report',

688. 'I simply dread': JTW to AEW, 4.8.19.
12. Stimulus for science: Schedvin, 14; *Calendar,* 1917, 587. GES research: Dawson, 161. Professiorial Board Minutes, 27/28.6.19 and printed report (7pp.). SUA. 'the idea of': quoted in Schedvin, 14. 'future prospects': Professiorial Board report, 28.6.16, 1. 'fuller acceptance': *ibid.,* 7.
13. Minutes: Professiorial Board, 30.7.17; Faculty of Medicine, 26.9.17. Postponed: *Calendar* Senate Report 1917, 617. 'each year's work': Senate Minutes, 30.7.17.
14. Pharmacology: *Centenary Book,* 234–45. On Chapman: R Teale, *ADB* 7; Senate Minutes, 2.7.17 and 10.12.17; JTW opinion, letter to Barff 28.2.21; *Centenary Book,* 243–5. 'intense objection': Burkitt to JTW, 5.6.34.
15. Warren proposal: Professiorial Board Minutes, 8.10.18; Senate Minutes, 14.10.18. Background: *Australia's First,* 246–55; 386–93. 'The Engineering School': Senate Minutes, 14.10.18.
16. JTW's Faculty organization: Senate Minutes, 4.11.18; Professiorial Board Minutes, 8.10.18 including typed papers by Warren and Wilson. All quotes from JTW paper in Professiorial Board Minutes.
17. Professiorial Board Minutes, 9.12.18, 28.7.19. Senate Minutes, 3.2.19.
18. Professiorial Board Minutes, 7.10, 11.11, 16.12.19. Senate Minutes, 7.8.19, 8.9.19. 'best methods': Senate Minutes, 7.8.19. Senate Report, *Calendar* 20, 698–90. Deans: Senate Minutes, 19.7.20. *Australia's First,* 439–40.
19. Application of Bequest: Senate Reports, *Calendars* 1920 to 1922. Professiorial Board Report 27.4.20: Senate Minutes, 27.4.20.
20. Positions: *Australia's First,* 435–9. Biology, offer to Hill: Senate Minutes, 17.5.17.
21. Five grades: Senate Minutes, 10.5.20. 'possibly in': *ibid.*
22. 'swords before breakfast': Burkitt to JTW, 21.2.39. Fights: Carslaw to John Read, 26.7.42. 'in spite of': JTW to J, 20.11.29. Reader position: *Australia's First,* 607.
23. On Piddington: M Roe, *ADB,* 11. Laudable actions: Senate Minutes, 1918–20. Entomology lectureship: Senate Minutes, 27.4.20 and 7.6.20. 'I have seen': JTW to J, 26.6.35.
24. Faculty of Medicine, Professiorial Board and Senate Minutes for 1917 to 1919.
25. 'an anxious gloom' and Chair of Medicine: *Centenary Book,* 364.
26. Anderson Stuart: Epps, 58, 159; Scot Skirving ms, 118 Vol. 4; Last lecture: interview with Grace Cuthbert Browne; *Senior Year Book* 1922, 9; Blackburn, 129.
27. JTW tribute: ms, 1920. 'For Australia': Dart, in *Nature,* 27.1.1923, 111.

28. 'it was of the': JTW memo of 19 April 1920, Faculty of Medicine Minutes.
29. *Ibid.*
30. Clinical teaching: *Centenary Book*, 201. Student complaints and hopes: Report, Faculty of Medicine to Senate, 21.9.17.'
31. 'Mills-Hinder': AMacC to JTW, 26.12.41. 'That Dr Mills': 11–12 *SUMJ*, Oct. 1920.
32. On Schlink: R Teale, *ADB* 11 and Maddox Ch. 3. L.O.G. case: Moran 1939, 104–5.
33. Epps to JTW, 31.5.20. *MJA*, 3.4.20, 325–6. 'the destiny': *SUMJ*, Nov. 1912, 2.
34. JTW to GES, 4.8.19.
35. *Ibid.*
36. GES to JTW, 15.9.19.
37. 'pseudo-intriguing' and attitude clear: GES to JTW, 27.1.20 and 27.2.20. GES/JPH/WHRR cable to JTW, 10.5.20.
38. 'like a sack': KR to author. 'I am so': MMW to JTW, 28(?).5.20. 'Of couse I': JTW to J D Stewart, 2.6.20, Stewart Papers, SUA [Wilson wrote to J B Peden in similar terms: Peden Papers, SUA]. Louise and Dorette with Massons: LH to author.
39. P Giles (V-C, Cambridge) to JTW: letter 28.5.20; cable 10/11.6.20; letter 6.7.20. Maguire: *Centenary Book*, 285–6, 399.
40. Senate Committee: Senate Minutes, 5 and 19 July 1920. 'he is worthy': Maguire's oration on Hunter, quoted 289 *Centenary Book*.
41. On Wood Jones: M MacCallum, *ADB* 9; JTW to JPH, 1.11.33; JPH to JTW, 4.3.38.
42. Letters of congratulation to JTW, June 1920.
43. *Ibid.* Holme to JTW, 25.6.23.
44. Editorial, *SMH* 5.6.20, written by Mungo MacCallum II: MWM to JTW, 8.6.20.
45. Conference of Australian Universities, May 26–9, 1920: *Abstract of Proceedings; Calendar* for 1921, 728–9; Senate Minutes, 12.4.20. Appointments to Universities Bureau: 458, *MJA* 13.11.20; Barff to JTW, 15.12.20; JTW to Barff, 28.2.21; JTW to J, 23.3.21.
46. Extensions to Medical School: Senate Report 1920, 732 *Calendar* 1921. J J Fletcher to JTW, June 1920. J G Legge to JTW, 1920.
47. Farewell functions: *SMH* late July 1920; *SUMJ* Oct. 1920, 5–8, 17–18.
48. 'my predominant feeling': JTW Notes, address to Uni. Med. Soc. dinner. WP.
49. The last lecture: *DT,* 30.7.20.
50. 'I feel as though': *The Scotsman*, 15.6.26.

13

Cambridge and British Anatomy

The SS *Miltiades* of the Aberdeen line was not as large or as smart as ships of the P & O or Orient Lines, but comfortable and friendly. The Wilsons settled down to a leisurely voyage around the Cape. Wilson's three attractive daughters and three lively sons, all excited about the new turn their lives were taking, presented him with an awkward job in general surveillance, especially in ports. 'Personally I would prefer to omit the ports altogether' he wrote to Jeanie as the ship approached its third landfall, Durban, 'but I daresay the family think otherwise.' He participated in the usual shipboard recreations with marked enthusiasm, taking first prize at the ship's fancy dress party as a distraught passenger facing imminent shipwreck. With hair tousled, clothes askew, a life buoy around his neck, all evening he kept up a portrayal of agitation, harassing passengers and crew with questions about lifeboats, provisions, the behaviour of the sea and the chances of rescue. It was not a difficult role; he had merely to discard the cloak to his more or less constant state of anxiety.[1]

Wilson had a lot on his mind. He discharged his last official act as a Sydney Professor in a letter to Barff from Perth on 1 September while trying to come to grips with his new job via letters and cabled correspondence with the Vice-Chancellor at Cambridge, and the acting professor of anatomy, W L H Duckworth. At Durban they were caught up in a coal strike which delayed the voyage by more than a week. Wilson was going to be late for the start of Michaelmas Term on 8 October and he hated being late for anything. He was however, preparing himself for Cambridge with some heavy reading in physiology and biological chemistry as well as in lighter literature like Quiller-Couch's essays. When the ship turned its nose northward after the Cape he started work on his Inaugural Lecture.

As a Scot and a colonial it is not surprising that he approached exalted Cambridge with trepidation. He knew furthermore that his appointment was controversial.[2]

In Cambridge W L H Duckworth had seemed to be Alexander Macalister's natural successor. A distinguished Cambridge graduate, Bursar and later Master of Jesus College, 'Duckers' and Cambridge Anatomy were synonymous for medical students. But formidable forces were ranged against him as one of the selectors, Arthur Keith the Conservator of the Museum of the Royal College of Surgeons, later revealed:

> The physiologists of Cambridge ... were of the opinion that the Chair should be filled by one conversant with the latest methods of anatomical inquiry, one who could introduce a new tradition in Anatomy. Elliot Smith also took this point of view, and induced his old master, Professor J T Wilson, FRS, of Sydney University, to become an applicant. I, too, had the highest opinion of Wilson, both as a man and as an anatomist: he had proved at Sydney that he was a begetter of anatomists. My heart was with Duckworth, but my head was with Cambridge University, and when it came to voting, my heart had to give way.[3]

Elliot Smith had played a pivotal role in Wilson's appointment. Ever since 1909 he had kept before Wilson the prospect of returning to Britain and in January 1919 he had raised the question once more.

> Now that the War is over and ideas of reconstruction are fermenting in all our universities I have been wondering a good deal of late what your feelings are in the matter of taking some part in reshaping things 'to our heart's desire'.... Anxious as I am to get to London, I am even more so to see you in this country where things anatomical badly want stirring up...[4]

Beside the ferment of reconstruction there were three other circumstances influencing the outcome. The first was the driving ambition of the physiologist, Professor E H Starling at University College London, to establish an Institute of the Medical Sciences at University College. Private philanthropy had funded the Physiology Institute opened in 1907 and the Pharmacology Institute opened in 1912; after the war Starling was looking to complete his grand project with the Anatomy Institute. The second was the advent of two vacant anatomy chairs in 1919, at University College by the retirement of Sir George Thane in June, and at Cambridge by the death of Sir Alexander Macalister in September. The third was the arrival in

England at the end of 1919 of two representatives of the Rockefeller Foundation to identify suitable targets for its largesse. Before the war the Foundation had promoted public health campaigns against hookworm and yellow fever. Now the Foundation's policy was to promote education and research in the biomedical sciences and to do it by investing in people and institutions with a record of success. 'Make the peaks higher', went the adage, and emulation and competition will do the rest. Both University College and Cambridge sought Grafton Elliot Smith for their chairs and it was widely assumed that he would take the latter, but Starling persuaded him to settle for London. His appointment at the end of 1919 carried the certain prospect of College funds to build up its Anatomy Department and a Rockefeller grant of 1,205,000 pounds for the College's medical school and hospital, the largest single benefaction till then to any educational institution in Great Britain; 370,000 pounds of it was to be spent on buildings for anatomy, histology and embryology. The grant probably depended on London having Elliot Smith as one of the peaks Rockefeller was prepared to back. Towards Cambridge, which wanted him for the same reason, Elliot Smith adopted an ambiguous stance with a view to getting Wilson appointed. On 9 October 1919 he had reported to Wilson that

> ...nothing official has yet been done with reference to the Cambridge Chair; but I understand a good deal is happening unofficially. To prevent any hasty decisions being made, such as might permit support to crystallise in favour of undesirable persons, I have adopted the attitude of indecision as to what I propose to do, while putting forward quite confidentially with certain of the more influential and discreet people a presentment of your claims. But quite another group of people, who merely suppose that I am wavering or waiting for better conditions, are now pushing for an extension of the department to include Vertebrate Anatomy and a corresponding improvement of the financial conditions. What will be the outcome of this complex situation remains to be seen. My difficulty is that, while I am quite content to remain here and am most anxious for you to go to Cambridge, there is a danger of the C. enthusiasts making their job something vastly different from the comfortable haven of refuge you want in this country, and the situation is too delicate for me to attempt to put a break upon their efforts. You will understand then something of the difficulty of my position: but I hope to be able to continue walking the tight rope long enough to save the situation for you. I shall of course keep you

fully informed of the progress of events, which will probably be very rapid in a fortnight hence.[5]

In February 1920 the Cambridge University Senate had redefined the subjects assigned to the Chair of Anatomy to include vertebrate anatomy and embryology as well as human anatomy, and by a Grace (decision) of 12 March this designation of the chair was decreed and its stipend raised from 600 pounds to 850 pounds. A further 350 pounds from the Department made a total of 1,200 pounds a year. No retirement age was specified. More than two months elapsed before Wilson was elected, Elliot Smith acknowledging

> ....very great relief and satisfaction on May 28th when we learned that the Cambridge Electors did the proper thing for the University. I cannot tell you how delighted we are at the prospect of having you here and of getting your help in putting some life into Anatomy here.

The Senate had also created a Readership in Anatomy for Duckworth, who was to have charge of human or topographical anatomy, so relieving Wilson of the grind of vocational teaching for medical students.[6]

In a characteristic state of chaos that belied a very orderly mind, Elliot Smith was busy with ambitious plans. Huge post-war enrolments, a series of public lectures, the new Institute of Anatomy in which he proposed to install J P Hill as Professor of Embryology and Histology in a personal research chair to help speed up his work, and the dispatch of three post-graduate students – Wilson's former students Raymond Dart and Joseph Shellshear and the Melbourne-trained H H Woollard – for a year's training in methods in America, were his principal preoccupations at that time. He had become Britain's leading anatomist, but his dominant research interest from 1920 was cultural anthropology, or ethnology.[7]

During the 1920s and early 1930s Elliot Smith became a powerful figure in the medical politics of the Empire, and, on the international stage, a brilliant and popular propagandist for anthropology. Backed by Rockefeller funds he travelled extensively – in Europe, the United States, Australia, Java, China – promoting the study of physical and cultural anthropology. A Canadian disciple, Davidson Black, had gone to Peking in 1916 to accept a neurology chair and subsequently an anatomy chair, but his real interest was anthropology. Davidson Black became an ambassador for Elliot Smith from whom he had caught the passion for tracking primitive man; China, he was convinced, was the most likely place to find him. In 1922 Elliot Smith sent Raymond Dart (under protest) to the anatomy chair in Johannesburg, Joseph Shellshear in 1923 to the anatomy chair in Hong Kong and H H Woollard in 1928 to the anatomy chair in Adelaide. All pursued anthropology in those appointments, Dart winning fame for his discovery of the controversial man-ape fossil skull, *Australopithicus africanus* in 1924 and Davidson Black in 1927/8 for his discovery of Peking man *Sinanthropus pekinensis*. Elliot Smith in 1924 persuaded the Australian Prime Minister to establish a Department of Anthropology at Sydney University with Rockefeller money, and in October 1932 he appealed successfully to the Prime Minister to save it from extinction.[8]

The *Miltiades* arrived at Royal Victoria Dock on the Thames on 20 October, exactly two months after leaving Sydney, and while Mabel and the children settled into rooms in Kensington Wilson made a bee-line for University College

> ... to Hill's room & found him with Elliot Smith & D. M. S. Watson together. We talked hard together & Hill rang up Martin & Keith & arranged a dinner at the Univ. of London Club also in Gower St that evg. I then went off with E Smith & talked Cambridge with him hard till he had to go off to a meeting. I went part way with him & then off to the family for an hour or so & then back to Gower St where we had a delightful dinner-talk and I got further lights on the Cambridge situation & on other matters.[9]

The Fraternity of Duckmaloi had reassembled and in that heady moment it seemed that the embers of the old camps in the bush of New South Wales would be fanned to flames again. In November Wilson and Hill were discussing the joint editing of a book on mammalian embryology, begun but not completed by the late Richard Assheton of Cambridge. A contract with Macmillan was signed in March 1921 but Wilson was not enthusiastic, as he wrote to Jeanie:

> I am rather loath to undertake work of this kind in the early future but Hill says he wont go in unless I join him & Elliot Smith says we must both do it. Fortunately the work will be close along the lines of what is likely to be one of my main lines of teaching in Cambridge.[10]

They were soon sparring again. At a meeting of the Anatomical Society on 19 November Wilson felt compelled to 'partly' disagree with a paper Hill presented, a 'little scrap' they continued at the next meeting 'to the amusement of the others'. He managed, however, to 'overlook a good deal of immaturity' in the observations and theories of Raymond Dart and Joseph Shellshear from the USA, communicated to the meeting by Elliot Smith. Sydney was well to the fore at this meeting and so too were the Scots: Arthur Keith was in the chair and also present were three Scottish professors: Bryce of Glasgow, Waterston of St Andrews and Arthur Robinson of Edinburgh, all Edinburgh-trained, Robinson having graduated with Wilson in Edinburgh on 1 August 1883.[11]

There were prominent compatriots in Cambridge too. Wilson was delighted to discover that the Vice-Chancellor, Giles of Emmanuel College, was a plain Scotsman from Aberdeen. Old Edinburgh friends like W R Sorley in the philosophy chair, German Sims Woodhead in the pathology chair and the theologian Anderson Scott were there to greet him, as well as many old and new acquaintances: A C Haddon the ethnologist, J N Langley and H K Anderson physiologists, G H F Nuttall the parasitologist, Stanley Gardiner the zoologist, Holland Rose the biographer of Napoleon, Sir Joseph Larmor the mathematician, Sir William Pope the chemist. Most helpful of all was the anthropologist W H R Rivers. With Mabel's sister Lilian, Rivers had arranged housing and other practicalities for the Wilsons.[12]

By 29 October Wilson had been formally admitted as a member of the University and as Professor of Anatomy, and had received the usual honorary MA given to new teachers. His admission on 4 November to fellowship of St John's College, however, was not *ex officio* but a matter of personal recognition. The quaint ceremonial tickled his fancy:

> I have to read a lengthy promise or oath in Latin (!) and then I kneel down before the Master of the College, fold my hands as in the attitude of prayer, place them between his hands, when he will repeat the Latin formula of admission. Then after signing my name in sundry places I am a pukka Don of St Johns.[13]

The Wilsons were lucky with their houses. For six months they rented Croft Cottage in Barton Road, an interesting old place with odd corners and hidden stairs as well as a beautiful garden, from the theologian Baron von Hügel. Wilson appreciated particularly the Baron's books. Finding their own home did not entail the bother of house hunting. The owner of 31 Grange Road, needing a quick sale, sought them out to offer them the house. 'Would it be impertinent to ask the price?' ventured Mabel. Around 2,200 pounds was the answer, so unbelievably cheap for that location that they felt they should have sealed the bargain on the spot without waiting even to inspect the place. It was a large three-storey red-brick house, rather ugly by comparison with Croft Cottage but soon transformed by Mabel's knowing hand, maintained by a domestic staff of two and a part-time gardener. For his study Wilson commandeered the best room on the first floor: sunny, booklined and warmly carpeted, dominated by a huge desk with reference shelves on top and five drawers beneath. In the attic floor above was his workshop.[14]

By Christmas 1920 all but one of the children were slotted into their educational grooves; John and Maxwell at King's College Choir School; Katharine enrolled at the Perse High School for girls. Two were away for the first time: Douglas was at Oundle, the best public school in all England in the opinion of Dr Rivers (it was strong on science) and Louise was at University College London continuing with architecture. Dorette was deflected from her chosen course: to continue with science she would have had to start again, and take Latin, so she opted instead to serve her father's considerable need for assistance in the Anatomy Department. Mabel was busy with home-making, bicycling around Cambridge paying calls and leaving cards according to local custom, enjoying the cool climate that was so good for her health. Even Wilson, who had a strong aversion to the cold, found that here he seemed to feel it no more than other people.[15]

Cambridge was buzzing with change and innovation reflecting a national mood to build a better world. There were disquieting flashes from Ireland and the suffragists and the trade unions were resurrecting their pre-war grievances. In Cambridge a large enrolment of ex-servicemen assisted by substantial government grants brought new verve, a jousting against tradition. Critical eyes focused on the University's severely strained finances (in contrast to the well-endowed colleges), its antiquated administration and teaching system. Strenuous building activity was soon under way to accommodate the increased demands of science: parasitology, biochemistry, pathology and low-temperature research were all housed in new buildings in the 1920s. Research gained higher status and science edged the classics out of their primacy, the general inclination being to study the living and not the dead. And that was the essence of Wilson's prescription for Cambridge anatomy.[16]

On 26 January 1921, in his Inaugural Lecture, Wilson opened his crusade for a new tradition in Cambridge anatomy. He welcomed the widened scope the University had given his subject as an endorsement of the claims of science against the narrow vocational objectives insistently being urged at that time. Clinical needs had to be met, but since that service had long dominated British schools of anatomy it was not likely to suffer neglect. Cambridge in particular had a higher mission – and here he spoke as a representative of medical teachers around the Empire – as a nursery of medical men with a strongly scientific outlook.[17]

A thorough grounding in the basic sciences of physics, chemistry and biology at the tertiary level was necessary, he argued. They were medicine's intellectual mainspring and no one could become a master of any branch of medicine without them. For anatomy he claimed a large province: the problems of structure in widely diverse forms, in changes induced by function, pathology, the environment and the developmental process from the embryo through to senescence. Indeed, to be really complete, the anatomist should pursue his interest back to the phenomena of heredity. His methods should draw from every one available: time-honoured dissection, frozen sections, X-rays, the hand lens, the camera and the compound microscope.

In British medical schools – and at that time in them alone – microscopical anatomy was mainly pursued in physiology departments. This accident of history had become a convention in which British anatomists had too-readily acquiesced, to the serious detriment of both research and teaching. For instance the accounts of the sympathetic nervous system in some anatomy texts were written as if the great contributions of the Cambridge physiologists Gaskell, Langley and Anderson had never been made. More recent editions were better but they still betrayed the fact that they were not written *from the inside*. Restriction to naked-eye anatomy had confined the intellectual development of British anatomists, and British anatomy was now distinctly behind the rest of the world.

Wilson was claiming equal rights for anatomists and physiologists in the same territory. The anatomists' concern, like the physiologists', was with the living body, though naturally and inevitably they studied it differently. Structure is not static, he insisted. It is extraordinarily plastic, a thing of labile character, fluctuating in its constitution in response to varying functional needs and varying environments. Understanding the wonderful capacity of the live organism for integration, self-regulation, adaptation and regeneration was of vital concern to anatomists and was expanding the comparatively new field of experimental anatomy which Wilson briefly reviewed. In this area Wilson saw opportunity for a rapprochement between the two disciplines to remove the grotesque theoretical schism which was detrimental to both, but more so to anatomy. Only by contributing on the structural side to the solution of the problems involved could anatomy vindicate her title to full rank and status as a truly biological science.

That was Wilson's policy statement for his discipline and it was a vast relief to have it over and done with. Anatomy was first and foremost a biological science. Whether it could be accommodated as such in Cambridge and leaven English anatomical traditions was problematical. In Cambridge – the university of Bacon, of Newton and of Darwin – the climate seemed appropriate. Significantly perhaps, Anatomy and Physiology were part of the Natural Sciences, not the Medical School. Also, since the Cambridge Medical School was a pre-clinical school (for their clinical training students went to hospitals elsewhere, usually London) it was reasonable to suppose, as Wilson did, that the pressures of clinical medicine could be held at bay.

But if there were favourable winds for Wilson's programme in Cambridge there were also unfavourable ones. The battle to reclaim histology from the physiologists in Cambridge was bound to be more difficult than anywhere else in Britain. The great Michael Foster – who in the late 1860s had built an early British course in histology as part of 'practical physiology' at University College London – appropriated histology in 1870 as a vital basis for his new, and soon to be famous, Cambridge Physiological Laboratory. By 1884 when Alexander Macalister, in his inaugural lecture as professor of anatomy in Cambridge, argued for the return of histology to the domain of structure, it was firmly entrenched with the physiologists who were then building their magnificent neurological monument on histological foundations. He continued to do so over the 36 years of his tenure of the anatomy chair. It was all to no avail.[18]

Primed by Elliot Smith and H K Anderson, the distinguished Cambridge physiologist and university administrator, Wilson was wary of Michael Foster's successor in the physiology chair, Professor J N Langley. After an exchange of hospitality Wilson recorded his thoughts:

> Langley is a very pleasant person socially. Academically he is a bit difficult. Very touchy on certain points and had a sort of standing feud with Macalister over the teaching of Microscopical Anatomy.

'However he seems well disposed towards me personally thus far', Wilson reflected with cautious optimism. The biochemist

F Gowland Hopkins could have enlightened Wilson on how well-disposed Langley could be personally while being implacably ill-disposed professionally, if he saw any threat to physiology's dominion. Frustrated for more than a decade before the war by Langley's ruthless self-interest and want of foresight, Hopkins found succour from the Medical Research Committee (established in 1913) and philanthropic bodies like the Beit Trustees until in 1920 his department was secured by the Dunn Bequest. Langley was as guarded toward biochemistry's aspirations to independence from physiology as he was toward anatomy's bid to reclaim histology.

All British physiologists did not agree with Langley, however. One who began his long and distinguished research career under Langley was in entire agreement with Wilson. A V Hill, who left Cambridge in 1920 to take the physiology chair at Manchester where he reorganized a large teaching department, before accepting the physiology chair at University College London in 1923, plainly stated his views on the proper jurisdictions of anatomy, physiology and biochemistry in his Inaugural Lecture on 16 October 1923. Histology, he maintained, belonged 'logically and naturally' to anatomy and it would be wise, just and advantageous to both sciences, as well as histology itself, if physiology were to relinquish the subject. Physiology had wide pretensions which, for its own good, needed to be kept within a reasonable compass. Whenever the business of a department becomes too large there is a tendency to cramp initiative and individuality and to adopt bureaucratic methods. And now that anatomists were adopting experimental methods to elucidate the microscopic structure of living tissue, it was no longer necessary for physiologists to plough that field. Histology was not the physiologist's proper job.[19]

Logic and nature, however, had nothing to do with the outcome in Cambridge. Histology had provided the basis for a distinctive physiological school which won international respect and attracted patronage. The traditional constitution of that school was jealously guarded. Both Langley and his successor in 1925, Joseph Barcroft, a Fosterian of the fourth generation, proved good caretakers: both presided over major expansions of the Physiological Laboratory, making it by 1933 'one of the most spacious and fully-equipped physiological institutes in the British Isles' and enabled physiology to reclaim from the Biochemical Department after 20 years, the first-year teaching of physiological chemistry. Discipline building is a political activity involving the demarcation of academic territory, the allocation of responsibilities and privileges, and the mounting of claims for resources. In Cambridge anatomy and physiology were rivals for the university's exceedingly scarce resources. There was no place in that arena for altruism. Cambridge physiologists had won ascendancy by the 1880s and never for a moment did they let go. They were rivals too for government funds administered by the Medical Grants Committee. The only other source of funds was private benefaction which usually went to new disciplines, as for a laboratory for parasitology opened in November 1921 when Wilson commented 'I wish some one would give my Dept a new building!'[20]

Wilson had also to deal with a peculiar and unwieldy organization. The faculty system had not yet been adopted in Cambridge. The Medical School, presided over by the Regius Professor of Physic, Sir Clifford Allbutt, included the departments of medicine, surgery and pathology, but not anatomy and physiology. They belonged to the Biology School. The Medical School had no control over clinical teaching and University departments had no real connection with collegiate teaching, the Colleges being autonomous. There was no adequate machinery for coordinating teaching appointments or courses. And University finances were straitened. For the first time in its history Cambridge in 1919 had to accept substantial government funding to meet the demand of record enrolments and the challenge of modernization. The Anatomy department's laboratories and dissecting rooms were unbelievably dingy and unsuited to their purpose; equipment was meagre, and there were skulls everywhere, reflecting Macalister's long passion for anthropology. Given the means, however, Wilson was confident he could make a great improvement relatively quickly.[21]

In November 1920 the Medical Grants Committee voted Wilson 500 pounds which was 50 per cent more than he had sought for equipment, a matter to which the physicist Sir Ernest Rutherford had given strong support. Till Christmas he was busy with structural alterations, better lighting, specifications for new equipment, and orders for books, periodicals and microscopes. Then he concentrated on establishing a library. Skulls were swept away and new shelving installed. It was a great day on 19 January when he unpacked his 34 cases of books which till then had cluttered the floor. Added to books bequeathed by Macalister, this collection and further purchases made an excellent and comprehensive departmental library.[22]

Servicing the library became an endless and tedious job for Dorette, occupied day in and day out for months in a dusty corner where no one ever came, cataloguing books and pamphlets and binding periodicals. Wilson at 60 was as energetic and demanding as ever and Mabel, after being recruited to the cataloguing task, interceded on Dorette's behalf to ensure she had one afternoon a week for fresh air and exercise. During vacations Louise, Katharine and Douglas helped as well so the anatomy library became a family affair, especially while Dorette was mastering shorthand and typing to become Wilson's secretary.[23]

Wilson turned his attention to the curricula. The Cambridge medical school was a pre-clinical school. It prepared students for the first MB examination in the basic sciences, usually requiring one year's work, and for the second MB examination in the medical sciences, usually requiring three year's work. For their clinical training for the third MB examination students went to hospitals, usually in London, for three or more years. The Cambridge medical courses were essentially the same as those of other British universities. They provided an 'adequate' technical training without the 'special merit' worthy of the reputation of the Cambridge medical school. That was supplied by the Natural Sciences Tripos which all medical students were encouraged to attempt. Tripos work was an opportunity for better quality training in the fundamental sciences, conducted over three years concurrently with the second MB programme.[24]

The Natural Sciences (Anatomy) Tripos was the vehicle by which Wilson planned to lift standards and interest in scientific anatomy. In May and June of 1921 he concentrated on its design, having difficulties with Professor Langley and the zoologist Professor Stanley Gardiner for inevitably his subject impinged on theirs; indeed by 1923 Wilson's Tripos Part I course, a wide-ranging programme in vertebrate morphology and embryology looked like taking over Zoology's vertebrate course. A first in Part I gave entry to Part II (Anatomy), an adventurous experiment for Wilson drawn from American practice. It involved no systematic instruction: students were free to pursue their own interests, consulting staff as they wished. Their only duty was to appear in Wilson's room for tea and biscuits on Tuesday and Thursday afternoons, 'perhaps the most illuminating experience of the whole year', remarked one student, 'and one we hated to miss'. It brought together those interested in human and non-human anatomy as well as senior students and staff. 'He impressed us all with the acuteness of his mind and the generosity (that is the only word) of his outlook on all problems presented to him whether anatomical or personal' wrote W A Fell, a 1923 Tripos Part II (Anatomy) student, later to become a demonstrator.[25]

This new scheme came into operation in Michaelmas Term 1921. Professor Stanley Gardiner remained aloof but Dr Hans Gadow, Reader in Zoology and Curator of the Zoology Museum was very receptive and it was through him that Wilson forged links with the Zoology Department. Gadow, who until then had taught old-fashioned comparative anatomy, with Cresswell Shearer and A B Appleton of Wilson's department organized the resources for this new Tripos Part I (Anatomy) programme. Appleton, a young enthusiast for this style of teaching, had responsibility for the adult vertebrate morphology part of the course and he introduced American ideas as well as experimental and radiological methods of investigation. Shearer, an experimental embryologist of some stature who transferred from the Zoology Department to Anatomy in 1922, had charge of embryology which was effectively a new subject for the Anatomy Department. Wilson was always available for consultation and advice and his enthusiasm gave a sense of spiritual revival. The numbers in Part II (Anatomy) were small but were to become the teachers of the future: Frank Goldby, Howard Green and W A Fell, were all from the first cohort.[26]

In the new regime Wilson did no pass teaching and he rarely entered the dissecting room. That basic service to medicine was in the charge of Duckworth, a loyal lieutenant despite his disappointment at not getting the chair. He was assisted by Drs Hopkinson, Pennell and Reid, who had a clinical orientation. For medical students 'Duckers' and Cambridge anatomy remained synonymous.[27]

Wilson lectured only to Tripos candidates on the central nervous system and the embryology of the higher vertebrates, for which he had to prepare new lectures and demonstration material at an advanced level. How he missed those lantern slides he left behind in Sydney! Louis sent some to him and the embryologist Walter Heape of Tunbridge Wells contributed slides and mole embryos in 1923, Professor Weed of Johns Hopkins sent excellent pig embryos in 1924 and some years later came material from the Bles collection returned by Professor Peter Greiswald in Germany. Wilson combined lectures with demonstrations in thrice-weekly sessions timed for 75 minutes, but often longer especially if his beloved embryo H67 was on display. One student recorded a session lasting 95 minutes. Usually starting at 5 p.m., they made a strenuous end to the working day but Wilson seemed unaware of the passage of time. That idiosyncrasy and his use of 'I say' like a comma were picked out for caricature in student doggerel.

Professor I Saye is a wonderful man,
at a quarter to twelve the Great Sentence began,
with an odd er-um it onward ran,
and was still going strong when we left to a man
at ten past one in the morning.[28]

There were times in his first year at Cambridge when Wilson longed
for the familiar grind of Sydney but after he settled in he found his
new headquarters profoundly congenial. He revised his opinion that
Oxford was vastly superior, for instance in College architecture: 'We
have nothing quite comparable to the Magdalen buildings or
Christchurch. But they have not a Kings Coll. Chapel.' Oxford was
'a more metropolitan place' with 'far more spacious streets & more
imposing shops' but he preferred Cambridge: 'It is less hidebound
& conventional'. Cambridge bookshops he noticed usually carried
the latest publications even in his own special line and the
Cambridge University Library was a joy. 'I have hardly yet got used
to feeling that one can as a rule look up all the references to
authorities that one finds necessary. In Sydney one was always being
pulled up short by the absence of more or less important books &
periodicals', he wrote in April 1921. He was 'extraordinarily busy'
with even less leisure than he had had in Sydney, but he had
experienced as he had hoped, 'a new access of vigour'.[29]

Grafton Elliot Smith's concept of Wilson's role was that 'you can
do as much or as little formal work as you like, for in Cambridge a
professor does his best for the place by means of social intercourse
with students and dons'. Wilson was quickly inducted into
professional and professorial networks to perform that role. Three
times a week he dined in Hall, as required, and on feast days he took
guests to experience the enchantments of St Johns' famous dinners by
candlelight. Twice a term he dined with The Society, a group of 12
senior dons who took turns and infinite pains as host. They included
Sir Arthur Quiller-Couch, Peter Giles (Master of Emmanuel), A B
Ramsay (Master of Magdalene), G D Liveing (Senior Fellow of St
John's), H R Dean (Professor of Pathology), Louis Clarke (Director
of the Fitzwilliam Museum) and Sir Charles Darwin (Master of
Christ's). He joined the Cambridge Philosophical Society (serving as
President from 1924 to 1926) and addressed them in May 1925 on
'Evolution'; and before the irreverent 'Heretics' club in March 1922
he defended the proposition 'that the world of our experience is not
ultimately unintelligible'. He joined the Cambridge Natural History
Society, the Folk Lore Society, the Zoological Society, the Royal

Anthropological Society, the Atheneum Club, and was the inaugural President of the Cambridge branch of the British Universities Australian Association. He belonged also to two book clubs which met monthly. On Sunday mornings the family attended St Columba's Presbyterian Church and every Sunday afternoon they entertained groups of staff, students and friends, including in particular many Australians.[30]

Business took Wilson to London about once a week. In November 1921 he was elected to the Council of the Royal Society – 'an honour I could gladly have dispensed with but cannot graciously decline' – and served on its Grants Committee, where he pushed the idea of leave/research grants for professors (like Edgeworth David) who had in hand fruitful lines of research. A Councillor of the Anatomical Society during 1921 to 1923, he was elected unanimously as President in 1922, a circumstance which in C S Sherrington's opinion reflected well on the Royal Society as parent. Wilson arranged and hosted a highly successful Summer Meeting of the Anatomical Society in 1923. Obituarists observed that he brought learning, charm and urbanity to this office. Arthur Keith said he had the mental qualities of a statesman. At regular meetings he was probably better remembered for his 'scraps' with Hill and the force of his criticisms, as a Sydney visitor observed at one meeting when

> ...two intrepid young men presented a paper of a most imaginative and heterodox nature on the innervation of muscle. There was some desultory discussion for a while, until Wilson could contain himself no longer. After a period in which the characteristic fidgeting of his shoulders increased, with a voice that shook the rafters he proceeded to demolish the anatomical house of cards erected by the young authors. After a categorical denial of every conclusion they propounded, he thundered: 'But of course, I am not dogmatic.' He did not quite understand the laughter which greeted this statement, but the new theory was not heard of again.

He was President for two years and subsequently, from 1926 to 1935, served on the Editorial Committee of the *Journal of Anatomy*.[31]

Then there were his London and Edinburgh meetings for the Carnegie Trust. In February 1923 he was recruited to the Carnegie Trust for Scottish Universities as an expert in medical biology to advise on applications for grants, scholarships and fellowships for research. Each April and October a large bundle of applicants' files would arrive on his desk and he would go to Edinburgh to interview candidates, and sometimes to inspect a research centre, sending in his reports by the end of May and November. For four months each year it was a heavy part-time job, but a congenial opportunity in company with eminent Scots including John Buchan, J M Barrie, Sir George Adam Smith, Lord MacMillan and Lord Sands to help 'a great Scottish enterprise'. And unlike his work for the Royal Society, the Anatomical Society and various boards of advice for university appointments, it carried an honorarium of 150 pounds per year plus expenses.[32]

Much of Wilson's London business concerned Australia. Especially in the early twenties he sat on many Home selection committees for senior Sydney University positions, in company sometimes with Martin. In March 1921 he was elected by the Australian Universities to replace Sir William Bragg in representing them on the executive committee of the Universities Bureau of the British Empire; he also represented them on the Committee of Vice-Chancellors and Principals of British Universities held on the eve of those Bureau executive meetings. The Bureau had been founded in 1912, largely through the efforts of Donald MacAlister, the Principal of Glasgow University, who was also a driving force in the Carnegie Trust. Many of the people Wilson met through the Bureau were Carnegie Trust men, and this meshing of Scottish and Australian education interests in the broad context of Empire he found most agreeable. The Bureau arranged five-yearly congresses of Empire Universities, ceremonious proceedings with entertainments for delegates that swept like a royal progress through several universities. The main business of the second congress was conducted in Oxford in July 1921, with Lord Curzon, the University Chancellor, presiding. As a delegate for Sydney University Wilson gave a paper on the sabbatical year for professors, a custom Sydney had developed further than other empire universities. He stayed at Christ Church (the Haldanes being away) and once again met Professor Woodhouse, Professor Mackie and his wife and Professor Carslaw who were also representing Sydney.[33]

There were many Scots in Wilson's circle of acquaintances, but of the friends who called him 'Jim' – pre-eminently Jim Smith and John Haldane – he saw little. Family connections kept him in touch with the Lorrain Smiths, and if Jeanie had accompanied the family to Cambridge they might have been closer. Jim Smith was as busy in Edinburgh as Wilson was in Cambridge; the Wilsons saw more of his sisters Annie and Maggie who were in London. Wilson's friendship with John Haldane might have revived to intimacy had

311

Wilson gone to Oxford and not Cambridge. But, though he maintained his home in Oxford and remained a Fellow of New College, Haldane's work-base from 1913 was the mining research laboratory at Bentley Colliery near Doncaster, moving in 1921 to Birmingham University. Over the years that Haldane's son Jack was in Cambridge with Gowland Hopkins at the Biochemistry Department (1923 to 1932) family intercourse might have been renewed – Jack's work on the intricacies of the mechanisms of evolution would have fascinated Wilson – had Jack been other than he was: a confirmed and at times offensive authority-baiter. He preferred not to be called 'Jack' by his friends because his family and people he disliked did so. The challenge he threw down to the Vice-Chancellor and the Sex Viri ('meaning the six men, not the sex weary', Jack quipped) in 1925–6 over the divorce case of his future wife Charlotte Burghes, and the left-wing and non-conformist fraternity he established in his home, Roebuck House, would not have appealed to Wilson, however enlightened Jack's intentions. Wilson thought him 'clever – sometimes too clever not always profound, & frequently wrongheaded & bitter'.[34]

Wilson, Lorrain Smith and Haldane had drifted apart. If together they might have done great things, as Wilson felt at the outset of their careers, separately their achievements had not been negligible as he had feared. They had all won distinction. Haldane made a profound impact on pure and applied physiology in the fields of respiration and body temperature, and by 1913 when he resigned his Readership his work had established a reputation for Oxford as a vigorous school of a new physiology. Always alert to the amelioration of public health problems, after 1913 his contributions to the improvement in working conditions, disease prevention and safety for miners were very great; in recognition he was elected in 1924 President of the Institution of Mining Engineers. Lorrain Smith, who had collaborated with Haldane for ten years in physiological research, committed himself to pathology on being appointed in 1895 as lecturer in that discipline at Queen's University Belfast. It became a chair in 1897. In 1904 he accepted the pathology chair in Manchester and in 1912 the Edinburgh pathology chair, becoming also Dean of Medicine in 1919. He influenced significantly the teaching of pathology by correlating the pathological with the clinical aspects of disease, and in Edinburgh he crafted a better coordination of the medical curriculum. His research was in diverse fields: studies of the pathological effects of high oxygen pressures on lungs, and of blood colour and volume in pathological states, both extensions of his work with Haldane; bacteriological work on typhoid fever and Bright's disease; the wartime problems of poison gas, trench-foot and antisepsis; and a long series of studies of fats and lipoids which, taken together, made a valuable and original contribution to the understanding of the inner workings of cells, especially in reference to the processes of oxidation. In Haldane and Lorrain Smith, as in Wilson, their philosophy influenced their science and their teaching – it pushed them towards fundamentals – and made them attentive as professionals to social problems.[35]

While at his busiest with the reorganization of his Department Wilson was drawn into a neurological controversy early in 1921. On February 16 he attended a lecture in London by the neuro-anatomist Professor T Boeke of Amsterdam on the dual innervation of striated (or striped) muscle, published in *Brain* the following April. Wilson was familiar with the subject – he had opened his research career in the 1880s with studies of nerve/muscle relationships – and of Boeke's contributions to it, so at the request of Sir Henry Head, editor of *Brain*, he wrote a critical morphological review of the literature, published in *Brain's* July issue.[36]

Boeke's investigations, especially his experiments on the eye muscle of the cat, had led him to conclude that certain muscles are innervated by fine unmyelinated motor nerve fibres of sympathetic origin – he called it an 'accessory' system – in addition to and separate from the ordinary motor nerve fibres of cerebro-spinal origin. The idea was not new: Wilson's summary of work on it went back to 1882, but only in the last 20 years had histological technique supplied the means to gather reliable evidence and only with Boeke's work since 1909 had the hypothesis gained ground. Boeke laid stress on the characteristic endings of the nerve fibres of this 'accessory' system and their hypolemmal position (lying under a muscle fibre), often in intimate association with the terminations of the ordinary myelinated motor nerve fibres; outward conduction of impulses was indicated. Some physiologists were drawn to the theory because it suggested an anatomical base which certain physiological phenomena seemed to demand, such as the control of muscle 'tonus'. The neurophysiologist E D Adrian, however, was convinced that the sympathetic nervous system could have nothing to do with muscle tone.[37]

Wilson found the physiological evidence 'equivocal' and Boeke's interpretation of his evidence 'open to grave criticism in more than one direction'. But he also found in the evidence that Boeke

313

assembled, and in the results of similar investigations of the limb muscles of the cat by E Agduhr of Sweden, strong indications for corroboration of Boeke's hypothesis. The state of the case, however, was inconclusive: there was 'no stringent proof that true sympathetic fibres in the case of the eye-muscles do actually innervate accessory end-plates in muscle-fibres'.[38]

Boeke's lecture and subsequent demonstrations of his preparations at University College London aroused the interest of Nicholas Kultchitsky the eminent histologist and refugee from Bolshevik Russia whom Elliot Smith had secured for his staff in June 1921. More correctly, it re-aroused his interest, for the innervation of striated muscle had been his first research subject in 1881. He produced a superb series of gold chloride preparations of python muscle demonstrating the presence of two distinct types of nerve endings, one connected to unmyelinated fibres which he thought could be sympathetic in origin. Kulchitsky was working on this when from Australia came Johnny Hunter in mid-October, at the beginning of his *Wanderjahr,* and it triggered his interest. The innervation of striated muscle was to become Hunter's dominant research interest.[39]

Johnny Hunter's inaugural year as Associate Professor in Sydney had been impressive. He had borne with apparent ease the heavy burdens of teaching, administration and ceremonial duties, and had got down to research in not one but several areas: one was an embryological study of a specimen of ovarian pregnancy which Wilson had given him; another was an anthropological study with Burkitt on the Neanderthal characteristics of the Australian Aborigine; yet another, at the instigation of A E Mills and in collaboration with the orthopaedic surgeon Norman Royle, was an experimental study of injury to the spinal cord: they set out to test a theoretical suggestion of Wilson's that vascular disturbances at the site of spinal cord lesions may play a part in the symptomatology of 'spinal shock'. Their results showed that to some extent they did.[40]

Hunter arrived in Cambridge for the best part of a week in October, about the same time as Dart and Shellshear came back from America. Also visiting the Wilsons were Sir Arthur and Lady Keith, and Ralph Noble, a former Sydney student of Wilson's now studying neuro-psychiatry in London, who brought Louise home for the weekend on his motorbike. The Wilson household was renowned for its hospitality. Just then Wilson was 'so loaded up with things to do that I cant quite see my way through' but he was able to make arrangements for Hunter to begin work at University

College London without delay. He arranged also for Hunter to work for a time under Arthur Keith at the Royal College of Surgeons: 'a very fine chance' Wilson commented. On returning to London, Hunter found accommodation in the same house with Ralph Noble. Johnny, reported Wilson to Jeanie, 'is very busy & very happy now I believe. Everyone is trying to help him to make the best use of his time'. A month later Wilson watched over Hunter as he made his debut before the Anatomical Society.

> H. was quite equal to the occasion. He gave a splendid demonstration of his lantern slides with no obvious nervousness and with quite conspicuous ability. He quite established his reputation & justified the rather flattering judgement of him that I had been conveying to my friends.[41]

Hunter had had the best possible introduction to British anatomy. In company with Elliot Smith he impressed a wider audience. London journalists took them to lunch and reported:

> Both are famous in the scientific world for their uncanny knowledge of anatomy. Elliot Smith likes his bones a few thousand years old, and served in mummy cerements: Johnnie Hunter likes his with the marrow warm in them, and amenable to reform. Elliot Smith is middle-aged, thick-thighed, heavy torsoed, an old Roman type. Hunter is dark-haired, slender, with a wide laughing mouth, is an amazing 24 and looks 19. In a pre-scientific world he'd have probably filled in time crusading or being a troubadour.[42]

Between November and the following October when he left for North America Hunter worked at neurology and anthropology in London, presented another three papers to the Anatomical Society and spent a month at the Central Institute of Brain Research in Amsterdam with Ariens Kappers working on the preserved brain of a kiwi provided by Elliot Smith, which was to win him the MD of the University of Sydney in 1924. There followed a hectic tour of Canadian and American medical schools and research institutions including the Rockefeller Foundation before his triumphal return in mid-February 1923 to Sydney University and the laurel crown of Challis Professor of Anatomy.[43]

The old order was changing at Sydney University. MacCallum retired at the end of 1920 and Francis Anderson at the end of 1921. Edgeworth David relinquished his teaching duties at the end of 1922 to concentrate on his account of the geology of Australia and retired at the end of 1924. With the unveiling during 'Commem' in

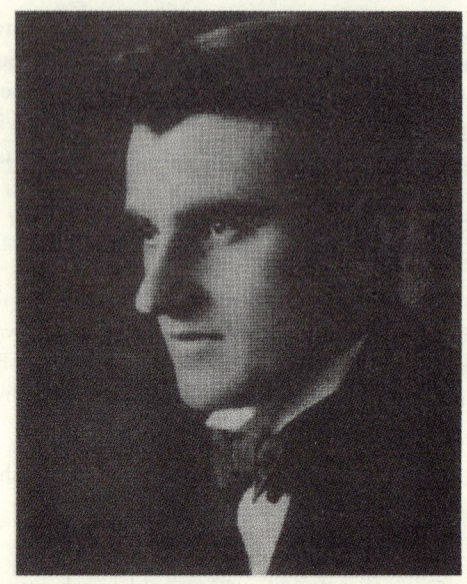

John Irvine Hunter   Photo: courtesy SUMJ.

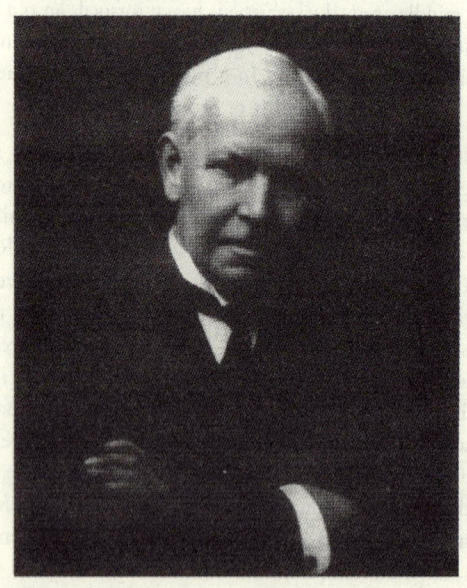

Grafton Elliot Smith Photo: from Dawson.

316

May 1923 of portraits of Wilson, Edgeworth David and Barff, the staff of Sydney University saluted the passing of the old guard. The choice of David's successor was contentious, both sides confiding in Wilson in personal correspondence. David strenuously backed Leo Cotton of his Department against Douglas Mawson who was recommended by Wilson and the English committee, MacCallum and half the Senate. David's will prevailed, much to the disgust of Carslaw who had argued for Mawson because he had the greater reputation: since 'Wilson had gone, MacCallum was no longer a teacher and T.W.E.D. was going', the University needed 'a Person – with a large P'.[44]

Also, H E Barff was going. Barff's authority was far greater than the titles of his offices, Warden and Registrar, suggest. For more than forty years he had steered the University through many hazards. He was more like an executive Vice-Chancellor, and in fact his retirement gave rise to that new office. He had advised Wilson in September 1923 of his intention to retire and in December he wrote that in August 1924 he would in fact be leaving. He also informed Wilson unofficially of the Senate decision to create the new office of Vice-Chancellor which it proposed to fill by invitation: 'Your name came up & was heartily acclaimed on all sides'. He concluded with a plea: 'Think of all your colleagues here struggling in the dark & waiting for the light to shine on them. What a delight it would be to me personally to have you back I cannot say. It would mean a very great deal to the University.' In July 1924 Edgeworth David wrote Wilson a letter and MacCallum wrote three, one official and two unofficial, asking him to seriously consider the new position of executive Vice-Chancellor. Was Wilson interested? This offer was backed by the Chancellor, 'persons in authority' and many Senators, and no immediate move was necessary as a Bill had to be enacted by Parliament. Meanwhile, MacCallum wrote, he was prepared to take the Wardenship until the end of 1924, and even be a stop-gap Vice-Chancellor for 1925 if Wilson could take over at the beginning of 1926. Wilson would be 65 in 1926, the usual age of retirement.[45]

Wilson had had plenty of time to think it over. He replied promptly with a cable 'Do not count upon me in the matter raised in your letters' and in a letter of 19 September 1924 he declined the honour explaining that a combination of family reasons (especially with regard to the younger members), his wife's health and his departmental obligations – 'I should feel something of a deserter if I were to leave at this juncture or in the immediate future' – prevented him from doing so.[46]

317

At that time there was a huge increase in the number of academic positions for which many current staff and Sydney graduates were preferred, some of them for senior posts advertised overseas. Johnny Hunter was a conspicuous example. Others were Professor E R Holme and J Le Gay Brereton in English, Bernard Muscio in Philosophy, Tasman Lovell in Psychology, F A Todd in Latin, F P Sandes in Surgery, G G Nicholson in French, H G Chapman and Henry Priestley in Physiology, R Reading in Dentistry, Christopher Brennan in German and Comparative Literature, T Griffith Taylor in Geography, J P V Madsden in Electrical Engineering, O U Vonwiller in Physics. Sydney University was recognising her own. Heavy reliance was placed on Wilson's advice via the 'home' selection committees and informally in letters. He maintained correspondence with MacCallum, Mills, Barff, Edgeworth David, Selle, Carslaw and Purser.[47]

Wilson was in the unique position of knowing well the local conditions and candidates while assessing the claims of British candidates. He may have leaned toward local candidates but fitness for the job was his prime criterion. For instance he thought Nicholson, Chapman and Priestley 'foregone conclusions' but he demurred on Brereton. In Reading the University had a capable, agreeable man but he wondered whether his energy and capacity were equal to cleaning up the Augean stables of the Dental Hospital. The case of the new Psychiatry Chair was special. Wilson's advice to Barff in February 1921 was that it needed a man of exceptional calibre and qualifications and it were better that the position were not filled if a suitable man could not be found. A high salary, the right of private practice and adequate clinical assistants should be offered as inducements. The man appointed in 1922 on Wilson's recommendation was Sir John MacPherson MD, of Edinburgh. Aged 60, knighted just before sailing for Australia, MacPherson was an eminent psychiatrist who had been Commissioner for Lunacy in Scotland and Senior Assistant Physician at the Morningside Asylum. It was an unusual appointment which proved sound: before retiring in 1926 he established his discipline at Sydney University on strong foundations.[48]

The fortunes of Sydney's Medical School remained near to Wilson's heart. He watched developments closely in the early years of this second era of expansion. There were disappointments. Shortly after Wilson's departure in August 1920 the Senate abolished the Chair of Pharmacology and reestablished the lectureship in Materia Medica. Wilson was dismayed

I am bound to say I greatly regret the abolition of the Chair of Pharmacology. I never regarded it, as some people wished to make out, as a position established to make way for Chapman. There is really a great field for pharmacological research in Australia, and there is now no Chair in that subject to provide a fully competent investigator. It will be a reproach to the Australian Medical Science if that situation is allowed long to continue.

The situation remained unsatisfactory until 1948, and it was indeed a reproach to Australian medical science.[49]

Then, during Hunter's absence, Wilson's project for a new Institute of Anatomy was dismantled. During 1922 the Senate distributed 30,000 of the 50,000 pounds originally voted to build the Institute to the Departments of Geology, Architecture, Chemistry, Zoology and Veterinary Science. The 20,000 pounds remaining available to Anatomy should have enabled substantial improvements to that department but only a mezzanine floor to the Museum – now called the Wilson Museum – was provided, at a cost of 1,500 pounds. Hunter made no effective protest. This outcome was a severe disappointment for Wilson.[50]

There was a power vacuum in the Medical School, awaiting the emergence of a new authority, an interregnum that Wilson hoped would last till Hunter's stature increased sufficiently. There were old hands enough to maintain equilibrium: Mills as Dean in the new chair of Medicine, Welsh who was to remain in the Pathology chair until 1935, Chapman in the Physiology chair with Priestley as Associate Professor (Biochemistry) and Maguire an experienced hand in the Anatomy department. Difficulties with Maguire did arise; Hunter was hesitant in assuming leadership and in the opinion of Louis Schaeffer too easily persuaded against his judgement.[51]

Hunter was, however, shaping well. He scotched moves to make histology a separate department and embedded it securely in anatomy's teaching programme. With funds provided by G H Bosch, a wealthy Sydney merchant, he gave impetus to research: G H S Lightoller was working on facial musculature (for which Wilson was able to secure a Royal Society grant), Maguire on anatomical variations of the female pelvic organs, and T K Potts on the main peripheral connections of the human sympathetic nervous system. Most exciting was Hunter's work on the dual innervation of skeletal muscle, in which H J Wilkinson the demonstrator in histology and Oliver Latham of the pathology department became involved.[52]

Hunter joined forces with Norman Royle, with whom he had collaborated previously, in an arduous experimental investigation into the possibility that the sympathetic nervous system controls 'plastic' tone, and that consequently sympathetic ramisection might ameliorate spastic paralysis. They presented their first findings to a meeting of the NSW branch of the BMA in October 1923, and in November gave a paper and demonstration at the Australasian Medical Congress. In a series of papers in the *Medical Journal of Australia* in 1924 Hunter, in the words of his biographer, Michael J Blunt

> sought to define as a principle, that the action of the sympathetic component of the autonomic nervous system was fundamental and constant and that intermittent activity of the cerebrospinal system and the parasympathetic component of the autonomic was superimposed upon it. The principle was held to be true for voluntary muscle, blood vessels and certain hollow viscera.

Hunter was seeking to ascribe primacy to the peripheral over the central nervous system. This was highly speculative but, supported by Royle's testimony that 'unilateral sympathectomy of decerebrate animals reduced rigid paralytic extension of limb musculature on the operated side', it was plausible. Elliot Smith during a visit to Australia in August/September 1924 promoting anthropology saw the goats on which Hunter and Royle had experimented, and later declared that there could be no doubt about the validity of their findings. Hunter published the results of these experiments in *Brain* in 1924. The results of further experiments on the wing of a roosting fowl and the seagull's wing in flight which Hunter claimed supported his thesis were published in the *Medical Journal of Australia* in September 1924. The first clinical trial on a human subject by Royle (a new operation of unilateral sympathetic ramisection on a soldier with a bullet wound to the cerebral cortex causing a spastic condition of both legs) led to an apparent unilateral improvement in his spasticity and a cure of his constipation.[53]

Because this work raised hopes of a miracle cure for the paralysed, amongst whom were many ex-servicemen, it attracted wide media attention. At least five newspapers and the radio reported Hunter and Royle's presentation of November 1923. In April 1924 two visiting American surgeons raised larger hopes: spastic paraplegia, Little's disease and certain Parkinsonian syndromes might be alleviated. They addressed a large gathering of medical students in the Great Hall of the University and Hunter and Royle were invited to give the fifth J B Murphy Oration to the American College of Surgeons in New York in October. The Senate gave Hunter leave provided he completed his teaching programme beforehand, so in Trinity Term he gave five neurology lectures every week and all the neurology practical classes.[54]

From Cambridge Wilson was readied for assistance. Hunter must have written him of the early findings before their presentation to the BMA meeting in October 1923, for Wilson cabled Mills four days afterwards, urging publication of a preliminary note to be followed by the full paper in *Brain*. He consulted Adrian and Langley who were unmoved in their opposition to the hypothesis. On 18 August 1924 Hunter wrote an excited letter to Wilson detailing his own progress in research and Royle's in his clinic: 80 operations on patients with spastic paralysis. Elliot Smith invited Hunter to give three lectures at University College, after his American visit.[55]

By 1924 the Wilsons were well settled in Cambridge and Wilson's health, threatened by pressure of work in the first few years, was fully restored. In the summer of 1922, coinciding with a meeting of the BMA on 28 July in Glasgow, he took the whole family for a holiday in his native Glencairn where they rented a farmhouse called Coatston. Jeanie and five-year-old Patrick on a one-year's visit from Sydney, were with them (Jeanie studied social psychology under Professor F C Bartlett in Cambridge that year). Mabel added 'auld hen' to family menus and Wilson lapsed easily into the local dialect to the astonishment of his children. With them he had been strict about English usage. They explored Moniaive and cycled around the lovely valley of Glencairn and further afield to Annie Laurie's house at Maxwelton. Back in Cambridge Wilson cycled every day to work, occasionally went on a day-long ride with Mabel, and regularly played golf. Carslaw, for whom Cambridge was 'home', had initiated him to the Gogmagog Golf Club in June 1921.[56]

Most of Wilson's spare time was spent in his private laboratory in the department preparing demonstration material and lantern slides for lectures – he produced a huge amount – trying out new techniques and examining new specimens under his beloved binocular microscope. Working in the adjoining laboratory Howard Green was often summoned by a sudden 'Come and look at this, Green', and, reported Green, 'No matter whether it was a new silver preparation of nerve cells, a low-powered three dimensional view of thick slices of embryo, or naked-eye stained preparations of whole brain pieces, each was immensely exciting and stimulating.' Among many others Wilson's senior assistant Walter Calcott caught his enthusiasm: 'You see that! You see that!' he once barked at Wilson's youngest son, indicating a stained section of an embryo, 'I made that section; it's beautiful, isn't it? Your father couldn't have done it.'[57]

Wilson published accounts of three useful techniques. One described his new method of using Spalteholtz clearing fluid in the study of thick sections of embryos. While it was not suited to the high-powered magnification needed to see the finest detail, this procedure was useful in conveying 'a vivid stereognostic conception of structure'. He could for instance demonstrate with one specimen 'the entire system of bronchial buds in the lung of a mammalian embryo'. Another concerned the problem of uneven illumination of stereo pairs, for which he designed a simplified microscope table with a new lighting arrangement. A third gave an account of experiments, including the use of an ordinary bread slicing machine, to find the best way of cutting thin slices of whole brains embedded in gelatine.[58]

For the well-reviewed fifth edition of Cunningham's *Textbook of Anatomy* Wilson contributed the article on the ductless glands, a much expanded section because of much expanded knowledge in recent years. He also wrote up some research that went back to the early years of the war when Raymond Dart was his young collaborator, on the existence of hypoglossal ganglia in certain mammals especially in their embryonic stages. Wilson's work on a new-born calf with extra ganglia on one side led him to conclude that the single ganglion is a vestigial survivor of a series, thus supporting the interpretation that Froriep had given it in 1882. Thereafter it was named Froriep's Ganglion. With his major undertaking, the embryology textbook with Hill, Wilson was making little progress.[59]

Research output by the Department was impressive. Shearer made a series of researches on the effect of fertilization on the metabolism of sea-urchins, published in the *Philosophical Transactions of the Royal Society* between 1922 and 1924. Frank Goldby published a paper in the *Journal of Anatomy* on his work on the reptilian brain begun under Elliot Smith but much-assisted by Wilson. An American post-graduate student Marion Hines enjoyed some very productive years with Wilson working on the brain of *ornithorhynchus*, later published in the *Proceedings of the Royal Society*. Appleton's studies on the growth of bone won him the Horton-Smith prize for his MD thesis in 1922 and in 1923 the

Symington Prize in Anatomy; through teaching he soon became an authority on comparative myology. In September 1924 he turned down the offer of a chair in order to stay with Wilson.[60]

Johnny and Hazel Hunter arrived in London on 24 November. He was flushed with success from his American tour and 'brimming over with schemes for further investigation'. At the annual meeting of the Anatomical Society he gave two papers, one on behalf of T K Potts and another on his own account, while Elliot Smith delivered a paper for G H S Lightoller. After the meeting the Hunters went to the Wilsons in Cambridge where Hunter delivered his final paper – 'lucid and masterly in style' Wilson recorded – on 5 December. Hunter was unwell, the after-effects of seasickness he thought, but Hazel who was a trained nurse suspected something more sinister. In fact he had typhoid fever, probably contracted in the United States. The following day they left for London as Johnny was to deliver lectures at University College. His temperature rose to 105 degrees and he was admitted to University College Hospital. He died on 10 December, six weeks short of his 27th birthday.[61]

Hunter's death shattered Wilson. He mourned him as a son. At the funeral on 12 December he was too distressed even to speak to former Sydney students who were there. In Cambridge he took up his pen to write the story of Hunter's brief life and career for the *Journal of Anatomy*. His death was a bitter misfortune not only for Sydney University but for the science of anatomy in general and for British anatomy in particular. Wilson's thoughts were with his old department in Sydney and the traditions Hunter had upheld. All that remained was the hope that his memory and his inspiration would endure and be fruitful.[62]

Hunter and Royle's hypothesis of the dual innervation of striated muscle lost ground over the next several years, Wilson keeping an acute eye on the build-up of the evidence for and against. Morphological studies by H J Wilkinson and Oliver Latham of Sydney University and later by Marion Hines (another of Wilson's former students) and Sarah Tower of Johns Hopkins Medical School, together with physiological studies by Gilbert Phillips of Sydney demolished it by 1932 though some, like Boeke, adhered to it till 1940. The critical defect in Hunter and Royle's theory, surprisingly enough considering Hunter's morphological orientation, lay in their failure to establish the structural basis for dual innervation of muscle fibres.[63]

At the time of his death Hunter himself may have had reservations: more caution is evident in his last paper with Latham, published in the *Medical Journal of Australia* in 1925, and the 'brimming' ideas for further studies noted by Wilson could have included revisionary ideas. Anyway serendipity garnered an important clinical benefit in quite another field. With good results the Mayo Clinic in Rochester, Minnesota, applied Royle's technique of sympathetic ramisection to patients with vascular disturbances: it released vasomotor tone with flushing and warmth in the limbs. It rapidly became an established treatment procedure, the most famous patient being King George VI in 1949.

In Australia Hunter's death caught and held the public imagination, and it gave rise to a myth of quite ridiculous proportions. By 1933, when the Medical School celebrated its Jubilee, Hunter had become 'probably the greatest genius of our race': 'a second Shakespeare in intellect'; in neurology he had been far in advance of Wilson his teacher 'such as enabled him to detect any inaccuracy slight or great, that the Professor might make during his lectures, although he himself was taking them for the first time'; and on his first trip abroad he had been recognized as a world authority in anatomy, neurology and embryology. These opinions were authored by Walter J Hull, MB, BS, BSc and the Challis Professor of Anatomy, A N St G H Burkitt, MB, BSc writing in the *Sydney University Medical Journal* Jubilee Issue (September 1933). They had weight. Burkitt wrote to Wilson apologizing for its 'extravagance and stupidity' and disclaimimg a share in it. But he published no disclaimer. It was all a storm in a teacup, said Burkitt.[64]

In Cambridge Wilson read these absurdities, professed a thick hide and dismissed them with contempt. However, he took the trouble to refute one of the more extravagant claims of Hull and Burkitt in the Jubilee issue of the *Sydney University Medical Journal*: that Hunter had written 'his lucid and concise description of Neurology, the most difficult of all anatomical subjects, before Professor J. T. Wilson had completed his lectures on it', by sending Burkitt a carbon copy of Hunter's notes on Wilson's Neurology lectures, a copy of which Hunter had presented to Wilson in 1920. 'These notes', wrote Wilson, 'were undoubtedly the basis of Johnny's teaching of Neurology to which so much reference was made in that article'.[65]

The myth prospered. In 1939 a Sydney radio broadcast, purporting to be an interview with John Hunter, cast Wilson in the role of a satellite. Wilson read the typescript with disgust.

> I consider it an impertinence to have brought me into it and to put
> in my mouth statements quite alien to my thought, representing

324

me as a satellite of J.H. whom I loved & admired, but the extravagance of the estimates of his achievements revolt me. No one had the right to put words in my mouth and I heartily resent it. A lot of nonsense has been talked of Johnny which he himself would have been the first to repudiate.[66]

What was it that gave rise to this legend that so distorted Sydney's memory of both Hunter and Wilson? Perhaps Johnny represented that generation, marvellous in promise, that was destroyed in war. Mungo MacCallum in his first Commemoration Address as Vice-Chancellor in May 1925 made that link:

...like him [Hunter] almost all of them were mown down in their springtide, their lives unlived, their opportunities brought to nought. Sorrow for blighted promise, such as we yield to him, is also due to them.

National sorrow was mixed with a great surge of national pride. Australians now had the image of Anzacs, General Monash was 'the best man in France', and as a result of their contributions to victory Australia had taken her place on the international stage. Altered significantly were Australia's relations with Britain, now the target of criticism for the conduct of the war and the magnitude of Australian losses. In this feverish post-war mood Sydney University appointed a surprisingly large number of its own graduates to its much-expanded staff establishment. Native sons, of whom Hunter was the most gifted and the most popular, were coming into their own while their British 'foster fathers' receded appropriately into the background. Johnny had been a local hero long before he succeeded to the Challis Chair and during his short occupancy of it he had been applauded for his work by international audiences. He represented unalloyed native genius. With his sudden death in London the Hunter legend became not so much a measure of Johnny's abilities, impressive though these were, as a grossly inflated estimation of the national character: young, vital, intrepid, destined for greatness and ill-used by the old world. The legend received fresh stimulus from another burst of unbridled chauvinism during the depression of the thirties. In the popular mind the government's British advisers were to blame for Australia's financial and economic predicament.[67]

A year after Hunter's death the Wilsons were dealt another blow. One January afternoon in 1926 while taking tea with a friend, Mabel suffered a cerebral haemorrhage. For about a fortnight she was unconscious. The prognosis was poor, but the doctor noticed a

325

flicker of one eyelid indicating that 'something was there'. So the girls took turns to sit with her, reading aloud Jane Austen's *Pride and Prejudice* in the hope that she could hear. She did hear, but could make no sign, and commented later when she had recovered all her senses, 'Oh! You girls read so badly!'

Dorette was recalled from London where three months before she had begun a nursing course, and a night nurse was engaged until Mabel became convalescent, then replaced by an extra maid. A 'wireless set' was bought and a car, which at 65 Wilson learned to drive but had little liking for, especially after hitting a bridge. As soon as his competence was acknowledged he thankfully gave up the wheel to younger hands and became the proverbial back-seat driver.

With characteristic spirit Mabel took up the challenge of hemiplegia. Her left leg and left arm were paralysed but by persistent effort she recovered her independence. Her long hair was cut, requiring only her useful hand to arrange it, and all her frocks were made to fasten at the front. She was able to darn socks using a wooden egg, but could not manage to sew on buttons. With her handbag hooked over her left arm she went shopping regularly, and to London occasionally, alone. She remained the mistress of her household, she was zealous in her work for the church and as her family grew up and scattered she became a prodigious letter writer. The comment 'One never thought of her as disabled', indicates the measure of her success. Frustration, however, induced a change of temperament. There were moments of despair, moments of anger, moments of tactlessness. She hated to be helped yet needed help, and Wilson gave it as tactfully as possible. She was now his 'dear invalid', yet still his 'mainstay and mainspring'.[68]

For the third time in his life Wilson faced and weathered the shock of bereavement for his dearest companion, though this time the loss was not total. Photographs show a change. His figure became fuller and more rounded, substantial and solid looking and his demeanour mellowed. There was now a certain resignation in his expression.

Notes

1. 'Personally I': JTW to J, 16.9.20. JTW at fancy dress party: KR, LH, JMGW to author.
2. On board SS *Miltiades:* JTW to J, especially 1.9, 16.9, 22.9.20; JTW to P de B, 18.9.20.
3. Cambridge Anatomy: Green in *The Cambridge Review*, 10.11.45, 84; JTW to J, 17.11.20. 'The physiologists': Keith, 1950, 391–2.
4. 'Now that the War': GES to JTW, 25.1.19, quoted in Dawson, 73–4.
5. Three circumstances: H A Harris in Dawson, 170–3. Starling: CJM in *BMJ* 14.5.27, 941. Rockefeller targeting: Kohler, 90. Grant dependence: GES to JTW, 20.1.20. GES' appointment: Dawson, 172–3. 'nothing official': GES to JTW, 9.10.19.
6. Chair of Anatomy: Fozzard, 61. 'very great relief': GES to JTW, 6.6.20.
7. GES' plans: Dawson, 77–110; Dart 1973, 419; GES on Davidson Black, RSO 1932–5.
8. Dawson, in Dawson (ed.), Ch. I.
9. '...to Hill's room': JTW to J, 3.11.20.
10. 'I am rather': JTW to J, 21.11.20. A contract to write the book on mammalian embryology was signed March 1921: JTW to J, 9.3.21.
11. 'little scrap' etc.: JTW to J, 21.11.20 and 1.3.21.
12. Cambridge acquaintances: JTW to J, 3.11.20, 17.11.20, 21.11.20.
13. 'I have to read': JTW to J, 3.11.20.
14. Wilson houses: KR and LH to author; JTW to J, 11.1.21, 8.5.21; J to MMW, 25.2.21.
15. Family activities: JTW to J, 19.12.20, 11.1.21.
16. Cambridge activity: Howarth, 76, 84–7, 91.
17. Wilson's Inaugural Lecture: JTW typescript 1921; JTW to J, 2.2.21. [And next three paras.]
18. Michael Foster: Geison, 68–71. Macalister: JTW, farewell speech to Anat. Dept, 1934.
19. Wilson's priming: JTW to J, 3.11.20. 'Langley is a': JTW to J, 1.3.21. Hopkins' experience: Kohler, 49–52, 81. Funding supports for Hopkins: Mark Weatherall of Cambridge to author, 1995. 'logically and': A V Hill, 18–20.
20. On Langley: Geison, *DSB*. On Barcroft: Roughton, *RSO* 6. 'one of the': Roughton, 326. Discipline-building: Kohler, 1. Ascendancy of physiologists: Mark Ridley in Horder *et al.*, 49. 'I wish some one': JTW to J, 29.11.21.
21. Anatomy Dept : JTW to J, 3.11.20, 19.12.20, 19.1.21.
22. Rutherford's support: JTW to J, 19.12.20.

23. Library: JTW to J, 19.1.21; DC to author; Obituaries on JTW by H
    Green in *The Cambridge Review*, 10.11.45, 84 and by MH in *The
    Eagle*, 52 (1941–6) 390–1.
24. Cambridge medical and Tripos (Anatomy) courses: *Cambridge
    University Reporter*, 2.10.32, 145.
25. Natural Sciences Tripos: JTW to J, May 1921, 5.6.21, Willmott
    Dobbie to JMGW, 15.11.78 and H Green interview with JMGW,
    1.12.78. Take over Zoology: Gadow to JTW, 4.7.23. 'perhaps the
    most': Willmott Dobbie to JMGW. Staff teas: JTW to J, 2.11.21.
    Frank Goldby to JMGW, 1.12.78. 'He impressed': W A Fell to
    JMGW, 30.11.78.
26. New scheme: JTW to J, 19.10.21; Gadow to JTW, 4.7.23. Shearer:
    RSO Nov. 1942, 15–19; Ridley in Horder *et al.*, 49. Appleton: *J of A*
    1950, 397. Green & Goldby to JMGW, 1.12.78.
27. JMGW to author.
28. JTW lectures: W A Fell to JMGW, 30.11.78; Willmott Dobbie to
    JMGW, 15.11.78. Slides: J/JTW corresp. ; Heape to JTW, 13.10.23.
    Pig embryos: L Weed to JTW, 26.1.24. Bles' material: JTW to Karl
    Peter, Anatomische Anstalt, Greiswald, 8.6.33. 'Professor I Say': J
    Swift Joly to author 11.5.78.
29. 'We have nothing' etc.: JTW to J, 1.3.21. 'I have hardly': JTW to J,
    6.4.21. 'extraordinarily': JTW to Barff, 28.2.21. 'a new access': JTW,
    Inaugural Lecture.
30. 'you can do': GES to JTW, 15.9.19. The Society: Brittain 1947, 105;
    JTW to J (*passim*), 1921–2. 'Evolution': JTW typescript 31.5.25.
    Heretics: Howarth, 50; JTW typescript 12.3.22.
31. 'an honour': JTW to J, 29.11.21. Leave/research grants: JTW to
    TWED, 27.3.23. Sherrington opinion: CSC to JTW, 2.12.23.
    Qualities as Pres.: *RSO* on JTW, 657. 'two intrepid': SAS, 11–12.
32. Carnegie Trust: Edith MacAlister, 187, 345–6. Sir Donald
    MacAlister to JTW, 14.2.23. 'a great Scottish': JTW's reply of
    15.2.23.
33. Universities Bureau: MacAlister, 190–3. JTW was first elected to
    represent Sydney a year earlier (*SMH* 3.11.20). Sabbatical paper:
    JTW to J, 13.7.21.
34. Jack Haldane: Ronald Clark, 73–80. 'clever – sometimes': JTW to J,
    29.5.35.
35. John Haldane: C G Douglas, *RSO* 1936. James Lorrain Smith: J S
    Haldane and R Muir, *RSO* 1931.
36. Boeke Lecture: JTW to J, 1.3.21. Head to JTW, 5.3.21.
37. Boeke, *J of A* Pt I Vol. 44, 1–22. JTW, 1921. Adrian's view: Blunt,
    98.

38. 'equivocal', 'open to' and 'no stringent': JTW 1921, 242, 243, 244 resp.

39. Kultchitsky: JPH obituary on Kultchitsky, *J of A* Vol. 59, 336–9.

40. JTW 1925a, obituary on Hunter, 341.

41. 'so loaded' and 'a very fine': JTW to J, 19.10.21. 'is very' and 'H. was quite': JTW to J, 2.11 and 29.11.21.

42. 'Both are famous': Report of London Institute of Journalists, quoted · in Brett, 60.

43. Hunter's tour: Blunt, 49–52, 64–76.

44. Fund set up 1921 to commission three portraits: two by John Longstaff, Wilson's (in England) by William Nicholson. (Letters JTW to J, 5.6.21, 7.9.21, and J to JTW, 17.5.23.) David's successor: MWM to JTW, 6.7.24. 'Wilson had gone': Carslaw to JTW, 30.12.24.

45. Barff's retirement and the V-C'ship: Barff to JTW, 14.12.23; MWM to JTW, 6.7.24 and 9.7.24.

46. JTW to MWM, 19.9.24.

47. Appointments in Sydney: Turney *et al.*, 437–8. Wilson's advice: e.g. JTW to Barff, 28.2.21. [Appreciation of JTW's 'home' role: by Holme, J to JTW, July 1924; TWED to JTW 1.11.23.]

48. JTW to Barff, 28.2.21. On MacPherson: *Centenary Book*, 271.

49. Pharmacology decision: *Centenary Book*, 196, incorrectly attributes this move to Wilson. 'I am bound': JTW to Barff, 28.2.21. Unsatisfactory situation: *Australia' First*, 552–3.

50. Dismantling of Institute: Blunt, 80. Wilson's disappointment: JTW to Barff, 28.7.21.

51. Sydney Medical School: *Centenary Book*, Ch. 4. Difficulties with Maguire: Blunt, 80. Hunter too pliable: Louis Schaeffer to JTW, 14.12.24.

52. Blunt, 81.

53. Hunter's work: Blunt 97–9; Cleland, 288; JTW 1925a, 343; Hoets, *MJA*, 13.12.47. Clinical trial: *Centenary Book*, 290. 'sought to define' and 'unilateral sympathectomy': Blunt, 97, 98.

54. Blunt, 89.

55. Wilson cable: Blunt, 97. Adrian to JTW, MS 35/4, WP. Hunter to JTW, Blunt, 89.

56. Holiday in Scotland: KR Notes.

57. 'Come and look': Howard Green to MW, 8.11.78. 'You see': JMGW Note in interview report with H Green, 1.12.78.

58. JTW, 1924 and 1928a.

59. *Cunningham's Anatomy* review articles: *BMJ*, 26.5.23, 899–900; *J of A* Vol. 57 (1922–3), 390–1. Hypoglossal ganglia: JTW, 1925b;

JPH, *RSO* 652–3.

60. Shearer: *RSO*, Nov. 1942, 17–19. Goldby: *J of A* 1924–5, 301; Goldby to JMGW, 14.10.85. Hines-Loeb: corresp. with JTW. Appleton: *J of A* 1950, 397–9; JTW to MWM, 19.9.24.

61. 'lucid and masterly': JTW 1925a, 343. Hunter's illness: Brett, 66–71; LH to author; Blunt 90–2.

62. Hunter's death & JTW: LH and KR to author; Cooper to author, 30.5.78. JTW 1925a.

63. [And next para] Blunt, 100–3, 108; Hunter, *Brain* 1924, 261–74; Royle *ibid.* 275–92; Wilkinson, *Journal of Comparative Neurology,* 1930, 129–51 and 1934, 221–38; Boeke, *ibid.* 1930, 299–309; Phillips, *Brain* 1931, 320–9.

64. 'probably the greatest genius', etc.: Hull & Burkitt, 'John Irvine .Hunter', *SUMJ* Jubilee Issue, Sept. 1933, 78–82. Burkitt apology and 'extravagance and stupidity': JTW to J, 14.11.34.

65. 'These notes': JTW to J, 14.11.34; JTW to Burkitt, 14.11.34.

66. 'I consider it': JTW to J, 18.7.39.

67. 'like him [Hunter]': MWM, V-C's Address, May 1925. Nationalism: Souter, 266; Berlin, 246.

68. Mabel's stroke: family communications to author. 'dear invalid': Mary David to author.

14

'I am become two bands'

1926 was an eventful year. In Britain it was the year of the Great
Strike and in Australia the year of the Great Drought. In October, at
the Imperial Conference in London, the Empire passed another
evolutionary (or devolutionary) political milestone with the
enunciation of the formal definition of Dominions as autonomous,
free and equal members of the British Commonwealth of Nations,
united only by a common allegiance to the Crown. Cultural bonds,
however, remained strong.

For the Wilsons it was the year that unequivocally divided the
family. Jeanie was settled in Sydney and seemed content to be so,
even after her divorce from Tom de Burgh in 1923 following her
return from her year in Cambridge. In 1924, when Barff and
MacCallum sought to bring Wilson back as Vice-Chancellor of
Sydney University, Jeanie knew for a certainty and accepted with
equanimity that Wilson would refuse. With some financial
assistance from her father she managed to support herself and
Patrick by various means: by living in a boarding house and renting
her house and sometimes the holiday house at Bayview; by writing
occasional articles for the press; by jobs Professor E R Holme
directed her way like private coaching, marking intermediate
examination papers in English and acting as secretary to the
Australian English Society; and from 1924 as a lecturer in
psychology and English literature for the Workers Education
Association. Wilson's long arm was protective. From the respect in
which he was held by many people in Sydney flowed concern and
help for his daughter. Her divorce case for instance was not the
ordeal she had expected. Lady MacCallum accompanied her to the
court hearings and the barrister H G Edwards, who had served

under Wilson in the Australian Intelligence Corps and the Censor's Office, made her part 'quite easy': he said 'he was glad to do anything for me as he owed more to Father than anyone'. And when, in January 1929, Jeanie married Alan Clunies Ross at the beautiful Kater family home near Moss Vale, Dr Norman Kater expressed similar sentiments.[1]

On 14 March 1926 after an engagement of two years Louise set sail for Sydney to marry Lloyd Hutchinson, a struggling young barrister. Lloyd, as secretary of the local branch of the British Universities Australian Association, had welcomed the Wilsons to Cambridge in 1920. Mabel's beautiful and talented first-born – Louise was 'more hers than anyone else's' she insisted – had become her close companion, recreating the sort of relationship that Mabel had enjoyed with her own mother. She had been dismayed by Louise's engagement in 1924. 'It is rather hard', she had written at the time, 'that we should bring you heart whole from Australia only to lose you back to that country again.' Louise's departure, so soon after her stroke, Mabel found especially hard to bear. For the occasion Wilson composed a special prayer. Like Jeanie, Louise was to need Wilson's financial help until Lloyd established himself. Although he had served on Gallipoli and in France during the war his legal practice suffered from the professional discrimination in favour of AIF returned men, an option denied him in Britain in 1914 by the Australian rule forbidding recruitment to the AIF from outside Australia.[2]

Romance deprived the Wilsons of yet another daughter after Katharine became re-acquainted with Thyne Reid in 1926. The Reids, of Scottish stock, were old friends of the Wilsons in Sydney and Thyne, then adding experience in Sheffield to his Sydney engineering degree, was a frequent visitor at 31 Grange Road. In December 1926, four days after Louise and Lloyd were married at Woollahra Presbyterian Church in Sydney, Katharine married Thyne in a quiet ceremony at St Columba's Presbyterian Church, Cambridge. Shortly afterwards they left for Sydney. Wilson consoled himself and Mabel with the thought that the three sisters would be a comfort and a help to each other in Sydney. Love, Wilson never tired of telling his children, is the greatest thing in the world, but sometimes it must have seemed to him a complicated blessing.

In 1926, the bicentenary year of Edinburgh University's Medical School, Wilson was honoured by his Alma Mater. On 14 June at a ceremony attended by delegates from British, Continental, American and Dominion Universities, among ten of Edinburgh's distinguished medical graduates including George Newman of London, Robert

Howden of Durham, William Jolly of Capetown, Alexander
Primrose of Toronto and Arthur Logan Turner (son of Sir William),
Wilson received the honorary Doctorate of Laws. Sir George
Newman, an eminent medical educationist, then addressed the
assembly on the traditions the Edinburgh Medical School had given
the world, traditions inspired by Boerhaave of Leyden who had
taught Alexander Monro and his pilgrim companions in 1718. There
were three essential ideas said Newman: that great teachers, not
methods, make great teaching; that medicine is a science; and that
clinical teaching is best provided by a hospital subservient to the use
of the university. Edinburgh still prided itself on its cosmopolitanism
and the pervasive influence of its graduates in education centres
around the world. Sydney University, a prime example, was built
largely by 'the Big Four', claimed *The Scotsman* next day: Anderson
Stuart, Mungo MacCallum, Francis Anderson and J T Wilson, all
Scots and two of them Edinburgh men. Wilson's mark was that of 'a
man with a moral ascendancy over the students of all Faculties such
as no other man, possibly, ever had in the history of the University'.³

But Edinburgh University was not so cosmopolitan as it was in
Sir William Turner's heyday. New Universities in Britain, the
Dominions and America had deprived Edinburgh of most of her
foreign clientele. Nor was Scottish education so distinctive. A quiet
revolution dating from the last two decades of the nineteenth century
had brought it more into line with English traditions. More specialist
studies, notably in science, and the introduction of a matriculation
examination which raised the age of entry by two years amounted, in
the opinion of some, to the betrayal of Scotland's democratic liberal-
education principles. As for anatomy, the supremacy Edinburgh had
enjoyed with William Turner and D J Cunningham now resided in
London, associated as it was with Elliot Smith, Arthur Keith, J P Hill
and H H Woollard, an Australian pioneer in experimental anatomy
at University College. The bearers of this hegemony were Scottish or
Australian or a mixture of both, with Wilson – an archetype of the
breed – in the background at Cambridge.⁴

Retirement is often associated with such honours as the LLD.
They are valedictories, an acknowledgment of achievement and a
hint that it is time to pass the torch to younger runners, who by and
large keep a keen eye on that prospect. An age limit of 65 for all
teachers in Cambridge came into force in October 1926, part of a
major reorganization of its teaching and administrative systems. It
had been foreshadowed. In 1920 one of Elliot Smith's confidential
reports to Wilson had alluded to this aspect of the Cambridge chair:

the appointment will be for life: but the feeling is so strongly in favour of modifying this system that you would acquire great merit if you were to volunteer to transfer to a superannuation agreement, if and when it comes into force.

That idea had seemed reasonable to Wilson in 1920. 'I can give them five good years', he had remarked to the family. But there was one overriding condition for Wilson's retirement, as he had advised Elliot Smith in a letter of 4 August 1919:

> I shall not do so unless I find that the family resources are economically secure enough to allow me to be independent of an ordinary salaried appointment...[5]

Wilson would have welcomed relief from the administrative, teaching and ceremonial duties of his chair and the opportunity to concentrate on neurological and embryological questions which excited his interest, but he set his face against retirement. He was fit; there were no indications of failing powers. He probably felt that his new Tripos scheme still needed his personal attention. A more compelling reason was that he could not afford to retire. The family was at its most expensive stage of development with four daughters not fully launched and three sons fully dependent: Douglas doing medicine at Cambridge, John and Maxwell at Oundle. There were also the additional expenses entailed by Mabel's illness. It would not have been possible to fund all of these responsibilities on the reduced income of retirement which, as economic conditions deteriorated, receded further and further into the future.[6]

Mabel's illness wrought a fundamental change in Wilson's outlook. Her sunny disposition was now clouded by disability and intimations of mortality. At 52 and 13 years younger than Wilson she was now the more afflicted and dependent, her physical handicap requiring adjustments in all aspects of her life. There were times when she wished she had died in January 1926. She had been the perfect antidote to all the disturbances of Wilson's anxious nature; now her emotional need exceeded his. In response he grew in resilience and gave constant attention to her welfare. Instead of cycling trips they had outings in the car; a holiday in Switzerland in the summer of 1928 improved Mabel's powers of walking and for adventure they flew back from Paris to London. He worried that life without him would, for her, be bleak, not only for the want of his personal attention. The terms of his Australian pension made no provision for his dependents: it would cease when he died. The Cambridge 'supplementary' pension was probably uncertain, depending on how many years he served in his post. Wilson formed the determination to outlive his wife. His tendency to hypochondria became more marked.[7]

It is likely that Wilson's disinclination to retire displeased Elliot Smith. A J E Cave, another of Elliot Smith's young protégés, recalled hearsay on the matter among the anatomical fraternity:

> I gathered from my seniors (when a young man learning my trade) that Wilson had been appointed to Cambridge on a more or less temporary basis, but had subsequently held on for a decade or more. How true this may be I cannot say, but certainly Wilson kept finance to the fore and did pretty well for himself during his Cambridge days.

The substance of this piece of gossip has enough accuracy to suggest that it originated with Grafton Elliot Smith. While its derisory tone contrasts sharply with Elliot Smith's fulsome expressions of respect for Wilson in his letters, the theatrical language and mock modesty he employed in this personal correspondence implies at least a lack of sincerity, perhaps even duplicity. Elliot Smith's reminiscences during tea breaks were evidently entertaining for young protégés, and at times libellous, with figures of authority as favoured targets. In 1918 he had publicly aired his enduring grievance toward Wilson regarding his boring osteology lectures, a bitter pill 'sugared' with a compliment to the perpetrator ('one of the most clear-sighted and inspiring teachers') according to a formula he often employed in public lectures. It was a grievance that served well to emphasize his point that anatomy teaching should not be hung on the skeleton. There is testimony on both sides, however, that Elliot Smith and Wilson were 'great friends'. One thing is certain: Elliot Smith could not effect 'move on' powers with Wilson as he could with Raymond Dart, Joseph Shellshear and H H Woollard.[8]

In late 1926 Wilson read an article in the *Transactions of the Royal Society, Edinburgh* which aroused his critical instincts. An anatomist, Dr Norman MacLaren of Glasgow University had given an account of the implantation of the blastocyst (a hollow sphere of cells containing a knob of cells destined to become the embryo) in the wall of the guinea-pig (*Cavia*) uterus, which contradicted the 'classic' accounts in the 1880s of Emil Selenka, a distinguished German embryologist, and M Duval a French authority. The salient point was: does the blastocyst at any time have an outer layer of trophoblastic ectoderm [nutritional epithelium]? Selenka and Duval found that it did while MacLaren, endorsing the view of another German authority F Graf Spee of 1901 (which had been reproduced in most recent textbooks), found that it did not. There was a fundamental incompatibility in the two findings.[9]

In rejecting Selenka's and Duval's view MacLaren and Spee were also rejecting Selenka's widely accepted interpretation of the guinea-pig's implantation process which was distinguished by the 'inversion of germ layers' or 'entypy'; and to do so they implied quite extraordinary events like the sudden disappearance of the blastocyst cavity and the rapid transformation of the blastocyst's atrophic wall into a layer of active, well-formed cells. Wilson found this proposition untenable. After a masterly critique of the published descriptions and figures of Selenka, Spee and MacLaren to which he added his own study of serial sections of the guinea-pig material in the Walter Heape embryological collection in his department, he presented an interpretation of the structure of the guinea-pig's blastocyst which brought it into line with other 'entypical' rodents. As corroborative evidence Wilson drew on the work of J P Hill's colleague at University College, G S Sansom, on the implantation of the blastocyst in the vole (*Arvicola*), another 'entypical' rodent. Sansom's illustrations showed a strong resemblance to Spee's on the implantation process in the guinea-pig but their interpretations were different. Wilson argued that Sansom's was 'the true reading', thereby reinstating the classic interpretations of Selenka and Duval.[10]

Wilson presented this work to a large and distinguished audience, a joint meeting of the French and British anatomical societies in London in April 1927 under the presidency of Elliot Smith and Professor A A T Brachet, where it created much interest. It was subsequently published in the *Journal of Anatomy*. Norman MacLaren in Glasgow was not persuaded however and nor was his chief Professor Bryce, as the American neuro-embryologist George Streeter reported to Wilson in September 1928; 'but they will certainly have to come to it' Streeter concluded. J P Hill was appreciative for it clarified an issue that had a bearing on his long investigation into the phylogeny of the primates. He needed to establish whether the *cavia* blastocyst's mechanism of implantation (inversion of the germ layers) represented a primitive condition, as prevailing embryological opinion held, or was a secondary or 'specialized' development. Hill and Sansom therefore studied the *cavia* implantation process directly, taking account also of descriptions of the process in other 'entypical' rodents. They confirmed Wilson's interpretation, also Spee's finding

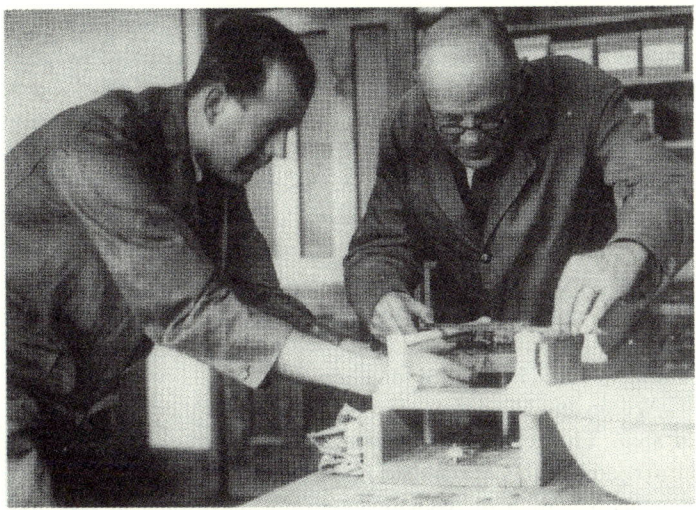

Wilson slicing brains in the Anatomy Laboratory, Cambridge with Simpkin, laboratory assistant, c.1933.

that the *cavia* implantation was interstitial (precocious lodgement of the blastocyst in maternal tissue) and discovered that in three cases of 'rodents with inversion' the process was contrived in three separate ways. This satisfied Hill that 'entypy', far from being a primitive condition, was a highly 'specialized' device independently contrived by some rodents. He was now confident that the early development of the cat, which for a decade Hill had been closely investigating – he made out a cell lineage as far as the 63-cell stage – is the basic, or primitive, eutherian pattern.[11]

On 21 November 1929 J P Hill gave the Croonian Lecture to the Royal Society on 'The Developmental History of the Primates', reporting on an investigation begun 35 years before, almost to the day. On 28 November 1894 with C J Martin he had delivered in Sydney to the Linnean Society of New South Wales a paper giving the first precise description of the platypus embryo and its foetal membranes. In that paper they set forth the view that the basic pattern of foetal membrane development is phylogenetically instructive. In his Croonian Lecture Hill marshalled the results of his long labours in the intervening years to trace the phylogeny of the primates through four developmental stages – the lemuroid, tarsioid, pithecoid and anthropoid – by an entirely new line of evidence: the constitution of the blastocyst, the type of implantation, the origin

337

and mode of formation of the mesoderm, the formation of the amnion and the structure of the placenta. He demonstrated not only the general plan of monotremes, marsupials and mammals, but also established that certain details in the early development of each stage can only be explained by derivation from the development of the preceding stage. Hill recognized that there were many matters both of fact and theory still to be elucidated before the phylogeny of the primates could be satisfactorily established but he had shown – it was his main theme – 'that the data of Embryology, properly interpreted can and do furnish striking and demonstrative evidences of genetic relationships'. That question, in the opinion of D M S Watson writing in 1955, Hill settled for all time.[12]

Wilson and Hill's ideas were in harmony but their work was out of step. The textbook on mammalian embryology that they contracted with MacMillan and Company in 1921 never materialized. Richard Assheton's widow looked for it in vain and that thought burdened Wilson's conscience for more than a decade. He worked at it fitfully, as did Hill – given their other commitments they could hardly have done otherwise – but their efforts did not coincide. 'Very glad to hear you are making some progress with the C.N.S. [central nervous system]' Hill wrote in July 1928. 'I have been so occupied clearing up to get away that I haven't had time to look up Robb's & van Beneden's figs. So meantime you must gang yr ain gate!' Hill just then was in the grip of his thesis on primate phylogeny. At the end of 1931 they resolved to make one more attempt, but that also foundered. In 1939 Hill's successor at University College, Gavin de Beer thought of completing it. 'He doesn't know what he is up against,' wrote Hill to Wilson, 'but he has plenty of self-confidence .... I feel inclined to let him try as I would like to see the job done.' De Beer did not succeed either.[13]

Wilson was given to chiding himself with laziness, which was manifestly untrue as everyone who worked with him could testify. Hill too was diligent: he worked from 9 a.m. to 6 p.m. in his department every day except Saturday when he left at midday, and frequently in the evenings at home. But he was dilatory: he had absolutely no sense of urgency, deadlines being deferred from year to year and some projects like this textbook never achieved. What he did produce, as with Wilson, was of superb quality. It is doubtful that either of them was suited to this extended kind of literary labour. As descriptive biologists wrestling with new and controversial facts and concepts, writing was an important part of their craft and both were particular about producing, as economically as possible, an exact correspondence of word with thought and word with observed fact. Wilson also addressed broader issues like philosophy, to which he directed the same meticulous care. Both wrote well but Wilson – and probably Hill too – did not enjoy the writing process and was only too aware of his want of facility with words. Both Wilson and Hill much preferred bench work with their beloved microscopes, the excitement of discovery and the wrangling about interpretation that went with it. To write a textbook this original work would have had to be put aside.

Research in Wilson's department was ticking over satisfactorily. Beside his paper on the *Cavia* blastocyst Wilson demonstrated maternal haemopoiesis in the rat placenta to the joint meeting of English and French anatomists in April 1927 to which A B Appleton also delivered a substantial paper, later published in two parts in the *Journal of Anatomy*, on the phylogeny of the sacrotuberous ligament and certain mammalian thigh muscles. At a meeting of the Royal Microscopical Society in February 1928 Wilson described his convenient table for microscopy. Appleton turned his hand to editing with J F Gaskell *The Evolution of the Vertebral Column*, a book by Hans Gadow whose death in 1928 was a great loss for the Tripos programme. In 1929 Appleton published *A Guide to Vertebrate Dissection for Students*, based essentially on the Tripos practical work on vertebrate types ranging from cyclostomes to mammals, and about 1930 he began to develop an interest in radiological anatomy which resulted some years later in another book. Frank Goldby turned out a short paper for the *Journal of Anatomy* in 1928 on a series of ectodermal placodes in the head region of a sparrow embryo while Cresswell Shearer contributed a paper on metabolic gradients to the *Journal of Experimental Biology* in 1930. In 1927 under Wilson's supervision Howard Green embarked on a long investigation into the development of teeth in the platypus embryo, taking up where Wilson and Hill left off in 1907. For this – and for work of his own on the platypus brain – Wilson was able to borrow excellent material from Sydney's anatomy department which had been given the abundant Harrison collection of platypus material in 1928. So Green with 11 platypus foetuses – Wilson and Hill had had only two – was able to work out the full dental formula in the platypus embryo, published in the *Philosophical Transactions of the Royal Society* in 1937.[14]

There was irony in that transaction. Launcelot Harrison the Professor of Zoology in Sydney, and Harry Burrell an enthusiastic field naturalist and a collector for the University and for the

Commonwealth National Museum whose book *Platypus* Wilson favourably reviewed for *Nature* in 1927, had collected the foetal material over many years. When Harrison died in February 1928 his widow gave the collection to the Sydney anatomy department, expressing the view that Wilson was the most desirable recipient but she did not want it to go to the Anatomy Department in Cambridge. In May 1928 Wilson was sufficiently moved to send her a cable and in August he found himself writing to Neville Burkitt a lengthy case for access to it for his own work and that of Green. He was given leave to borrow it. At that time no one in the Sydney department was working on platypus, and only H J Wilkinson and G H S Lightoller were working in the field of comparative anatomy. Research in Sydney's anatomy department had developed an almost exclusively clinical focus.[15]

In Britain's anatomical community during the 1920s, contention over its own language was becoming intolerable. Since the 1880s more ink, paper and hours of discussion had been spent on this subject than any other. The first opportunity to establish an agreed international anatomical nomenclature was lost by the opposition of Britain and France to a German production, the *Basle Nomina Anatomica* (*BNA*) of 1895, which was acclaimed in America and the British colonies; Wilson introduced it in his Sydney department in 1897. For the next 30 years a sequence of Revision Committees of the British Anatomical Society, aiming to stabilize a 'recognized medium of description', foundered on the rocks of European dissension, diehard allegiance to the old nomenclature, or the 'co-ordination' of several specialist committees. A revision of the *BNA* published in America in 1927 triggered a battle royal in June 1928 at the Anatomical Society's Summer Meeting in Manchester and resulted in the defeat of the diehards by a younger generation free of undue reverence for traditional usage. Led by T B Johnston, Professor of Anatomy at Guy's Hospital Medical School, London, a three-member committee undertook a British revision of anatomical nomenclature which lifted the question above the general babble of contention, carrying enough momentum to achieve a result. The committee completed its monumental revisionary labours by the summer of 1933 when the Anatomical Society, meeting in Birmingham, approved the committee's *Birmingham Revision* (*BR*). International discussions followed – other countries, notably Germany, had been conducting revisions also – and an international agreement was finally reached at Jena in 1936 with the production of the *Jena Nomina Anatomica* (*JNA*).[16]

Wilson did not attend the Manchester meeting of June 1928 but he sent some literature on neural terms and a letter from Franz Keibel of Freiburg about proposals for an international congress on nomenclature – which he also discussed with George Streeter about that time – to Professor J C Brash of Birmingham who subsequently reported the outcome to him. Wilson was opposed to individual attempts to introduce changes which were not absolutely necessary in advance of collective consideration at international level. Capricious change would result in anarchy.[17]

He was only too aware of the unsatisfactory state of neural terminology due to rapid advances in knowledge and the framing of important new concepts in neurology. Many anatomical neologisms were born in this burgeoning field but only a few achieved preferred status. Waldeyer coined 'neuron', Sherrington 'synapsis', Langley 'autonomic', terms which stuck. Wilson proposed the replacement of 'cerebrospinal' and 'sympathetic' with 'medullary' and 'ganglionic', terms which did not, unlike the term 'omphalopleure' he coined in 1898 for an embryonic membrane, which did stick. As prolific as anyone in the creation of new terminology was Grafton Elliot Smith. The iconoclastic novelty of his researches on the mammalian brain induced the change and invention of many terms to define or re-define precisely his observation of the facts of brain structure and to render intelligible the revolutionary interpretations he derived from them. He also changed his own names as his understanding of the brain grew. In 1896 for instance, on a certain region of the brain he bestowed the name 'area praecommissuralis', which in 1897 became 'corpus praecommissurale', in 1899 'corpus paracommissurale' and in 1903 he settled on 'corpus paraterminale'. To the same region T B Johnston – who in 1928 took charge of the Anatomical Society's Revision Committee – subsequently applied the term 'parolfactory area'. Johnston liked terms which carried a definite meaning, especially for students, in this case identifying an area of the brain with its sensory function. In another instance he created confusion by designating a region of the brain 'primordium hypocampi', a term which Elliot Smith much earlier (1903) had used to designate a specific primordial brain structure. That, in Wilson's view, was 'a confusing misuse of a previously current designation' and an alternative term for Johnston's designation was 'highly desirable'. Since by the 1920s Johnston's 'misused' term had gained recognition in Holland and the United States it seems, as Wilson argued, that only an agreed international nomenclature would solve the problem.[18]

Not infrequently neurological researchers got stuck in a bibliographical quagmire, trying to establish by searching the literature which terms had priority, preferred status, or appropriateness. Early in 1928 Wilson found himself in this predicament on behalf of one of his students. Marion Hines was an American PhD graduate of Chicago University who in the early 1920s began research on the platypus brain with Elliot Smith at University College London, and later with Wilson at Cambridge. She was teaching in the Anatomy Department of Johns Hopkins Medical School in Baltimore when her important paper on the adult platypus brain was accepted for publication by the Royal Society London, provided she made corrections to her terminology. Her 'errors' surprised her for she had tried hard to use the right terms, and for additional insurance had consulted Wilson who had, she believed, 'the most critical mind in all neurology': 'And you were so critical of my terminology.' The issue, she soon realized, was that she had alighted on a few of Elliot Smith's 'terminological aversions'. She conceded the trivial objections – 'fibre' instead of 'fiber' – but held out for others, like 'area subcommissuralis'. The problem was resolved by detailed explanatory footnotes for the disputed terms. This exchange with Wilson was wrapped in banter:

> M H, 4.2.28: There is not a little humor (rather I suppose humour) in a situation that requires a change of fiber to the French spelling fibre for publication in England.

> JTW, 19.4.28: 'Fibre' and 'centre' are not merely French but *English* spellings! The weak point about the American breakaway is that it is such a feeble one!... Why do you not write (rite) trubble and blu and reeson, and why oh why 'graciously', as in your letter, surely 'grashusly' would be far better American! Gracious humor!!!

> M H, 27.10.28: ...although you won with the respected .... Oxford dictionary as authority on the spelling of fibre, that great tome cannot keep up with us.[19]

Marion Hines was one of several American neurologists who became involved in the controversial theory of the double innervation of striated (or skeletal) muscle. The question was: do sympathetic nerve fibres innervate skeletal muscle in addition to the ordinary motor nerve fibres of cerebro-spinal origin, as J Boeke of Utrecht supported by E Agduhr of Uppsala hypothesized? Johnny Hunter's fervent belief that they did had brought him fame, and Wilson would have loved to see that faith vindicated but, as he noted in March 1928, the evidence against was becoming formidable. At Johns Hopkins Medical School Marion Hines and her friend Sarah Tower conducted some important experiments which helped to contradict Boeke's thesis. They found that different staining techniques produced different findings, and published a paper on this in 1928. Marion Hines wrote to Wilson in February of that year

> I have never seen a nonmedullated nerve as Boeke described terminating on such a fiber in the small muscles of the kitten's foot, using the methylene blue technique; but in the Bielschowsky silver preparations of the same muscles, I have seen a few small loops & whorls similar to Boeke's description.[20]

Another group of interested neurologists congregated at the new Institute of Neurology, Northwestern University, Chicago, most notably John Hinsey who in 1927 published findings of experiments using the pyridin-silver technique which also contradicted Boeke. In late 1929 Hinsey was joined by Boeke's main adversary, a former student of Johnny Hunter, H J Wilkinson of Sydney. Wilkinson's interest in the subject had its origin in an unsatisfactory answer Hunter had given to a question Wilkinson had put to him. As a Rockefeller Scholar Wilkinson in early 1929 had visited the laboratories of Boeke in Utrecht and Agduhr in Uppsala to examine the evidence of their findings; he had also visited Bielschowsky in Berlin to consult on staining methods. At the Chicago Institute where he was accorded generous laboratory assistance, Wilkinson established by careful and thorough experimental studies that there was no histological evidence for Boeke's hypothesis and that Boeke's 'evidence' for it was probably an artefact produced by his fixing and staining methods. Wilkinson's work was well vetted by the distinguished neurologists Dr S W Ranson, Director of the Institute, and Dr C Judson Herrick of the University of Chicago and it won him distinction. In 1930 Wilkinson was appointed Elder Professor of Anatomy and Histology in Adelaide (succeeding H H Woollard), where he established a department very much in Wilson's style. In 1936 he went to Brisbane to do likewise, as first Professor of Anatomy and Foundation Dean of Queensland University's new medical school. Wilson was for Wilkinson a 'mainstay' during his long public argument with Boeke and though Wilson never actually taught him, Wilkinson held Wilson in a kind of filial regard, which Wilson

343

reciprocated. Wilson kept a photograph of Wilkinson on the wall of his room in the anatomy department.[21]

Though he never visited the United States, Wilson enjoyed good rapport with American anatomists, embryologists and neurologists. At the invitation of Carl Huber of Ann Arbor, Michigan, Wilson had become a member of the American Association of Anatomists in 1913. George Streeter of the Carnegie Institution in Washington was an old friend whom Wilson first met at the Geneva Congress of Anatomists in 1905. Over Rockefeller business in Cambridge he became acquainted with C Judson Herrick and his colleague S W Ranson; in *loco parentis* Wilson took care of Herrick's protégé, G E Coghill of Philadelphia, for his lecturing debut in London in December 1928. Memories of Johnny Hunter prompted correspondence with Frederic Lewes of Harvard Medical School. Herbert Evans of California and George Corner of New York sought meetings with Wilson to 'talk shop'. Wingate Todd, who was actually a Scot trained by Elliot Smith in Manchester before going to Western Reserve University in Cleveland, Ohio, kept a photograph of Wilson on his desk. At the request of Marion Hines, Lewis Weed of Johns Hopkins sent Wilson some excellent pig embryos to add to his slender Cambridge collection. Travelling Americans seemed to delight in the Cambridge experience, especially if they stayed in Wilson's rooms at St John's as was frequently the case. It gave 'insight into the intimate life of the Colleges' wrote Herrick, while Streeter deemed it 'a great thrill to get that touch of your fine old university'.[22]

Wilson would have been welcomed by these Americans, and especially by Marion Hines, in 1928 in place of the editor of the *Lancet* who was then ruffling the feathers of American medical educationists. On October 27 she wrote to Wilson:

> The editor of the Lancet has been making a tour of inspection of medical schools in Canada and the U.S.A. What he will write puzzles us, because he has failed to understand the chief characteristics of medical education on this side of the Atlantic. He was unable, at least yesterday after four weeks over here, to comprehend our idea of a medical school as a part of a University. He came with an idea about us and he has it yet. He can see no value in the independence of each medical school, when in England the curriculum, so he says, is prescribed by an act of Parliament. Why is it, that so many Englishmen can never see virtue outside of England? ... I am still hoping that something will bring you to this

country, for then … we might receive a fair criticism and a friendly comprehension from your lips.[23]

Marion Hines may have been oversensitive, or Sir Squire Sprigge lacking in diplomacy, for Sir Squire came not to find fault, or so he averred, but to appraise the American system of undergraduate medical education against the British system with the idea of promoting reciprocity in medicine, or 'a larger fusion'. He claimed impartiality but Marion Hines was probably correct in assuming that Wilson would have found otherwise on the two most important differences Sprigge identified: responsibility for educational standards, and control of clinical training. In these two characteristics American medical education stood in the Scottish tradition. Wilson as a Scot and Sprigge as an Englishman would most likely have leaned in opposite directions on the relative merits of the indirect control of standards by external authority, as in Britain (the General Medical Council) which tended to produce homogeneity, or by the internal authority of individual medical schools as in America which tended to produce variety. The principle of variety in medical education had been defended by William Turner in 1881 to safeguard the integrity of the Scottish system and Wilson had argued for it in 1921 to give the Cambridge course a stronger scientific emphasis. Likewise on the second question, of whether it was better for the school to own the hospital as in America, or the other way around as in Britain (or more accurately London): Sir George Newman as recently as 1926 had identified the 'subservience' of the hospital to the school as a hallmark of the Scottish system. The traditional differences between Scotland and England had persisted, despite the reforms initiated by Lord Haldane to bring medical education in London within the jurisdiction of the Universities, and the closer alignment of the Scottish to the English system from about 1880. There was a world of difference between the medical scientist who thought primarily as a biologist and the one who thought primarily as a clinician. It was a difference in the very mode of thought.[24]

Sir Squire's mission in visiting North America was also a sign of the times. European hegemony in the medical sciences had not survived the war. Like the balance of power it had shifted to the United States where the doctrine of self determination – inimical to the idea of Empire – held sway. As Britain lost her hold on the Empire she looked towards the United States to promote the idea of a Special Relationship. As Sir Squire put it: 'fulness of understanding between the English-speaking peoples in all departments of life must make for the happiness of a world that is so permeated with their energies'. In America, he observed, money seemed to flow 'as naturally for hospitals and laboratories as gold flowed in mediaeval Europe for the great cathedrals', while in Britain there was 'too little money but greater experience and greater right to rely upon precedent'. This implied that the hospital-based English system was wiser for being older, and that the American schools had too much money for their own good. Strangely, he made no reference to the extraordinarily generous investment in British medical education by the Carnegie and Rockefeller Foundations. It was mainly American money for example that had built Starling's fabulous Institute of the Medical Sciences at University College London. But perhaps that was the point: did Sir Squire not approve of the funding of universities rather than hospitals for medical education? Anyway Marion Hines' impressions were justified. It is hard to imagine that Sir Squire's tour or his report would have done anything to promote 'fulness of understanding'.[25]

By the end of the twenties Wilson was approaching 70 and ailments were beginning to accumulate. Dyspepsia, an old enemy, he kept at bay by careful dieting assisted by golf and the occasional brief holiday, often at The Lizard in Cornwall. Bacillus coli was another persistent problem, the remedy causing 'ghastly nausea' for 48 hours. His teeth were giving him more trouble than they were worth so he bade a glad farewell to his last stump in 1933. Teeth, he declared, were one of nature's – or rather civilization's – failures. His most worrying symptom was a chronic hoarseness of the throat, which from 1928 required periodic radiological treatment. A long holiday was indicated.

In January 1930, after an engagement of four years, Dorette married Leslie Cuthbert, a former student of Wilson's, at St Columba's Church in Cambridge. When they sailed to Australia for their honeymoon they began a commuting tradition for which the Wilson family was to become renowned. For most of March the four sisters rejoiced in their first Sydney reunion in a decade, engrossed in the 'little unimportant details that no one would bother to write' of three new households: of Jeanie and Allan Clunies Ross, with Patrick de Burgh, now a teenager; of Louise and Lloyd Hutchinson who now had two children, Mary born in 1928 and Edwin born in early March 1930, only days before the Cuthberts arrived; and of Katharine and Thyne Reid of Carlingford – then an outer Sydney suburb, almost in the bush – with whom they stayed. The visitors returned home via New Zealand and America to Leslie's general practice in Stirling, Scotland, and at the end of the year Helen, the first of their four daughters, was born to them. As his family multiplied Wilson grew patriarchal in the style of biblical Jacob, whose words he recalled: 'with my staff I passed over this Jordan and now I am become two bands'.[26]

After ten years in Cambridge the Wilsons senior took a long Australian holiday, leaving London in mid-June on the SS *Oronsay*. In Adelaide they were entertained by Professor and Mrs Wilkinson who mustered old friends – including the Vice-Chancellor Sir William Mitchell, an Edinburgh contemporary, and former Sydney students Professors Cleland and Harvey Johnston – to a memorable morning tea, after which Wilson went through a series of Wilkinson's preparations relating to the innervation of striated muscle. Arriving in Sydney in mid-July, their visit, Wilson made clear, was private: they wanted to relax with their family and become familiar with their three new households, their new son-in-law and Louise's two babies. But there were numerous old friends they wanted to see – 'a formidable array' Jeanie discovered as she listed them. They observed a marked· change in both Wilsons. Mabel though lively and independent was now disabled. Wilson had grown more ample, benign-looking and urbane. The taut-framed man with lean face and piercing eyes had mellowed. He was fit and energetic as ever, though bothered to some extent by a bad bout of hoarseness. There was less of 'the mastiff about him' and a new serenity. He was a senior figure in the most hallowed of the Empire's universities and once again he had weathered, in the tragedies of Johnny Hunter's death and Mabel's illness, devastating personal upheavals. [27]

The Great Depression which was to disrupt the lives and careers of so many people – one of whom was Allan Clunies Ross, Jeanie's new husband – was beginning to affect staff and students of Sydney University. In 1931, one of the most difficult years in the history of the University according to the Vice-Chancellor, New South Wales Government funds were cut by 24 per cent. In fair-minded spirit University Staff accepted a salary cut of 10 percent in 1932. From early 1930 the Federal Labor Government was in dire financial straits – 'absolutely bankrupt' said the British Trade Commissioner in Sydney in August 1930 – and sought the advice of Sir Otto Niemeyer of the Bank of England who recommended austerity, an end to overseas borrowing and an end to the protection of Australia's growing manufactures – in other words a return to traditional Anglo-Australian trade. Niemeyer arrived in July and left in December 1930 having aroused a long-to-be-remembered political and popular storm, nowhere more bitter than in New South Wales. The Federal Labor

Government followed Niemeyer's advice in the main but the New south Wales Labor Government led by 'mad dog' J T Lang raised strong nationalist objections. When he defaulted on British war-loan repayments he provoked a crisis between the Federal and State governments and was dismissed by the British-appointed State Governor of New South Wales in May 1932. The imperial connection had already been tested in October 1930 at the Imperial Conference in London when Prime Minister Scullin claimed and won the right to appoint an Australian as Governor-General of Australia. Wilson followed the contest with keen interest. His erstwhile comrades-in-arms, Thomas Bavin in the NSW Parliament and John Latham in the Federal Parliament, both now prominent politicians, were in the forefront of opposition to Lang. The rift in Anglo-Australian relations spread from trade and diplomacy to cultural foundations when English cricketers under Douglas Jardine perpetrated 'bodyline' bowling on the Australian team during the 'Ashes' tour in the Australian summer of 1932–3. Imperial cricket, far from restoring harmony to imperial relations as many hoped, itself became a major imperial problem at the highest political level, and chauvinism had another season.[28]

The Medical School had a special claim on Wilson's attentions. Physically it had grown by the completion of the north wing and its entrance modified by a new and clever late-Elizabethan addition. Warmly greeted by his anatomy kin – Louis, 'the ever green', and Mills, Burkitt, Royle, Maguire and Lightoller – Wilson took a keen interest in current developments and future plans. The transfer of histology from the physiology department to anatomy had not been smooth, H J Wilkinson bearing most of the difficulties, but with the appointment of C W Stump an Adelaide-born, Edinburgh-trained man as associate professor of anatomy in 1926 histology's fortunes prospered, ultimately making it independent of both anatomy and physiology, a development Johnny Hunter had resisted in 1922. Stump had a Midas touch. He became associated with the Sydney merchant G H Bosch, who in 1924 had endowed the research of Hunter and Royle on spastic paralysis (which Royle was still pursuing). Money flowed for anatomical apparatus and a chair in histology and embryology to which Stump was appointed in 1928; for two full chairs in medicine and surgery and a chair in bacteriology; and in 1929 Stump and Bosch played an important part in negotiating a Rockefeller grant of 100,000 pounds for a new medical school building. In money terms the anatomy department was in excellent shape, but in research Wilson would have been less impressed. Research in anatomy now had a predominantly clinical

348

focus. However, Burkitt was generous with material for morphological studies: when Wilson left Sydney for the last time on the SS *Otranto* in mid-September he had some excellent marsupial and monotreme material, mainly on loan from the Harrison collection.[29]

The Cambridge household had now lost all its daughters and one by one the sons were taking off. By the end of 1931 Douglas had graduated in medicine and married Hazel Fulton. They honeymooned with a trip to Australia, spending Christmas at Bayview where on arrival Douglas jumped off the bus and made straight for the pier to gratify his nostalgia. By mid-1932 they were settled in London where Douglas made a start in general practice. John had by then completed an honours degree in law and was articled to a London firm of solicitors while Maxwell was in second year medicine at Cambridge.

Bayview

Wilson was never really at ease with his sons. His need for order and his exacting paternal authority raised barriers. On the observance of the Sabbath for instance, all three were aggrieved: they hated the morning church service and the afternoon passivity and each in turn defected. Wilson remained faithful to Idealism – an expression of radical philosophy and politics in his youth – but he could not interest his sons in the reality of Spirit and self-realization through citizenship, or that in some sense Time is an eternal Now. Under attack in Cambridge from G E Moore and Bertrand Russell, Idealism went out of fashion and materialism again took the ascendancy. Wilson's politics encompassed a belief in the Empire and responsible capitalism, conviction that religion is essential in the fabric of the state and that democratic government must be served and guarded by active citizens. Though he hated war he was no pacifist: war in some circumstances is the lesser of two evils. He had evolved into a robust Conservative but his sons like most of undergraduate Cambridge in the thirties veered to the left. Wilson's tolerance was stretched by his sons, but he remained tolerant nevertheless. Of the *New Statesman and Nation,* their preferred journal, he wrote: 'I confess I never read it myself. It is too left-wingish for my taste. But there are some good things in it all the same & the young men seem to like it.' However on Marxism, then commanding salvationist enthusiasm in some quarters, he was unequivocal: 'I do *not* agree on the value of Marx's "new outlook on history" nor with any view which pretends to find an adequate explanation of any humanist activity in merely environmental conditions, social or economic.' Firm, not to say dogmatic on principles, with his sons Wilson went to some lengths to break down the barriers. In the summer of 1927 with Douglas he made an extraordinary effort:

Idealism

we two went to Paris and walked it from end to end seeing the
sights but had no intimate conversation.... I remember one amusing
and rather touching episode in Paris. Being there, Father thought it
right to include seeing the Parisian sights a visit to the Folies
Bergeres. We both became more and more embarrassed at the sight
of so many high-kicking nude females so, to cover his
embarrassment, Father began pointing out to me the surface
markings and actions of the thighs and leg muscles. We left before
the end![30]

Wilson returned from Australia much refreshed. Lecturing thrice
weekly was no longer a strain and the old relish for the laboratory
returned. He worked away steadily, building his stock of vertebrate
brains which now included that of a bandicoot given him by Burkitt.
It was slow going, however, and he recognized that putting together
an adequate collection would take a long time. In vacations he worked
at it in his laboratory all day and every day, joined in the summer of
1932 by his brilliant Sydney prosector of 1910–11, T K Potts. Wilson
prevailed upon him to contribute one of his fine dissections to the
Cambridge collection. In 1933 Wilson reported with some
excitement that the brain-sectioning contraption he had rigged up
worked beautifully. It produced excellent serial sections of brains for
naked-eye teaching purposes. And when in August of 1933
physiology decamped from its lecture theatre to a new one, the
anatomy department with relief moved in, acquiring at the same time
some new and very superior Leitz micro projection equipment.[31]

There were trials to be borne in his last teaching years. In June
1932 he was depressed over 'a shockingly bad lot of exam. papers',
marked also by Elliot Smith. And in Michaelmas term of that year he
had only one enrolment for the Tripos Part II in anatomy. He had
hoped for two but one student opted for Part II in pathology 'which
has', he conceded, 'definite attraction for a medical [man]'. A year
later, however, he had several Part II students to whose work he
applied a stimulant: meetings with him, which had become
intermittent, were now to be twice weekly for each student. That put
quite a heavy burden upon himself, but he was fit and equal to it.[32]

Intimations of mortality were getting personal. Jim Lorrain
Smith died in January 1931 rather suddenly and his sister Maggie
two years later. Annie was now the only surviving Lorrain Smith of
that generation. In October 1933 in Sydney 'Boy' MacCallum died,
victim of a poisoned arm and the family disease, alcoholism. Sadness
at his death was compounded by the knowledge that he had not

realized the full measure of his talent. Edgeworth David died in August 1934 and was given a state funeral. Wilson himself had been sufficiently alarmed by a prostate malfunction in November 1932 to face squarely the prospect of his own death. That problem corrected itself. A month later Elliot Smith's health gave cause for alarm. Returning to London after examining in Cambridge he had a 'slight seizure' in the train and was taken to University College Hospital. It was a stroke. For Wilson, who was Elliot Smith's senior by ten years, it was 'a great blow to see him stricken'. The symptoms passed quickly, however, and hopes were high for a full recovery. But it was in fact the beginning of a slow and final decline. By the end of 1933 Wilfrid Le Gros Clark noted sadly, Elliot Smith had 'lost all his old fluency and facility of expression'. In June 1934 he was knighted.[33]

The most sustained trial of Wilson's last teaching years was the revision of the medical curriculum and its relationship to the Natural Sciences Tripos (honours BA degree), the conjunction of the two being the distinguishing feature of the Cambridge medical training. It began as a direct attack on Wilson's anatomy programme. Dr Clark-Kennedy, a Fellow and Medical Supervisor in physiology at Corpus Christi College, also a clinician at the London Hospital, fired the first shot in 1929 with a memorandum to the Regius Professor of Physic, Sir Humphry Rolleston, reporting the dissatisfaction of Cambridge medical students with their pre-clinical training. At Cambridge they were disadvantaged in competition with the non-medical science students in the Natural Sciences Tripos by having simultaneously to work for the second MB examinations at the end of the second and third years of medicine;[34] then, in London, they found themselves not as well prepared in bio-chemistry and pathology as students from London medical schools. There were two basic problems. Firstly there was the overcrowded MB curriculum, a recurrent problem caused by the pressure of new knowledge, particularly at that time in biochemistry, pharmacology, pathology and bacteriology. Secondly there was a lack of co-ordination of medical and Tripos courses and examinations which were controlled by five separate boards. The result was a tendency for medical students, including good ones, to drop the Tripos, so threatening the cherished Cambridge tradition of a broad and fundamental scientific education for medical students. Clark-Kennedy advocated the abolition of morphology and the reduction of embryology as compulsory subjects in the Tripos. On the other hand he had no objection to an increase in topographical human anatomy (general architecture of the human body, or 'medical' anatomy). He was a clinician, opposed to the 'academic' or 'scientific' scope and emphasis that Wilson had effected in Cambridge anatomy with his Tripos anatomy scheme.[35]

This memorandum gave rise to a Committee which for 18 months surveyed the problem, interviewing 22 Directors of Studies in medical subjects and Supervisors in Cambridge Colleges. This led, in turn, to the appointment in April 1931 of a Syndicate of the Vice-Chancellor and 11 teachers of medical students including Wilson – six of them, like him, heads of departments – to revise the medical courses and examinations of the University. Dr Clark-Kennedy was the Syndicate secretary. It sat in weekly session through many weary hours over 16 weary months and witnessed many heated exchanges. 'Indeed', remarked H R Dean the Professor of Pathology, 'on no other occasion, perhaps, did medical men devour one another with such hearty and voracious enjoyment as when they discussed the education of medical students'. Anatomy was a prime target for criticism. There was a strong demand for reducing the time given to anatomy, especially 'scientific' anatomy (morphology and embryology) in the Tripos. Wilson had a fight on his hands, particularly in the Syndicate's early meetings and towards the end in May 1932. He fought hard and effectively for his subject, supported by Appleton, taking what Clark-Kennedy disparaged as a 'reactionary hard-line attitude'. And, again according to Clark-Kennedy, Wilson won. In Wilson's own appraisal he secured 'a reasonable compromise'.[36]

The Syndicate reported to the Senate in June 1932. Its principal objectives were to maintain the broad scientific base of the Cambridge medical education, and to lighten the load of the medical student by making many changes: the compression of some subjects and the introduction of others like pathology and biochemistry as half-subjects in the Tripos; the reduction of examinations; and the better coordination of courses and examinations. For anatomy there would be one regular course combining topographical anatomy with morphology and embryology, a change which would ensure that all medical students, not just Tripos students, were instructed in morphology and embryology; as well there was to be an optional half-subject in anatomy (like pathology and biochemistry) in the Tripos along the lines of the current Tripos Part I (anatomy). The Tripos was to be obligatory and – this was the main proposal – it was to be a new Tripos, a Medical Sciences Tripos under a single Board on which all the sciences allied to medicine were represented.[37]

On 25 October the Report came before the Senate House for

discussion, and it was searching. The provision for anatomy provoked a broadside in the discussion from the physiologist Sir Walter Morley Fletcher, Secretary of the Medical Research Council. Plainly, he said, the Syndicate had evaded the crux of the problem – the inordinate time given to anatomy, both topographical and morphological – at a time when progressive schools in other civilized countries were making large reductions in time given to that subject. Reductions in topographical anatomy alone would largely solve the problem of the overcrowded curriculum and morphology overlapped zoology which had always included comparative anatomy. Moreover, he continued, according to the report:

> in almost all other countries histology or microscopic anatomy belonged to anatomy, whereas in England that burden was borne (rightly he thought) by physiology. That was an additional reason for not equating the claims of anatomy to those of physiology ... all would agree, he thought, that a training in morphology, in the powers of visual observation, was not so necessary with regard to its development in other directions in medical education, as training in the methods of experiment and in the judgment of evidence.[38]

This was rubbing salt into Wilson's wounds. Reclaiming histology from the Cambridge physiologists had been one of his prime objectives and his failure to do so one of his keenest disappointments. Morley Fletcher was also ignoring the fact that experimental anatomy was an established and expanding field which in Britain had been pirated by the physiologists, Cambridge neuro-physiologists prominent among them: Gaskell, Langley, Anderson and Sherrington had 'dissected' the nervous system by the experimental method. Younger anatomists like Henry Woollard were now undertaking experimental rather than descriptive anatomy. Morley Fletcher was seeking to declare the experimental method to be beyond the pale of anatomy and was forthright, indeed rude, in his assault. His perception of anatomy, like Clark-Kennedy's, was that of the clinical physiologist. Anatomy was no longer a vital force in medical education – that quality now belonged to physiology – nor was it an autonomous science: it had become merely a handmaiden to medicine. However, he had a point: anatomy did have a larger allocation of time in the curriculum than physiology, which therefore had less time to drill students in methods of experiment.[39]

But critics of Wilson's view were outweighed by its supporters, including three distinguished physiologists. A V Hill, Foulerton Research Professor of the Royal Society, endorsed Wilson's view exactly in arguing that a good general education at school and a good scientific education at the university were the best preparation for a medical career, and efforts to introduce professional subjects into the university years should be resisted. If that meant a struggle with the General Medical Council he would back certain persuasive university authorities to win. Professor Langdon-Brown the new Regius Professor of Physic 'could imagine few subjects more valuable than embryology to serve both as a general education and as a help to man's outlook on medicine', and Joseph Barcroft, the Professor of Physiology in Cambridge, added that all his instincts were against giving up the teaching of embryology which he for one had enjoyed enormously and, speaking without any vocational bias, he would be sorry that men should not have the chance of learning it now. As for topographical anatomy, Barcroft felt sure that first class surgeons in London would consider that it should not be curtailed.[40]

The proposal for a Medical Sciences Tripos aroused the strongest opposition on the grounds that it would promote vocationalism which, said Sir Walter Morley Fletcher, would be a disaster both for Cambridge medicine and Cambridge science – indeed 'a national disaster'. To segregate medical students in professional classes, added A V Hill, would be wilfully to throw away the unique advantage of the Cambridge medical school: the training of medical men in a general school of science. 'Reform the Natural Sciences Tripos, Part I, by all means', Hill concluded, 'but not by eliminating some of its more important subjects, and by giving the latter [medical subjects] an inferior intellectual standing in the University.' Support for these opinions was general. The Report went back to the Syndicate for amendment. Wilson, too ill on that day to attend all of the discussion, was back a week later at the same grind, protesting,

> I am sick of it as it probably means more fighting ! I am really beginning to long for my retirement from the hurly burly. But I must try & hang on for a year or two yet – at least till John is out of his articles.[41]

The proposal to create a Medical Sciences Tripos under a single faculty board was dropped. Alterations within the four corners of the Natural Sciences Tripos would meet the needs of medical students, it was decided. An honours standard was made a necessary qualification for admission to the final MB examination. Pathology and biochemistry were made half-subjects in Part I of the Tripos. The problem of anatomy – its wide scope – was met by cuts in both the vocational and scientific divisions. Topographical anatomy was to have less descriptive detail (though such detail was still required for the primary FRCS); and the optional half subject in anatomy on which Wilson had set his heart, was dropped. Wilson in consultation with his staff saved his subject by streamlining both elements and integrating them into one course as in Sydney, giving pass students as well as honours students instruction in morphology and embryology. No doubt he approved that principle: the artificial separation was the result of Elliot Smith's devious negotiations with the Cambridge Syndicate on the anatomy chair in 1919–20, when the Syndicate widened the scope of anatomy but divided it by creating a readership for Duckworth in the distinct domain of topographical anatomy. This division deprived first-year students of the inspiring influence of Wilson's fierce rendition of his subject, and it deprived Wilson of the opportunity to build among junior students a receptivity for his Tripos programme. Elliot Smith's scheme and Wilson's efforts had failed to establish in Cambridge a distinctively scientific anatomy school on equal terms with physiology. By the end of May 1933 the amended report was produced, and in October it passed the Senate with very little demur. It was 'a remarkable achievement to have obtained such unanimity' Wilson acknowledged, though implementation of the new scheme 'bristled with difficulties'. He was heartily glad that it would not fall to his lot to make it work. On the day the report was passed, 25 October, Wilson's notice of resignation for 30 September 1934 was published in the *Cambridge University Reporter*.[42]

Wilson had no say in the succession and he sought none, though he did confidentially discuss the question with Hill. The up-and-coming Wilfrid Le Gros Clark would not be interested he thought, being a candidate then for the Oxford chair, vacant by the retirement of Arthur Thomson. J S B Stopford might not be inclined to leave Manchester but would perhaps respond favourably to an offer. On his staff there was Duckworth, but at 63 his age was against him under the new retirement rules. Wilson thought well of Appleton's claims and sprang to his defence against negative opinions relayed by Hill:

> I cannot in the least agree with you about Appleton. He has been pulling more than his weight in the Department and I know that he has for a considerable time been engaged on a projected book on

Morphology which fully accounts for an apparent diminution in his output of work. But as a matter of fact he pursues his lines of investigation very diligently. And his range of knowledge of Anatomy in the broadest sense is most impressive. Your informants do not know what they are talking about.

But if a member of his staff was not to be preferred, Wilson favoured the Australian, H H Woollard, then in the Chair of Anatomy at Bart's Medical School, London.[43]

The choice was none of these, and something of a shock, as Wilson confided to Jeanie.

> It is a rather sore subject and I do not care to discuss it except in strict privacy.... I gather that there were only two applications one by Dr Appleton (Senior Lecturer here) and the other, H A Harris, Elliot Smith's junior colleague, as Prof of Clinical Anatomy, in U.C.L. Elliot Smith was on the Electoral Bd. as also was his colleague D M S Watson. They chose Harris over Appleton's head. In my opinion A.. is the better man & far more suitable to Cambridge. Harris I know & am quite friendly with, in fact he is very friendly to me, but he is a bit of a rough diamond and far better fitted for his present job than for the one here. However it is all over & we must make the best of it.

J P Hill summed up the matter crisply: 'it was the worst day's work E.S. ever did for Cambridge!'.[44]

Harris did not fit in with Cambridge traditions, as he himself acknowledged. 'No, Cambridge is not my Park', was his first response to Elliot Smith's proposition. He was a brusque Welshman, square-shaped, and with no pretence at culture. A J E Cave, another of Elliot Smith's protégés, described him as

> no profound anatomist, being entertaining rather than informative in exposition and sometimes specious in argument. None of us younger anatomists regarded him as scientifically sound no matter how amusing his discourse might be.

Elliot Smith's dictum, that 'In Cambridge a professor does his best for the place by means of social intercourse with students and dons', was not observed; nor was the primacy of scientific anatomy affirmed.[45]

Why then did Elliot Smith draft Harris? A J E Cave believed that 'this appointment was Elliot Smith's last "push" in academic politics made from a sense of indebtedness to Harris, who had constituted himself Elliot Smith's right hand man'. Cave also advanced other reasons, which may have reflected Elliot Smith's perceptions at that time: that 'Under Wilson Cambridge anatomy had slumbered'; that Harris who 'could at least teach anatomy' would revitalize the Cambridge school; and that Appleton, 'a smug and indolent character', would not have improved the situation. If Elliot Smith's selection of Harris had any professional principle at all it would have been to boost the interests of the clinicians, thus aligning himself with Wilson's 'progressive' critics in the Syndicate on the medical curriculum. Harris was a clinical anatomist, and Cave's remark that Harris 'could at least teach anatomy' sounds like the comment of a clinician who had no real interest in anatomy as a biological science. The appointment of Harris to the Cambridge chair was perhaps the ultimate rejection of Wilson's morphological concept of anatomy (now outmoded?) or, more simply, it may have been the act of an inveterate rebel. Elliot Smith was, wrote Harris, 'the staunchest supporter of the young man who took up the cudgels against any person or institution which supported *auctoritas* or authority – especially from the point of view of intellectual superiority'.[46]

Wilson's attention turned to securing the tenure of his staff. With his retirement in mind he had moved in August 1933 to promote Howard Green from a demonstratorship to a lectureship with Frank Goldby stepping into the vacancy, while Ruddell Shore was elected to another demonstratorship. This was all in accord with Wilson's plan. After the decision to appoint Harris to the chair, Wilson's concern focused on Appleton whose situation was now untenable. In June 1934, as a selector for the Anatomy Chair at St Thomas's Hospital, Wilson pushed and secured Appleton's appointment. Despite his best efforts, however, Wilson did not secure the tenure of two of his staff, Doctors Pennell and Reid.[47]

His final year in the Anatomy Chair was strenuous. Every lecture now was ticked off with the thought that he would not have to cover that ground again – 'And it does *not* make me sad.' – but it pleased him that his youngest son Maxwell was in those classes. In September 1933 in the company of Hill and Goodrich of Oxford he attended a meeting of the Hubrecht Institute of Embryology in Utrecht, of which he was a foundation member in 1911. It was a small organization but well housed and well funded as a legacy of its founder, A A W Hubrecht. Wilson met friends he had known since 1905 – George Streeter of Baltimore, Levi of Turin, Van den Broeke of Utrecht, Ariens Kappers of Amsterdam – and with Hill he spent an afternoon with the President of the Institute, Professor Boeke, looking through his fine preparations of nerve endings. 'I cant agree with his interpretation in many cases', Wilson noted, 'but his technique is superb.' Lavish meals brought on another bout of dyspepsia.[48]

October and November were burdened with a quinquennium report for the Carnegie Trust. And the routine pressures of teaching, examinations, visitors, meetings and boards of election continued. 'There maun aye be somethin' !' he wrote at the end of February 1934, when dyspepsia was giving him prolonged discomfort. In March he consulted an expert on the alimentary canal and had 'the curious experience of actually seeing my own heart, diaphragm, stomach & intestines all alive oh !' There was nothing organically wrong and he was exhorted not to worry.[49]

More remedial for Wilson's health than perhaps anything else at the time was Charlie Martin's decision to retire in Cambridge at the end of 1933. Knighted in 1927, Martin had retired from the Lister Institute a few days before his 65th birthday on 31 December 1930 to accept, at the request of David Rivett, the leadership of the division of animal nutrition in Australia's Council for Scientific and Industrial Research (CSIR) in Adelaide where he was also appointed professor of biochemistry and general physiology at the University. For nearly three years in Adelaide he assisted the fledgling division to recover from the untimely death of its brilliant young founder T Brailsford Robertson, and joined the hunt to discover the role of various minerals in sheep nutrition. Instead of fundamental research in physiology, Martin favoured an interdisciplinary approach, for which CSIR's structure was ideal. Success in solving, for instance, 'coast disease' – an anaemic, wasting condition of sheep grazed in certain coastal areas, later shown to be due to cobalt deficiency – could 'be expected only when the agrostologist, the soil chemist and the physiologist collaborate', said Martin prophetically. CSIR benefited from the prestige and wisdom of a world-ranking scientist, while Martin gratified again his abiding love for Australia. But for Lady Martin he might well have stayed. In retirement in Cambridge he continued to research animal nutrition for the CSIR and the Lister Institute.[50]

'I am so glad that the Martins are to be here permanently', Wilson wrote to Jeanie. 'Except for Dr Anderson Scott, whom I knew in Edin. Martin is the oldest friend I have here.' Memories of the early 1890s in the Sydney suburb of Stanmore where the two families had lived within 300 yards of each other flooded in on him. He recalled Jeanie's precarious infancy and Lady Martin's timely recommendation of a wet nurse; the years of intense fertile activity studying monotremes and marsupials far into the night, and the exploits of the Fraternity of Duckmaloi in the Australian bush. The Martins bought a rambling and ramshackle old inn Roebuck House from Jack Haldane, who had moved to London. They moved in just before Christmas 1933. At Wilson's suggestion St John's College invited Martin to become a member of the College.[51]

Events were driving his thoughts backwards. The Sydney Medical School's Jubilee in 1933 coincided with Edinburgh University's 350th anniversary, and the 50th anniversary of his own graduation on 1 August 1883. Early in May 1934 he attended the centenary of Liverpool's Medical School and discovered that his host, C Sydney Jones, was not only a Pro-Chancellor of the University but also a partner in the Blue Funnel Line. Wilson could introduce himself as an old employee. In August he was at the grand opening of the first international congress of anthropologists – 20 years in the making – in the Great Hall of University College London, to represent the Royal Society of New South Wales. Grafton Elliot Smith was there, now a sad figure enfeebled by diabetes in addition to the effects of his stroke, putting up a gallant effort as president of the anatomy section. In September 1934 for a meeting of the British Association Wilson was in Aberdeen, which he had last visited when his sister Helen was a student there in the 1870s.[52]

Wilson delivered his last lecture of a 50-year teaching career on 16 May 1934 and matter-of-factly turned his attention to the endless details of organizing the Summer Meeting of the Anatomical Society, set for Friday 22 and Saturday 23 June in Cambridge. He had also to prepare a paper and demonstrations of brain sections and embryo sections which in the event attracted much interest. The meeting went without a hitch, becoming a sort of finale to Wilson's official career. At the formal dinner on Friday evening he and Mabel were guests of honour, the second occasion only that the Society had paid such tribute to one of its members. The President, Professor Dixon of Ireland, in proposing the toast made a 'very eulogistic speech'. An immense luncheon party the next day was Wilson's salute to his peers.[53]

His contribution to the meeting's serious proceedings gave Wilson great satisfaction. It was a short paper on an unimportant but intriguing subject: the nature and mode of origin of the foramen of Magendie. This obscure opening in the fourth ventricle of the human brain had been the subject of debate for many years and Wilson had touched on it incidentally in his paper in 1906 on the anatomy of the calamus region of the human bulb. In 1930 two Cardiff men, Lambert Rogers and C M West, had disputed *inter alia* Wilson's

opinion of 1906 that the foramen was 'the imperfect representative of
an epithelial evagination of the cavity of the rhombencephalon',
concluding instead that it was 'a complete defect of the lower part of
the roof of the fourth ventricle'. Wilson, using his recently-devised
technique for cutting a continuous series of alternate thick and thin
sections of large embryos, displayed incontrovertible evidence
validating his opinion of 1906. Rogers and West, who were both·
present, had to climb down. 'I have settled it', he said emphatically.
Wilson's delight in controversy was as keen as ever.[54]

A farewell dinner on 14 August given by the teaching staff of the
anatomy department was a more intimate occasion. There were ten
guests, not including Appleton who had already left Cambridge.
Duckworth arranged an elegant dinner in a guest room of Jesus
College, and made a long and graceful speech. Wilson's reply was
'rather an ordeal'. He briefly reviewed a teaching career of 50 years
which had seen great changes in the medical sciences. In Britain in
the early 1880s, topographic anatomy, especially of the viscera, had
to be rewritten in the light of frozen sections; surgery, with its
Listerian enthusiasts, had just begun its triumphal march;
bacteriology which in Wilson's memory was born on 24 March
1882 (the day before his sister Helen's death) with the dramatic
announcement by Koch that he had isolated the tubercle bacillus;
Francis Balfour and others in Cambridge were rewriting embryology
with the aid of new serial paraffin sections; neurology was being
transformed by the work of Golgi, Kölliker and Ramon y Cajal; and
vertebrate morphology was still feeling the stimulus of Darwin,
Haeckel and Huxley. And now the medical sciences had to reckon
with all the new knowledge accumulated by the use of experimental
methods in anatomy and embryology, by radiology and by tissue
culture. Texts must again be rewritten.[55]

The teaching of anatomy in 1880 was still largely in the hands of
the surgeons but the great morphological tradition established by
John Hunter in Britain was safeguarded by Humphry of Cambridge
and Turner of Edinburgh who had established the *Journal of
Anatomy*. Scientific anatomy had made steady progress in his own
time though he was only too conscious of the discrepancy between
his personal aims and his achievements. The teaching of histology, to
mention his keenest disappointment in Cambridge, was still officially
with the physiologists. He had argued in his inaugural lecture in
1921, as had his predecessor Alexander Macalister in his inaugural
lecture in 1884, that the teaching of microscopical anatomy belonged
to the anatomists, but to no avail. Yet his aims had been right and

there had been gains: a good scientific foundation had been provided for the ordinary anatomy course for medical students in Cambridge and 'with your ever ready cooperation we have I think succeeded in developing the work of the School along certain fruitful lines ... appropriate to the scientific spirit of Cambridge'. Vocationalism he believed was distorting the university ideal, even in Cambridge with its collegiate organization and broad cultural traditions. Students could be unduly limited in their reading by technical work, and their personal development stunted by group or faculty bounds.

Wilson's 50 years' service had been guided by the ideal of a university as a school of character, culture and craftsmanship – in three universities of different organization and traditions but with that central purpose. As the University of Sydney coat of arms proclaims, 'Sidere mens eadem mutato': the selfsame spirit under different skies.[56]

Notes

1. 'quite easy': J to JTW, 23.8.1923. 'he was glad' and Kater sentiments: J to JTW, 8.1.1929.
2. 'more hers than': JTW to LH, 13.2.1921. 'It is rather': MMW to LH, May(?) 1924.
3. Edinburgh Medical School Bicentenary: *The Scotsman*, 15.6.1926. 'a man with': *ibid.*, 16.6.1926.
4. Shift toward English traditions: Sanderson, 186.
5. 'the appointment will': GES to JTW, 27.1.1920. 'I can give': KR to author. 'I shall not': JTW to GES, 4.8.1919.
6. Tripos: JTW to J, 29.8.1928. Retirement income: JTW to Allan Clunies Ross, 21.1.31.
7. Mabel's death wish: Lady Murray to author. Swiss holiday: J to MMW, 8.8.1928. Sydney pension: JTW to J, 19.7.33.
8. 'I gathered': Cave to author, 15.8.1984. GES 1918, 8.
9. JTW, 1928b. *J of A*, Vol. 61 (1926–7), 490.
10. Hill study: de Beer, *J of A*, Vol. 82 (1948), 6; Watson, *RSO* on Hill (1955).
11. Streeter to JTW, 12.9.28.
12. Croonian Lecture: JPH, *Philosophical Transactions*, Series B, Vol. 221, 45–178. 'that the data': *ibid.*, 45. Luckett, *passim.*
13. 'Very glad to hear': JPH to JTW, 29.7.1928. One more attempt: JPH to JTW, 23.11.1931. 'He doesn't know': JPH to JTW, 8.8.1939.
14. Table: JTW, 1928a. Hans Gadow's book: *J of A* review, Vol. 68, 1933–4, 575. Goldby paper; *J of A* Vol. 62, 135–8. Green's work: *Phil. Trans. B.* 228. 367; JPH on JTW, *RSO* 649.

15. Harrison collection: C W Stump to JTW, 24.5.28; JTW to Burkitt, 21.8.28. Clinical focus: 'Bibliographical Summaries' in U of S *Calendars* for 1927–33.

16. Anatomical revisions: Barclay Smith, 45–8. Wilson 1897: Binney. American publication: HAH, 'Review', *J of A*, Vol. 62, 362–3. C'ttee of 1928: J C Brash to JTW, 19.7.28. JNA: *J of A Index to the First 100 Years 1886–1966*, ix.

17. Wilson's views: JTW to John Anderson, 16.6.28. Keibel to JTW, 25.5.28. Discussion with Streeter: JTW to A J Bant, 12.6.28.

18. JTW on nomenclature: JTW to MH, 19.4.28 on footnotes for MH paper. 'a confusing': *ibid.* JTW and 'omphalopleure': JPH 1898, 396. Johnston's term: *J of A* 1928–9, 159.

19. MH-JTW correspondence, 1928. 'the most critical': MH to JTW, 4.2.28.

20. Evidence against: JTW to MH, 31.3.28.; *Bulletin of the Johns Hopkins Hospital*, No. 5, 264–307. 'I have never': MH to JTW, 4.2.28.

21. Wilkinson, 129–43. Interest in dual-innervation; Geoffrey Kenny to author, 7.12.93. His Obituary: *MJA*, Vol. 1 1963, 869. His courses: Adelaide, HJW to JTW, 8.3.33; Queensland, *University Calendars*. 'mainstay': Geoffrey Kenny to author, 16.7.93.

22. JTW and Americans, e.g. corresp.: Lewis Weed to JTW, 27.12.1923 and JTW reply, 26.1.1924. Judson Herrick to JTW, March 1928 and 4.6.1928. George Streeter to JTW, 12.9.1928. Ranson to JTW, 20.4.1932.

23. 'The editor of the Lancet': MH to JTW, 27.10.1928.

24. Sprigge Report. Scottish system; Newman, *The Scotsman*, 16 June 1926.

25. 'fulness of understanding' etc.; Sprigge Report.

26. 'with my staff': JTW to LH, 30.12.36.

27. Adelaide visit: JTW to J, 29.6.30.

28. Sissons, Ric & Stoddant, Brian: *Cricket and Empire. The 1932–33 Bodyline Tour of Australia.* Allen & Unwin. London 1984.

29. Medical School: *Centenary Book*, Ch. 10 and 312–15.

30. 'I confess': JTW to J, 3.4.1935. 'I do *not* agree': JTW to J, 16.6.1937. 'we two went' [dated by JTW list of holidays]: TDGW, in JMGW letter to author, 30.4.1983.

31. Lecturing and lab work: JTW to J, 29.10 and 23.12.1930, 2.3.1932. Potts: JTW to J, 13.7.1932. Leitz apparatus: JTW to J, 7.8.1933.

32. 'a shockingly': JTW to J, 15.6.32. 'which has': JTW to J, 12.10.32. Meetings for Part II: JTW to LH, 25.10 and 15.11.1933.

33. Lorrain Smiths: JTW to J, 24.4.33. MacCallum: JTW to J, 1.11.33. Prostate: JTW to J, 16.11.1932. 'slight seizure' and 'a great blow': JTW to J, 14.12.32; Dawson, 102–4; Le Gros Clark to JTW, 3.11.33.

34. Work for the MB Part III was done in Long Vac term (summer) of the final year, before going down. The Natural Sciences Tripos Part III was completed in the preceding 3 main terms: JMGW (a Tripos graduate, 1935) to author, 1994.

35. Problems with Cambridge Medical Course: Leslie Cole 271–3; Clark-Kennedy, interview with JMGW, 15.7.1984.

36. 'Indeed on no': Dean quoted in *Cambridge University Reporter,* 7.11.1932, 314. Wilson's fight: JTW to J, 25.5.1932. 'reactionary, hard-line': Clark-Kennedy to JMGW, 15.7.1984. 'a reasonable': JTW to J, 25.5.32.

37. Syndicate proposals: Cole, 271–3; *CUR,* 7.11.1932, 294–318.

38. 'in almost all other': Fletcher, reported in *CUR,* 7.11.32, 301.

39. 'dissected' nervous system: Keith, 1927/8, 242.

40. Supporters' views: A V Hill, *CUR,* 7.11.32, 303–5; Langdon-Brown, *CUR,* 7.11.32, 308–9; Barcroft, *CUR,* 7.11.32, 317–18.

41. 'a national': Fletcher, *CUR,* 7.11.32, 302. 'Reform the Natural': A V Hill, *CUR,* 7.11.32, 305. JTW too ill: JTW to J, 26.10.32; 'I am sick', 2.11.32.

42. 'a remarkable' and 'bristled with': JTW in report of discussion in the Senate, *CUR* 7.10.1933, 238. JTW letters to LH and J, 25.10.1933.

43. 'I cannot': JTW to JPH, 1.11.1933.

44. 'It is rather': JTW to J, 13.12.1933. 'it was the worst': JPH to JTW, 27.12.1933.

45. 'No, Cambridge': Harris, in Fozzard, 71. Views of Cave to author, 15.8.1984. 'In Cambridge': GES to JTW, 15.9.1919.

46. Cave to author, 15.8.84. Harris on GES: Dawson, 179.

47. Staff promotions: JTW to K, 7.8.33 and to J, 27.6.34.

48. Last lectures: JTW to J, 18.10.33, 17.1.34. Utrecht: JTW to J, 13.9.33.

49. 'There maun aye': JTW to LH, Feb. 1934. 'the curious experience': JTW to J, 4.4.1934.

50. Martin in Cambridge: JTW to J, 18.10 and 15.11.33. Martin in Australia: Chick *et al.*, *RSO*; Schedvin, 126–33. 'be expected': *ibid.* 129.

51. JTW to J, 18.10 and 15.11.33.

52. JTW to AEM, 1.1.1934 and JTW to J, 1934 letters.

53. 'very eulogistic': JTW to J, 27.6.34.

54. Foramen of Magendie: JTW, 1937b and 1906b. 'a complete defect': Rogers & West, in 'The Foramen of Magendie', *J of A*, Vol. LXV 1931, 457–67. 'I have settled it': JTW to J, 27.6.34.

55. 'rather an ordeal': JTW to J, 15.8.1934. Notes for farewell dinner, Anatomy Dept, 1934.

56. 'with your': *ibid.* University of Sydney motto: JTW version, in speech at St John's College 1941.

15

Resolution

The transfer of reins at the Anatomy Department was smooth. Though Wilson and Harris were as unlike as two men can be, they stepped carefully and cordially around each other exchanging polite gestures. In June 1934 Appleton had been appointed to the anatomy chair at St Thomas's Hospital, London, a move Wilson had pushed, so relieving the Cambridge situation of potential discord for the new professor. Harris visited Cambridge twice in 1934 before Wilson retired and once introductions in the Department were over Wilson left the business meetings to Harris and the gentlemanly Duckworth. For his part Harris invited Wilson to retain the use of his laboratory. Wilson formally handed over the charge of the Department on 30 September and on 16 October he attended Harris's inaugural lecture. Wilson on retirement became a Professor Emeritus of the University and a non-stipendiary Fellow of St John's, honours that were by no means automatic. In Cambridge he had found favour that was not to be accorded to Harris. Even Harris's election to a College was long delayed, till January 1937 when St John's did so. It was subsequent even to a member of his staff.[1]

The new professor and the new curriculum brought turbulence to Cambridge anatomy for about six years. There was a considerable increase in student enrolments due to the new course and considerable difficulties with the staff, who formed pro- and anti-Harris factions. Wilson's men were destabilized. Arthur Fell was given marching orders in 1935:

> I was summoned by Harris and told that I should apply for a six months tenure as Professor at Singapore, while [the incumbent] was

364

on leave. I was given no alternative – take it or leave it. So I took it. I was to save most of my salary in Singapore and use it for a stay in the Carnegie Institute in Baltimore to reconstruct and study an embryo H67 which [J T Wilson] kindly provided.... [Harris] never let you know what he had in mind, and everything done was in a devious way. In fact if I let my feelings go I should be an obscene ranter ... he was a so-and-so was HAH.

Fell was 'an expendable demonstrator'. Howard Green had a tussle with Harris too but, being a tenured lecturer, held his ground. Frank Goldby, on the advice of Wilson and H H Woollard, left in early 1937 to take the chair of anatomy in Adelaide vacated by H J Wilkinson when he accepted the Brisbane chair.[2]

Harris, however, did import some stimulating new blood, notably James Dixon Boyd, in 1935. He was an Irish-American, and a prize-winning graduate in both science and medicine, of the Queen's University in Belfast. His interest in embryology and his friendship with Wilson began in his demonstrator years from 1931 to 1934, when he consulted Wilson on the suckling mechanism of platypus. Awarded the MD with a Gold Medal by Queen's in 1934, he then spent a year at the Carnegie Institute in Baltimore where he came under the influence of George Streeter before moving to Cambridge. He was a man of broad interests and high scientific calibre. To Harris's bitter disappointment Dixon Boyd left in 1938 to accept the chair of anatomy at the London Hospital Medical School. He returned to Cambridge temporarily during the war when the London school relocated its pre-clinical departments there – Wilson saw a great deal of him then – and permanently in 1951 when he succeeded Harris in the Cambridge chair. He was to establish a regime in the tradition of Wilson who had assisted him in various ways: 'a splendid chap in every sense' Wilson noted in 1944, his dominant interests being embryology, neurology and developmental biology. He died in 1968 lamenting that there was no full-blooded embryologist in his department.[3]

Much of Harris's first four years went into the planning and building of a new anatomy school, in 'a truly contemporary idiom', toward which Harris adopted – as had Anderson Stuart in Sydney – a strongly proprietorial attitude. The main front door entrance was permanently locked except on the day of the Linacre Lecture. He abhorred the disrespect of students who whistled as they ascended the three floors of stairs outside his office, and would call them down with instructions to 'Go right down to the basement and walk up quietly.' Opened in the autumn of 1938 at the time of the

Munich crisis, funds dried up before the modern equipment the building was meant to house could be bought, and before projected research programmes could get under way. The grand new anatomy school was but an empty shell.[4]

In his laboratory at the old school, at the end of 1934 Wilson took stock of a large accumulation of embryological and neurological material that he had never been able to give time to. There was no end of work to be done but, as ever, the distraction and pressure of other matters eroded his time and energy for it. He spent long sessions over the microscope – 'till my back nearly broke' he recorded one day in February 1935 – but they were fitful, try though he did to establish a daily half-day-in-the-laboratory routine. It was not until June 1937 that he published his account of the question he had so emphatically settled at the Cambridge meeting of the Anatomical Society in June 1934. It was his last scientific paper. By then he was 77 and finding laboratory work a strain.[5]

The calendar for 1935 was dominated by a long family reunion. In May came an influx from the Antipodes – Katharine, Louise and the three Hutchinson grandchildren Mary, Teddy and Susan (born in October 1933) – and for four months the grandparents endured the clamour of the clan at its Cambridge headquarters. For the month of July it moved to a seaside station, a large house at West Runton in Norfolk where the Cuthberts with their two daughters, Helen and Katharine, joined them. Bathing, golfing and billiards were the staple pastimes, to which Wilson added stereo-photography, and reading Dickens and Shakespeare. A car tour of Scandinavia in August came to a sudden end for Wilson and Mabel when the car overturned into a ditch between Stockholm and Uppsala. There were no injuries and Wilson was cool enough to record the episode on film. It featured in both the Stockholm and Cambridge news. Katharine, Louise and John continued on, none the worse, but their parents returned home. Late in September, a tense time in the Mediterranean with Mussolini's troops invading Abyssinia, Louise and her children returned to Australia via Panama, and Katharine followed in the new year.[6]

Wilson and Mabel never saw their Australian grandchildren again, but through letters, photographs and all kinds of mementoes they followed every detail of their lives. Correspondence held a wonderful place in the Wilson family. Mabel's contribution was prolific; she wrote at length by seamail and more economically by airmail every week to each of her daughters in Australia, and Wilson added his 'scraps' to these budgets. He hated writing letters, having neither the patience nor the resource he complained, but he yearned for 'the feeling of warm and intimate association' with his scattered flock. Mabel 'lived her life largely for Louise's letters' one of her daughters-in-law observed, 'she fell on them every week and pored over them for hours'. Wilson doted on Jeanie's letters; he enjoyed – indeed he envied – her facility and adventure with words. Through her Workers' Educational Association work and special connections with Gerald Portus, Professor Carslaw, Professor Mills, Professor Holme, the MacCallums, the Barffs, the Edgeworth Davids and others she sent him news, and stories behind the news, of Sydney University affairs.[7]

From 1934, when he entered the Medical School, Patrick made another vital family connection with Sydney University. He was warmly welcomed, especially by Louis. Like his grandfather, Patrick was scientifically inclined and clever with both his head and his hands, talents which Wilson promoted by giving him a microscope and sending on copies of the *English Mechanic* to which Wilson subscribed for many years. The well-equipped workshop at Bayview was a stimulus too. In 1935, when Patrick became interested in neurology, Wilson was delighted. In 1938, when Patrick was considering his career options, Wilson's advice revealed his disappointment with the condition of anatomy:

> I should like to think of Patrick carrying on the tradition of academic teaching. But I should not advise Anatomy much as I value it as a biological science. But in these days it is rather the physiological group of subjects which have the most vital appeal and are closer to the professional interests of medicine as well. I include of course pathology in this group of subjects as well as biochemistry and physics.

After war service, which tested his powers of invention in the improvisation of apparatus, Patrick decided to become a bacteriologist. In 1952 he became the third Bosch Professor of Bacteriology.[8]

On 30 June 1936 the Sydney Medical School marked the 50th anniversary of the legendary Louis Schaeffer's appointment with a ceremonial presentation to Louis by Professor Burkitt. In a large gathering of graduates and students Louis was particularly pleased that Jeanie and Patrick attended to represent Wilson, who in Cambridge reflected on the development of 'a small common-looking boy of 14 or thereabout .... into a splendid man, gifted in various ways, very wise & level-headed and devoted to the School & Department'. He sent his congratulations, which Louis prized above all others. Louis, assailed by nostalgia, reflected on the 'divine inspiration' Wilson had given to generations of students. 'It is only plain truth to say that your influence has changed the minds of hundreds of young men, shaped their destinies and given them ideals in life that were unknown before contact with you.' He concluded with his usual incisive report on the state of the Department.[9]

In the summer of 1936 Cambridge hosted the Fifth Congress of the Universities of the British Empire. Wilson was one of the organizers, being a Cambridge-based member of the Executive Council of the Universities Bureau. Among the delegates from Sydney was W J Dakin, the Professor of Zoology and a man after Wilson's own style, who stayed with the Wilsons for the congress week. Proceedings began with welcoming parties for seven different academic groups on the afternoon of Monday 13 July, the Wilsons hosting 150 medical and biological scientists in the Combination Room at St John's. That evening the Vice-Chancellor gave a formal reception in the newly restored and imposing rooms of the Old School, and for the first time academic dress was worn 'without hoods'. Congress proceedings included secondary education, physical education, teacher training, universities in Canadian national life, and a question of perennial interest: provision for post-graduate studies in Great Britain. Lord Rutherford reviewed the Cambridge experience with the PhD degree since it began in 1920, noting that of the 365 research students currently registered there, nearly 70 per cent were in science. Growth in research student numbers, mainly from British Universities, was taxing the resources of Cambridge. The PhD scheme had failed to achieve its purpose of attracting overseas graduates in significant numbers, or even of keeping Britain's best: according to J A Ryle, Regius Professor of Medicine at Cambridge, keen British graduates who had gone to European research centres before the war now went to the United States.[10]

For Wilson the highlight was Chancellor Stanley Baldwin's address as President of the Congress. He spoke of the university ideal which had flowered throughout the Empire, diversely, he emphasized, because freedom was 'the very breath of our being'. Expansion to meet the needs of the modern world was costly, a point he commended to the notice of wealthy citizens. There were certain differences of value: when Rutherford wanted to do a few experiments he required an elephant house and large sums of money; the poet on the other hand – and Cambridge had produced great poets as well as great mathematicians and scientists – how cheap was his apparatus! A few sheets of paper and a pencil. To Baldwin's way of thinking our poets had served us better. Science had been put to evil purposes, but poetry harmed no one. Produce poets, he enjoined his audience, who will inspire Europe and the world with a sense of unity, and a sense of freedom. This was fine as a university ideal, but it was not a reassuring message at that time from the lips of the Prime Minister.[11]

The fact is, international affairs were not Baldwin's strong point and, for him as for most of his generation, the very idea of war was almost obscene. Poetry had no hope of solving Europe's problems. Tough measures against Italy in 1935 and Germany in 1936 might have done so, but the guilt of Versailles had robbed Britain and France of the will for that course. It was fortunate for the Cambridge physicists, and perhaps for the free world, that private funds amounting to a quarter of a million pounds had already been pledged to their atom-splitting experiments. It was Baldwin, as Chancellor of Cambridge University, who had announced the bequest a few months earlier.[12]

For European freedom, 1936 was a critical year. In March Hitler occupied the Rhineland, in May Mussolini defeated the Abyssinians and in July, as the Universities Congress concluded, the Spanish Civil War broke out. 'Public affairs are a nightmare' wrote Wilson in September. 'God help us all in this distressful epoch!' He reduced to 'the narrowest dimensions' his reading of newspapers with their grim catalogue of horrors, turning instead to an old interest, medieval history. The past was 'much less exasperating, though the records are full of misdoings & cruelty oppression & wrong. But at least it is past & the sufferers are at rest'. He relied on *The Round Table* to keep himself informed on current affairs. Disappointed by the failure of the League of Nations and appalled by the behaviour of Europe's three 'full-blown tyrannies', he welcomed rearmament and any show of resolution in British policy. But the Empire, to which the world was looking for leadership – so said Baldwin – was weathering its own constitutional crisis culminating in the abdication of Edward VIII in December. Wilson did not seem to notice that crisis, perhaps because the British press maintained silence until its last days. More debilitating for the British people and Baldwin's National Government was the crisis of opinion about the Spanish Civil War, which destroyed Spanish freedom and brought the international conflict between democracy and dictatorship to a new pitch of intensity.[13]

In August 1936 Wilson was supervising the final act of moving from 31 Grange Road – sold the previous November when Wilson and Mabel took a rented house – into their new house at 24 Millington Road. For years they had been designing this smaller house and garden and now, with their children more or less launched, they realized it. It had involved a radical reduction of chattels, and of Wilson's vast accumulation of paper. The extent of his correspondence with family, friends and colleagues in Australia, Europe, the United States and Britain astonished him. He made the painful decision to burn most of it, virtually without review. 'I could never wade through it all' he decided. However he kept some old family letters and papers, John Haldane's older letters, a few of Jim Lorrain Smith's, some of his correspondence over many years with Hill, Martin, Elliot Smith, MacCallum, Holme, Mills, Carslaw, Purser as well as 'a few selected specimens' of other correspondence. On Christmas Eve 1935 a treasury went up in smoke.[14]

Number 24 Millington Road had two storeys with bathroom and bedrooms upstairs, and dining and drawing rooms plus Wilson's combined study-bedroom, downstairs. It was serviced by two maids, Maud and May. Wilson's study was warmed in winter by a gas fire and central heating to a temperature few visitors could stand for long. He created 'a ghastly fug' in there and would be annoyed at the loss of expensive heat if the maid left a window open. It had a door to the downstairs cloakroom and another to the garage, to the outfitting of which he devoted considerable attention and ingenuity. In his time it never housed a car, being instead an efficient combination of laboratory, workshop and darkroom, all meticulously planned, organized and labelled. 'Everything has fitted in well,' he reported on 26 August 1936, 'and I am far more conveniently fixed up than ever I have been before. It is a pity that I am so old!'[15]

Their quarter acre had magnificent garden soil, a deep loam which had been producing vegetables for them since the summer of 1934. Well before the house was finished two closely-planted rows of cordon apples and pears were established along the back fence, and eight plum bushes. With the assistance of Canwell, a jobbing gardener, Wilson laid out an orderly garden: lavender hedges along a gravel path to the front door between two square beds of roses under-planted with pansies, geometry softened by a large romneya with its great white paper flowers outside the garage door (never opened) and a fine clematis to climb over Mabel's upstairs balcony. A little greenhouse in the back garden became a horticultural laboratory where he cultivated various plants, noting in his diaries the chequered fortunes of all of them. He spent hours studying gardening manuals and plant catalogues, and many a session in the new University Library researching particular interests like iris, lilacs and lilies. There were always flowers in the house.[16]

Carnegie work regulated the Wilsons' year. Every spring they both went north for the Edinburgh interviews, combining duty with a holiday at the Cuthberts in Stirling. It was work Wilson took very seriously as a service to Scottish youth, mindful that careers in scientific research might depend on his recommendations. With his teaching career concluded it maintained his involvement with students and with developments across the biological and medical sciences: zoology, botany, anatomy, embryology, physiology, pathology and clinical medicine. Expert in some areas, he performed in others 'as an intelligent juryman or sometimes as a critic from a merely administrative point of view'; surprisingly often he found himself at the interviews in Edinburgh discussing work which chimed in with his own current interests. 'There were a lot of budding botanists this time,' he noted in April 1937, and some of them had 'the genuine itch for scientific research'. Not that he had time to dally: in one day in 1935 he packed in 18 interviews. Complain though he regularly did, when it came to the long and tedious business of writing his reports, especially in quinquennial years like 1938, Wilson enjoyed it all and it kept him young.[17]

Between the ebb and flow of Carnegie files he had the occasional thesis to examine and the occasional article to write or to evaluate for publication, even after retiring from the editorial board of the *Journal of Anatomy* in 1936. Frequent calls were made on him by colleagues and former students for advice, criticism, testimonials, and encouragement, a natural consequence observed one of them, Standish Lightoller of Sydney, of his influence as a teacher:

> I feel very guilty to trouble you thus [with a very long paper on the comparative anatomy of facial musculature] but, indirectly or even directly, you are reaping the whirlwind of sowing the wind of anatomical interest. Had any other of my teachers shown such disinterested enthusiasm for his subject I might have been pestering them instead of you.

Lightoller, one of Wilson's demonstrators in 1907–8, and later Mungo MacCallum's son-in-law, took up research and demonstrating again in the Sydney Anatomy Department in 1920, combining it successfully with a busy medical practice. He made notable contributions to morphology on facial musculature. Wilson successfully sponsored Lightoller's paper for publication in the *Transactions of the Zoological Society of London* in 1940.[18]

One of Wilson's saddest experiences was to witness the demise of his most famous former pupil. He had not seen Grafton Elliot Smith for about a year when they met at St John's College 'Port Latin Feast' in May 1935. Grafton was accompanied by his brother S A Smith. At dessert in the beautiful Combination Room Wilson sat between them. He was shocked by Grafton's appearance:

> He looks old now – he is about 10 years younger than I and I really think he looks 10 years older. But he seems fairly well although slightly crippled. Mentally he is quite all right.[19]

There followed a series of calamities. In October 1935 Grafton suffered another stroke which further disabled him: his speech was affected and in November his Huxley Memorial Lecture to the Royal Anthropological Institute (associated with its award of the Huxley Medal) had to be read for him. The year ended with the tragic death of his youngest son and the new year began with a domestic accident in which his wife, Kathleen, was severely burned. She was confined to hospital until October when she was moved to a nursing home at Broadstairs in Kent. Shortly after Kathleen's accident the lease of their London house expired and Grafton was required to vacate it immediately. He entered a nursing home, Queen Mary's Hospital in Sidcup, Kent. Officially he retired from his chair in September, as required by statute, and was showered with honours. He found occupation, which seemed to lift his spirits, in writing his autobiography. It was one more of several distinct beginnings and only a few pages was written. Just before Christmas he was taken to Broadstairs for a family reunion. He died there on New Year's Day 1937 and the news flashed around the world. A A Abbie, his youngest Australian disciple, heard it by wireless news aboard a ship bound for Hong Kong.[20] At the funeral on 5 January at Golders Green in London, Wilson represented the Royal Society and the Master and Fellows of St John's College; H A Harris represented Cambridge University – a self-appointment Wilson thought – and Elliot Smith's niece Ellice Nosworthy represented the University of Sydney.[21]

Wilson's last labours for Elliot Smith were elegiac. They had begun some months before his death, with the decision of the editors of the *Journal of Anatomy* to dedicate the October 1936 issue to him. Wilson was asked to contribute a biographical article. Out of his own recollections and some early letters from Elliot Smith in England, Wilson sketched the beginnings of his career, from 1888 to 1900, giving an account of the facts known only to the pair of them. Here Wilson was filling a significant gap, for it was generally believed that Elliot Smith's career was strange in having no apparent formative stage. Their association from the outset was 'of the happiest', wrote Wilson. Elliot Smith was a distinguished student, though lacking, it seemed, the urge to 'seek supremacy' in his studies and resistant initially to Wilson's recommendation of a life in scientific research. [His resistance to exploring technique – extraordinary for a neuromorphologist – persisted despite Wilson's most persuasive efforts.] Elliot Smith had an attractive personality, with a precocious, original mind and an emphatically independent style, whose very first contributions to neuromorphology were of fundamental importance and won him international recognition. Favourable circumstances assisted the launch: the research vigour in Sydney University's young medical school and science departments; the stimulus of colleagues of the calibre of Almroth Wright, C J Martin who had pushed him towards Australian fauna and J P Hill with whom he formed lasting and useful friendships; an abundance of monotreme and marsupial brain material, in both fresh and appropriately fixed and preserved condition; the fortuitous travelling scholarship; the credentials which opened doors of opportunity in Edinburgh, Cambridge and London.[22]

Wilson felt it a duty to set down these facts and he tried to be 'as objective as possible'. With the honesty and generosity to others for which he was renowned, he represented Elliot Smith's originality of mind by an invidious comparison with himself in 1894: 'I can even now recall the somewhat disconcerting impact of his fresh reading of some anatomical features of brain structure upon my own perhaps more traditional outlook.' Exercising restraint, Wilson claimed some credit for guiding Elliot Smith's first steps in research, but not for deciding the area of his research focus. Wilson's initial and most enduring research interest was the peripheral nervous system and the transitional area between the brain and the spinal cord (*medulla oblongata*); Elliot Smith's was always the brain in all three fields to which he contributed: neuromorphology, physical anthropology and cultural anthropology. Metaphorically these pre-occupations are reflected in their career paths: Wilson cultivated British ideals and traditions in an outpost on the Imperial periphery while maintaining vital connections with its centre; Elliot Smith seemed drawn inexorably to the Empire's intellectual, cultural and political centre. His controversial 'diffusion of culture' thesis – that human civilization took its origin from one centre, Egypt, from whence it flowed around the globe – never gained general acceptance among anthropologists, especially not the Americans who took an equally dogmatic stand for independent cultural origination. Their new world was not tainted by the sins of the old. A favourite of the Americans in 1920, by the mid-thirties Elliot Smith was on the discard. H H Woollard was disappointed that no Americans contributed to the Elliot Smith memorial volume in which was published Wilson's last scientific paper, on the origin of the foramen of Magendie.[23]

H H Woollard, acting editor of the *Journal of Anatomy*, inferred from Wilson's focus on the years 1888 to 1900 (the years devoted exclusively to neuromorphology) a judgement that they were his best years, or of greater scientific significance than his later work in anthropology. That was Woollard's view: 'His involvement in Egyptology is quite understandable but really unfortunate. 1900 was his critical year.' But Wilson had not meant to give this impression and in the obituary he wrote on Elliot Smith for the Royal Society, published in 1938, he gave this rebuttal:

> .... his fundamental preoccupation with neurology was far too profound to be overlaid by his manifold later interests. His interpretation of the facts of the structure and evolution of the brain became clearer, and riper as time went on. His 'Arris and Gale' lectures of 1909 may be taken as a landmark of the progress of his neurological thinking, embodying, as they do, an illuminating interpretation of the essential factors in cerebral evolution and morphology. From this period onwards his attention was focused less on the intimate structural detail of the brain, but rather on the brain, human or mammalian, as an index of evolutionary status.

Nor could he accept without reservation the most fierce criticism, relayed by Woollard, that Elliot Smith used the work of other men without making adequate acknowledgment. On good authority Woollard believed that Cunningham, Campbell and Symington had been offended in this way. Wilson's response was philosophical:

> The difficulty is, of course, to disentangle the individual contribution of any one man – even the greatest [to achievements of fundamental importance].... Elliot Smith naturally made use of

whatever material, in the way of fact and interpretation [that] was available from any source – and there were many – in the building up of his own constructive conceptions.... But what he borrowed he passed through the crucible of his own penetrating perceptions.[24]

Wilson had only one criticism of Elliot Smith: his indulgence in polemics.

He became .... a most vigorous controversialist who rather relished the joy of battle. One cannot but regret that at times his lucid thought was apt to express itself in a somewhat overforceful and pungent style, so that those to whom he was personally unknown could hardly be expected to discern the thoroughly genial and friendly personality concealed by the trenchant language of the acute and unsparing critic.[25]

The biographical sketch of October 1936, which Elliot Smith had acknowledged 'treated me with great kindness', became the basis of two obituaries Wilson wrote in 1937, one for the Royal Society and the other for the Johnian magazine *The Eagle*. He grumbled that he was not competent to review or evaluate Elliot Smith's contributions to cultural anthropology to which, he pointed out, Elliot Smith might have attached the most importance. But after some procrastination he did some research and wrote them. The original sketch was reproduced in a book, *Sir Grafton Elliot Smith*, edited by Warren Dawson and published by Jonathan Cape in 1938. For this Wilson also contributed a photograph of Elliot Smith, Hill and Wilson. Captioned *'Hunting for Platypus: In camp on the Duckmaloi River, Blue Mountains, N.S.W. September, 1895'*, it attracted interest and some demand for copies. George Streeter commissioned his daughter Sally to pick up 'a camp photograph' Wilson had promised him and in July 1939 Hill drove her to Cambridge to get it. Wilson's final public tribute to Elliot Smith was the unveiling of a bronze bust at a small ceremony in the Thane Library of the Faculty of Medical Sciences, University College London, on 3 May 1938. His throat was again giving him trouble but on the day his voice was in excellent condition for the short speech he delivered.[26]

Elliot Smith's family expressed gratitude for Wilson's efforts. Lady Kathleen Elliot Smith wrote

You were the inspiration of his early days – an influence which he carried with him all his life – which helped him to reach the position he attained in scientific research – and I shall always be grateful to you for the wise guidance and encouragement you gave him at all times.[27]

S A Smith, in acknowledging receipt of the Royal Society obituary, wrote from Sydney

> I have only one criticism to make viz that you failed to indicate the supreme importance of your influence upon his life and work. This, no doubt, is due to your modesty; and yet we all (just as Graf. himself did) fully recognise that without your kindly guidance, influence and support he could never have attained his standing in the world of science. The record of this must be left to others and we hope it will be more & more stressed in such accounts of his life as are published. We are all most grateful to you.[28]

But by another two decades that record was being buried beneath the monument of a figure larger than life. Revisionists were writing Wilson out of Elliot Smith's story. In 1959, when A A Abbie delivered an oration on Grafton Elliot Smith at Sydney University, he found it appropriate to record these words:

> Dr S A Smith (personal communication) tells me that his brother had no particular encouragement from his Sydney colleagues to study neurology and Wilson, who was deeply interested in techniques was always at him to try new staining methods. The methods then available satisfied Elliot Smith's requirements, however, and he rightly felt it a waste of time to get too involved in technique – which should remain a servant, never become a master.[29]

As with Johnny Hunter, Wilson's reputation in Sydney was diminished to build the arrogant myth of unassisted native genius.

Wilson's contemporaries were dropping off. Obituary columns, he remarked wryly, were becoming altogether too interesting. Ernest Rutherford, hale and hearty at Elliot Smith's funeral in January 1937, was dead before the year was out, his passing marked by a 'really beautiful ceremony' in Westminster Abbey at which Wilson, as an FRS, joined the procession of mourners. W R Sorley had died in July 1935, John Haldane in June 1936, and in September 1937 his sister-in-law Annie died, the last Lorrain Smith of her generation. Wilson was 'a confirmed old optimist' in his own opinion – and on life's broad issues that was so – but concerning his own health he was a confirmed worrier. He had a growing list of complaints: a treacherous memory, uncomfortable dentures, two pairs of spectacles, impaired hearing, bouts of dyspepsia, lumbago, an a-rhythmic heart, urinary trouble, fibrositis and, more sinister as he well appreciated, a chronic cough and husky throat condition for which, early in 1938, he had lengthy radiation treatment. It was pronounced perfect by the radiologist ffrancon Roberts in June 1938 but had to be periodically checked by Dr Walford at Addenbrooke's Hospital. There were numerous 'cancer scares' – he was mindful that both of his parents had died of cancer – which one or other of his two medical sons investigated and allayed. He was an established hypochondriac, but not a dispirited one. For the maintenance of health his standard resource was golf. In September 1938, at the time of his 40th wedding anniversary, he beat both Dorette and Leslie Cuthbert 'by a fair margin' and that, he declared, was a better index of his physical integrity than his memory, his hearing or his teeth. As for Mabel, she was an inspiration in the way she kept active and occupied despite her disability.[30]

Professionally Wilson was still very serviceable and after the death of Elliot Smith a few more briefs came his way, an important one in August 1938 from Robert Broom. This eccentric Glasgow-trained doctor, who had become associated with the Fraternity of Duckmaloi in 1895 when he was searching for the origin of mammals among the monotremes and marsupials in outback New South Wales before shifting his search to fossil reptiles in the Karroo region of South Africa, had in 1936 when aged 70, launched himself on another quest, the origin of man. 'I ... thought it would be worthwhile to hunt for an adult specimen of the Taungs ape', he later recorded. In August 1936, within weeks of starting to fossick in the dolomite caves of Sterkfontein near Johannesburg, he found such a specimen, a complete adult australopithecine skull, much to the jubilation of Raymond Dart and his following at the University of Witwatersrand in Johannesburg. Raymond Dart's controversial interpretation in late 1924 of the Taungs skull, as an ancestor of man, seemed at last to be vindicated. Two years later, in June 1938 at a farm at Kromdraai only two miles from the Sterkfontein site, Broom found fragments of the skull and teeth of another ape-man, which he reconstructed. His description of this find was the subject of a paper Wilson was charged with delivering to the Cambridge meeting of the British Association in August 1938. The difference of opinion it educed, reported an Australian journalist, contributed 'the only aggressive note' in an 'eminently decorous' gathering. Arthur Keith, in the chair, was the chief commentator.[31]

Raymond Dart had opened a new chapter in the saga of man's ancestry with his account in *Nature* on 7 February 1925 of the 'Taungs baby', the fossil skull of a primate about five years old with facial features and dentition intermediate between ape and man; the brain was small as with apes but somewhat human in configuration; and its posture was upright. This was an exquisite 'missing link' in Dart's opinion, an ape-like creature showing signs of having evolved in a hominid (or human) direction and he claimed for it a new genus and new species, with the designation of *Australopithecus africanus*. Robert Broom was quick to examine the skull and support Dart's interpretation but European, especially British, authorities including Arthur Smith Woodward, Arthur Keith, W L H Duckworth and Elliot Smith gave it a cool reception: Dart was probably justified in creating a new genus and species was the general opinion, but it was more akin to a gorilla or chimpanzee than man, and, said Arthur Keith, the discovery of an adult form of *Australopithecus* would prove this. More precise evidence was needed of its geological age, provenance and dentition said Elliot Smith.[32]

There were professional reasons for their scepticism: anthropologists of the time expected to find evidence of primitive man not in Africa but in the continent of Eurasia, and they expected all hominids to be large-brained as in Neanderthal man and Java man. There were also personal reasons: Raymond Dart had a reputation for rashness. Arthur Keith described him as

> ...another of J T Wilson's brilliant Australian pupils.... Of his knowledge, his power of intellect, and of imagination there could be no question; what rather frightened me was his flightiness, his scorn for accepted opinion, the unorthodoxy of his outlook.

Wilson knew that Dart could exhibit 'a good deal of immaturity' for in 1921 he and Shellshear had challenged Wilhelm His's doctrine that the neural tube and crest give origin to all the nerve cells in the human body, proposing instead that nerve cells in all animal tissues have a peripheral origin: this was akin to Johnny Hunter's subsequent thesis ascribing fundamental importance to the peripheral rather than the central nervous system. They were shameless colonials. Dart had also incurred the wrath of Elliot Smith for a misguided article published in the *Journal of Anatomy* in 1921 on the misuse of the term 'visceral'. Dart went to the new and raw medical faculty in Johannesburg in early 1923 under protest, believing he was being banished for misdemeanour by Elliot Smith, backed by Wilson and Keith. He may well have been. Davidson Black's anthropological finds in Peking in 1927–8 – one tooth, fragments of two jaws in association with pieces of brain cases from which he devised a new genus and species, *Sinanthropus pekinensis* –

378

T Thomson Flynn had been appointed to the zoology chair in Belfast, bringing with him an enormous collection of monotreme eggs and embryos. These were added to Hill's own large collection and Flynn and Hill in collaboration set out to extend and amplify the work of 'Wilson and Hill, 1907'. The problem of distance between Belfast and London was met by an exchange of visits for 3 or 4 weeks during vacations when the two men put in long and intensive work sessions. This was to be Hill's last major contribution to embryology and it occupied him for almost 20 years.

Hill's first work-in-progress report was given to the Anatomical Society in June 1934: a series of slides illustrating the processes of cleavage and germ layer formation in the monotreme egg. Wilson proclaimed it a 'triumph of technique' showing the significant events which bridge the gap between reptilian and avian development.[35] By 1939 Hill and Flynn had completed a minutely detailed description of oogenesis, maturation and early cleavage in 200 pages of print with 19 plates, published in December 1939 in the *Transactions of the Zoological Society of London*. Reviewing it for *Nature*, Wilson gave it perceptive praise and expressed an eagerness for the 'future elucidation of the succeeding stages of development and above all the beginnings of germ layer differentiation'. He added:

> Only those with some experience of the technical difficulties involved in the collection, preparation and sectioning of material at once both rare and refractory to treatment can fully appreciate the success with which those difficulties have been surmounted, as well as the excellence of the figures with which the memoir is so abundantly adorned.[36]

Hill and Flynn uncovered some remarkable developments in the monotreme egg, but none more intriguing for Hill than the formation of the germ layers. On 24 February 1940 he wrote to Wilson

> I've got on to the blastoderm stages & the first appearance of the primitive endoderm cells & the latter are hard to trace. At the moment I don't see why the blastodisc should transform into a unilaminar blastoderm composed of ectoderm & future endoderm cells. The latter should be marked out very early & why couldn't they stay below & save the trouble of crawling out again?!

Two months later he was still

> ...plodding thro' series after series, hunting the wily endoderm & trying to find out when it first becomes visibly determined. It is

remarkable that in its history it should agree so closely with that of the marsupial & that in both a unilaminar blastoderm should supervene.

By July he was satisfied.

I worked thro' the later stages up to the first appearance of the primitive endoderm. The 4–5 cell thick blastodisc becomes converted into a unilaminar blastoderm & the pre-endoderm cells migrate below just as in the marsupial.

The fundamental and almost identical agreement of the mode of primary germ layer formation in the Monotremata and the Marsupialia was the most interesting revelation of the whole investigation. That settled, only the tedium of minute description confronted Hill. It was 'slave labour' he complained, doing the same thing day in day out. For relief he pottered in his vegetable garden. In this unspectacular, painstaking fashion J P Hill achieved international stature as an embryologist. He built what is essentially all that is known of the early development of the monotreme and marsupial animals, and he established beyond dispute that Monotreme, Marsupial and Eutherian strategies are definite evolutionary stages through which the higher mammals have passed.[37]

Hill's retirement in September 1938, and a year later the outbreak of war, seriously interfered with his work. Publication of the second instalment of the long monotreme study by Flynn and Hill, completed in 1944, was not published till 1947, by which time Hill in collaboration with G R de Beer was working on a third instalment, published in 1950. Hill needed funds to house his extensive and irreplaceable embryological collection, which he hoped would form the nucleus of a British collection like that in the Hubrecht Laboratory in the Netherlands. He applied without success to the Rockefeller Foundation and the Bernhard Baron Trust for the establishment of such a laboratory at University College or the Royal College of Surgeons.[38] In mid-1939 with his collection he decamped to quarters in the Royal College of Surgeons, but in September when the RCS was evacuated the material he was working on went to his home in Finchley and the best of his slides and spirit material to the Rothschild Museum at Tring in Buckinghamshire; four months later he was feeling the frustration of not being able to consult it, and he contemplated moving to the Tring locality himself. The remainder, left in the Anatomy Department of the College, was subjected to 'absolutely unnecessary vandalism' Hill reported to Wilson in 1943, when the premises were taken over by the Infestation Department of the Food Ministry. 'What is going to happen to all my precious material when I go under the sod worries me.' In 1966 Hill's collection – 50 crates, 17 cartons and 6 metal cabinets – went to the Hubrecht Laboratory, whence in 1986 the survivals of Wilson's collection were transferred from Cambridge.[39]

Seeking a grant to enable him to continue his research, Hill applied in late 1938 for a Leverhulme Fellowship which was turned down. He then applied to the Royal Society Council for a research grant, threatening to 'go Bolshy' if it refused. The Council did refuse, on the grounds that it would be dangerous to establish the precedent of subsidizing the work of retired professors. Hill was angered to the point of considering resignation, particularly since the Council, quite recently and on poor authority, had offered a grant of 400 pounds to an American who did not want it. In 1940 the Council awarded Hill the Royal Society's Darwin Medal for work it had declined to support. Hill's third application, in April 1939 to the Halley Stewart Trust for a grant for three years, succeeded. After the war he received grants from the Wellcome Trust, which enabled him to work at his home and at the University College London Department of Anatomy until his death on 24 May 1954.[40]

Wilson was Hill's never-failing supporter. He praised Hill's work publicly, reviewed his papers authoritatively and wrote strong letters of support to prospective patrons like the Halley Stewart Trust. Hill's requests for assistance followed a certain pattern: respectful apologies for involving Wilson in 'money grubbing' which both found distasteful, followed by urgent exhortations to do what he suggested 'direct & soon' or 'please do this on receipt of this' or 'If you have any influence on the present Chairman I wish you would use it.'[41] Wilson, usually more restrained, at least in letters, could also be peremptory: 'Do, please, get the little Ornith. into acid as soon as you can!'[42] Their friendship, wrote D M S Watson, was 'delightful' and one of its beneficiaries was Gavin de Beer. It was at least partly due to Wilson's influence as an adviser on the Appointments Board that Hill secured de Beer as his preferred successor at University College London. Others at the College wanted Dixon Boyd and had gone to some lengths to secure his election, as Hill explained to Wilson: they downgraded the Chair to a Readership as a device to exclude de Beer, thinking presumably that he would not apply; but de Beer did apply and, wrote Hill, 'in face of his record I can't imagine any Board of Advisers passing him over – H.H.W. [Woollard] agrees.'[43] But Hill's debt to Wilson penetrated to a more profound level than the stratum of political backing:

...whatever I have been able to achieve in the way of scientific work is the outcome of the never failing help & encouragement Martin & you gave me in the days of long ago when I was a raw uncouth boy. Between you, you set me on my feet & gave me my chance in life & thro' out the long years. Your friendship has been to me as a sheet anchor & a lode star. What I owe to you, my dear old friend, words can never express.[44]

Of Martin, Wilson saw little in retirement, much to his disappointment. The honorary membership of St John's College which Wilson secured for him had scant use or observance. Martin never really retired. At the end of 1933 he returned from Australia with a brief from the Council of Scientific and Industrial Research to investigate *Myxomatosis cuniculi* with the idea of using this South American virus, lethal specifically to the European rabbit, to control rabbit plagues. Martin did the early experiments on transmission of the disease at the Cambridge Institute of Animal Pathology during 1934–5, and followed them with field trials on rabbits on Skolkholm Island off Pembrokeshire during the summers of 1936, 1937 and 1938. After further trials in Australia CSIR conducted the first effective epizootic in 1950–1. Martin served Australian interests as scientific adviser to the International Wool Secretariat from 1938 to 1949 by promoting fundamental research on wool and by his selection of research fellows. His influence on Australian science was so distinct that it was dubbed 'the Martin Spirit' and commemorated by the Australian National Health and Medical Research Council in 1951 by the creation of two Sir Charles James Martin Fellowships for overseas experience in medical science. Martin prized this honour above the many he received and was delighted to greet one of the first Fellows before he died on 15 February 1955.[45]

The hospitality of the Cambridge Institute of Animal Pathology (CIAP) prompted Martin to continue his long interest in nutrition. In 1936 to 1938 with colleagues from the Lister Institute he worked at the CIAP on pellagra induced in pigs by maize diets, and on the protein and vitamin requirements of swine. With the outbreak of war the Cambridge enterprise expanded. Martin's home, Roebuck House, once an inn, became the headquarters of the Lister Institute's Nutrition Division. The conservatory became a laboratory for rougher chemical work and preparation of food products, the office and library were accommodated in the house-proper and the outhouses took small animals. The CIAP housed the larger animals and the Biochemical School afforded facilities for finer chemical work. Martin, the Director of this 'institute-in-miniature' was also its 'chief technical assistant' and scientific consultant. Work was directed at improving the food supply of a nation at war, especially the potato as the most home-grown food, and wheat grain to enable the authorities to design the most nutritious 'National Loaf' of bread. In addition to these first-hand scientific labours Martin chaired, from 1934 to 1946, the governing body of the Dunn Nutritional Laboratory at Cambridge.[46]

Martin was often ill. He suffered chronic dyspepsia and the occasional bout of gastritis; he was always catching 'colds' and at least once, in February 1940, was seriously ill with pneumonia; he was prone to mishaps, like a 'bad thumb' which developed from a prick by a rose thorn to inflammation with a fever. 'He is terribly unlucky', observed Wilson, 'as he always gets something or other to knock him over.' When he was up he liked or felt obliged to work and his work sometimes threatened his health, like performing experiments on himself, or feeding pigs in the cold and wet of winter nights which he complained was 'a tough job for an old man', though he did it with punctilious precision. When Wilson called one day in November 1941, Martin in his sickbed refused to see him because of the risk of infection, so Wilson talked to Edith who

> got on to the subject of the occult and forced a little book on me to read which I took most unwillingly & found it almost unbelievably bad. It is about a 'spiritual healer' ... an enthusiastic eulogy of the man, who is clearly an arrant imposter. Imagine a concoction of all the hearsay testimony so familiar in quack advertisements. It is difficult to understand how anyone with the faintest glimmer of critical intelligence could tolerate stuff which is an insult to one's commonsense. Yet Edith laps it all up! She is a dear person in many ways, but her ideas of the intelligible world are idiotic. I have known her for over 50 years to be the ready prey to every fad & cult of a spurious and quasi-mysterious occult. and CJM is an embodiment of sanity & commonsense. They have evidently reached mutual toleration through the complete avoidance of all intercommunication on such topics.[47]

Wilson was not sociable when he was ill either. For one thing he lost his voice when he was having radiation treatment for his throat. Opportunities for meeting diminished further during the war, when petrol rationing put severe limits on both public and private transport: Wilson and Martin lived at opposite ends of Cambridge.

The two of them made special efforts to get together when Australian friends were visiting or if it would serve Australian interests. Their wives kept them up-to-date on each other's doings: by the late 1930s Mabel and Edith had established the practice of meeting for coffee at Matthew's Café on Wednesday mornings. They 'sat for hours, the cup of coffee well spun out', recorded a daughter-in-law, 'and as [Lady Martin] smoked Mother would also puff a cigarette, but only once a week.... It looked like her first smoke.'[48]

The crisis over Czechoslovakia at the end of 1938 threatened a visit, planned by Jeanie for early 1939 and coveted by Wilson: 'I had hardly dared to hope that I should yet have the opportunity again of seeing you, my darling daughter, face to face.' To his great relief the international crisis subsided and Jeanie arrived in early January for two months. The family was in an expansionist phase. Dorette had recently given birth to her third daughter, Bridget; John who had married Anne Colvin in July 1937 would have a daughter, Katharine, in October 1939; Maxwell having graduated in February 1938 was now a house-physician at University College Hospital under F M R Walshe the physician-neurologist and editor of *Brain* – a fine appointment 'very gratifying' for his father – and he would marry on the eve of war Vilma Mehner, an Austrian research chemist who shortly after war broke out went to the United States to work with the Du Pont organization. Jeanie's visit was a joyful reunion of father and first-born, tinged with sadness as always, and professionally purposeful: Wilson arranged for Jeanie to attend classes in social psychology by Professor Bartlett, under whom she had studied during her long visit in 1922. Katharine was the last of the Australian family to visit Cambridge before war began, and she seemed 'dearer and sweeter than ever' to Wilson. She came in March for five months. One of her kindnesses was to hire a car which facilitated more outings, and more meetings between Wilson and Martin.[49]

The Munich agreement of 29–30 September 1938, which sealed the fate of Czechoslovakia, heralded the end of Britain's policy of appeasement. Re-armament was accelerated, an inventory of the armed services was taken and the British people, while hoping for peace, confronted the implications of war. Forecasts were horrific: over 3,000 tons of high explosives might be dropped on London in the first 24 hours, causing 400,000 casualties. Air Raid Precaution (ARP) regulations were ordered, millions of gas masks distributed, miles of slit trenches dug, 'Anderson' shelters and the new 'Morrison' (ready in March 1941) were produced en masse. Plans were made for the evacuation from London of government departments, colleges, hospitals, and two million people, including half a million children. Even before the declaration of war, on 3 September 1939, evacuees began to flow into Cambridge. In August the Wilsons took in two young boys from London. Soon there was a flood. Students and cadet forces crowded the Colleges, raising the student population from 6,000 to 8,000; the Colleges also absorbed colonies of government departments and institutions like the Royal Society, which moved into Trinity College. Addenbrooke's Hospital overflowed into the Leys School to double its bed capacity. Wilson half expected to be recalled to teach anatomy, but the medical school's depleted staff managed to service a shortened medical course for its enlarged student numbers. The Cambridge community was well instructed and well drilled by the ARP: the blackout was instituted, sand bags filled, gas masks and ration books distributed, shelters organized and, added Wilson, 'An incendiary bomb I hope to be able to deal with!' He was astonished by the issue of a 'civilian pass' complete with photograph, for entry to St John's College. 'We are none of us nervous', he informed his daughters in Australia, 'We must just "dree our weird."' [50]

Life changed markedly. The war accelerated Wilson's disengagement with outside interests and social activities. He resigned from the Society in November 1939, meetings of the College Book Club were temporarily suspended and most evening occasions were precluded by the blackout and transport difficulties. He rarely dined in Hall. Home was now headquarters, Mabel his constant companion; unsure of her balance especially on wet or windy days, she ventured out less and seldom alone. The war was everyone's primary concern. Wilson's three sons were in uniform: Maxwell joined the RAMC and was attached to an artillery regiment; John became a gunner in an artillery regiment. Douglas was a surgeon with the Royal Navy Volunteer Reserve – he had actually joined in 1936 – on an armed merchant cruiser on convoys across the North Atlantic: dangerous work in a service that was 'neither fish nor fowl and very vulnerable', in J P Hill's words. The army was at a standstill during the winter of 1939–40, the months of what the Americans called 'the phoney war', but on the high seas there were great losses. In the first year of the war seven armed merchant cruisers were sunk. Attendance on the four daily news broadcasts became a ritual. 'We always get a pang when [the broadcast] begins "The Admiralty regret to announce", and when it begins to mention "the Armed Merchant Cruiser" we are very tense', wrote Wilson on 2 September 1940. 'The loss of the "Dunvegan Castle" announced yesterday gave us one of those moments of anxiety.' [51]

Concern for Douglas increased in 1941 and 1942. The 'bridge of ships' across the Atlantic, carrying vital supplies of arms and food to Britain from the United States, was seriously threatened: until 1943 British merchant ships were sunk faster than they could be replaced. Douglas's letters, however, did not reflect any sense of danger. He was, it seemed, bored for most of the time. His main concern was for the safety of his parents during the blitz of September 1940 to May 1941, when prolonged bombing raids shifted from airports to London and industrial centres. But only the occasional bomb fell on Cambridge. Thousands of civilians died and another wave of evacuees flowed out from London, including John's pregnant wife, Anne, and their small daughter Katharine who on 9 March came to the Wilsons 'for good', in fact for two years. For the birth in July of her second daughter, Joanna, Anne went to Stirling to be with Dorette whose fourth daughter, Jill, was also born in July. Dorette then made the hard decision to send her two elder daughters, Helen and Katharine, to Sydney for the duration of the war.

Wilson's demeanour, as revealed in his letters, remained calm and resolute. The constant drone of aircraft did not trouble him, the frequent 'alerts' were merely an inconvenience. He was purposefully occupied with his Carnegie work, review articles, letters to colleagues and family, and reading. Medieval history became a great interest, though as he conceded, 'useless'. As each theatre of war opened he bought maps and timetables of that region and followed the campaign as closely as possible. In the garden he attended particularly to vegetables, growing in 1941 16 different kinds. As part of the war effort they now had ascendancy over flowers: carrots replaced lavender, potatoes took over some of the lawn and more were grown on a rented allotment in an adjoining property. In his workshop he continued to produce useful household items like a book-holder for reading in bed, wooden blocks for his grandchildren, wire-netting screens for windows in case they were shattered by bomb-blasts, similar screens for bookshelves to frustrate the depredations of curious toddlers, and he took and processed innumerable family photographs. There were times when Wilson felt a 'useless log' or 'a mere cumberer of the ground', but since his main pension (Australian) would cease altogether when he died he could add: 'Fortunately, by merely living I am some use as a breadwinner.' His main contribution to the war effort was to give cheer and shelter to his family and maintain, for the benefit of all around him, a robust optimism about the ultimate 'triumph of truth and righteousness over wickedness, folly and ignorance', and a

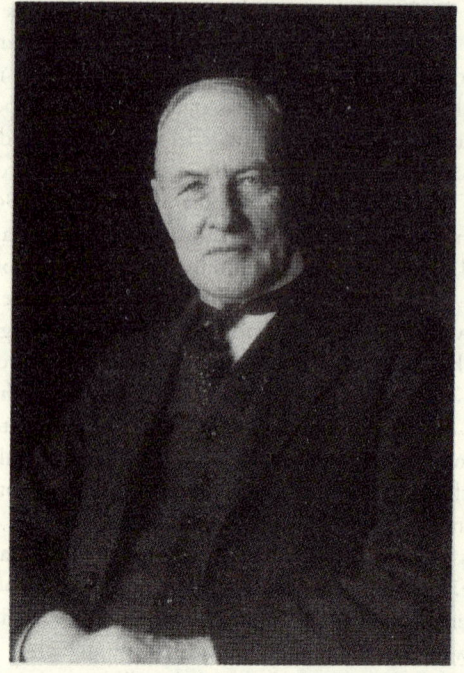

'The Nestor of British Anatomists'
Portrait by F J Pittock, J P Hill's technical assistant,
taken in 1934.
Reproduced in the Journal of Anatomy *Memorial*
Volume in Wilson's honour, October 1941.
Photo: Courtesy Wilson family.

fervent belief in 'Divine Reason which is, after all, the ground and source of all. In that faith I live and confidently "trust the larger hope".' He prayed that he might live long enough 'to see Peace in Israel and the divine judgement on the workers of iniquity'.[52]

Wilson celebrated his 80th birthday on 14 April 1941. The Anatomical Society honoured his 80 years by dedicating the October volume (76) of the *Journal of Anatomy* to him, as 'the Nestor of British Anatomists'. Among the articles was an excellent sketch of his career by J P Hill. Accurate, concise and authoritative as no one else could be of Wilson's scientific life, Hill indicated also the breadth of his non-scientific interests, the spiritual area of Wilson's striving intelligence where J P Hill, like most scientists,

388

rarely ventured. He had not, confessed Hill, the brains for it. For that dimension of Wilson's life he relied on the testimony of Wilson's oldest friend, Mungo MacCallum: Wilson came close to the impossible definition of a truly cultured man, of knowing everything of something and something of everything.[53]

St John's College marked Wilson's 80 years according to tradition by toasting his health at the Feast of St John the Evangelist on 27 December. There were tributes from colleagues like D M Blair of Glasgow, expressing gratitude for his example, kindness and inspiration. The American Association of Anatomists accorded him honorary membership. From Sydney came the felicitations of the Professorial Board and letters from old friends indulging in light-hearted reminiscences. Purser recalled the adventures of the Fraternity of Duckmaloi in the nineties; MacCormick savoured memories of sailing, particularly an occasion outside the Sydney Heads when Almroth Wright was sea-sick and accused MacCormick and Wilson of being drunk, and Wilson took shelter on the hatch under a tarpaulin and kept asking the time of day; Carslaw in rural Buradoo chortled over altercations in the Professorial Board with Wilson in his 'pre-Nestorian days'. Wilson's name seemed always to evoke affectionate laughter and an anecdote to tell. Mention of Wilson in the presence of Sydney men, a Cambridge colleague noticed, always elicited 'Oh, you mean "Jummy"', followed by 'a spontaneous fervour delightful to hear'. 'A splendid type is and was J.T.W.!', wrote Carslaw.[54]

Japan's assault on Pearl Harbor on 7 December 1941, and simultaneous thrust southwards through Malaya, shocked the world. The war now had global dimensions. Within weeks Hong Kong had fallen, Wake Island had fallen and Japan was in control of the vast North Pacific Ocean between the Hawaiian Islands and the Philippines. Australia's vulnerability was heavily on Wilson's mind when he replied to the toast to his health in St John's College on 27 December. He gave his familiar remarks on the British university ideal encapsulated in the Sydney University motto, "Sidere mens Eadem mutato", a new twist:

> ... *now* – at this fateful time when Australia is facing a menace of no lesser gravity to that which England had to meet when the Spanish Armada sailed against her – I do not doubt that the motto will still hold good when Australia is fighting for its life and for all it holds dear and that the 'selfsame spirit' which animated the men of England in 1588 will not fail under the Southern Cross.

There was nothing Britain could do. The fall of Singapore on 15 February 1942 was a humiliating defeat, exposing the Empire as an anachronism. On 19 February Darwin in Northern Australia suffered the first of many Japanese air raids. In May three Japanese midget submarines penetrated the defences of Sydney Harbour and sank a depot ship, the converted Sydney ferry HMAS *Kuttabul*, with the loss of 19 killed and 10 injured. For Australians this was the fulfilment of their worst nightmares of the 'Yellow Peril'. Wilson blamed Britain for the Singapore debacle, but Australia's extraordinary complacency about the Empire's protective capacity – in marked contrast to the outlook of the National Defence League in 1905 to 1909 – had made her no less culpable.[55]

The Wilsons in Britain experienced a long drawn-out anxiety about the Australian predicament, made all the more keen by an interruption of several weeks in the mails. In Stirling Dorette was in an agony of concern for her daughters in Sydney. She asked her father for his opinion of the likely developments. His almost formal reply, like an intelligence report, was that prospects in the short term were grave but in the long term excellent:

> ... invasion, in the sense of landings somewhere on the Aust. coasts and in more than one place are extremely probable – almost a certainty – but that invasion *in the sense of an overthrow or effective occupation of any considerable area is most unlikely* and that any such attempt would certainly fail and would afford the opportunity for smashing disaster to the enemy forces – both on the land and through attacks on their communications which are bound to be very vulnerable ... there may be raids ... on Aust. bigger coastal centres of population & industry [but] they will meet with effective resistance.... The reaction to these threats to Aust. security appears to be in the highest degree satisfactory ... the Japs are up against a far tougher problem than they have ever encountered so far. In [this] judgment I naturally take account of the obvious large scale assistance from U.S.A. that now seems actually in progress & certain in the near future.

This appraisal was similar to the official Australian military assessment of the time. Fear of invasion waned with the realization that Japan's savage attack on the United States rendered victory to the Allies a certainty, both in the Pacific and in Europe. That powerful 'slow-moving organism', in Wilson's words, had been abruptly provoked into total war.[56]

For most of 1942, however, the Allies had little to cheer about. The Japanese conquered the Philippines in April, Burma in May; in July they landed in the Buna-Gona area on the New Guinea northeast coast, and within a week advanced to the top of the Owen Stanley Range and seized Kokoda just north of Port Moresby, where for seven months Australian troops fought their way over the Kokoda Track in appalling tropical conditions to drive them back. A gleam of hope came from American naval victories in the Coral Sea in May – which thwarted a seaborne Japanese attack on Port Moresby – and off Midway Island in June. On the Russian front in September a desperate battle for Stalingrad was being waged in the streets. In North Africa, where Katharine's husband Thyne Reid was serving with the Australian Ninth Division, hope crumbled when Rommel checked a British offensive. The Australian Prime Minister, John Curtin, stood up to Churchill while ingratiating himself with the Americans and brought the Ninth Division home in January 1943 to defend Australia in New Guinea. In Britain tighter food and fuel rationing added to the privations of life in bomb-torn British cities. Australia introduced similar but less severe food, clothing and petrol rationing in late 1941.[57]

In Sydney everyone was preparing for blackouts and air raids. The government was talking about evacuating 100,000 children from Sydney. 'Of course it is right to be ready', Mungo MacCallum wrote to Wilson on 15 December 1941, 'but the feeling is that we may have air raids such as devastated London or Coventry, & that I can hardly believe.' In February 1942 Louise took her three children and Dorette's two daughters to a rural property near Yass in the New South Wales tablelands. They returned in October when the fear of invasion had subsided. Katharine was working full-time in munitions production. In July Allan Clunies Ross was commissioned as a Military Personnel Officer for scientists. Science in this war was everywhere a potent force, giving the decisive edge in many contests, and ultimate victory to the Allies over Japan. Patrick de Burgh, who had joined the Australia Army Medical Corps directly from his post as a resident medical officer at Sydney Hospital in 1939, organized a mobile laboratory unit and in September 1942 was sent north with it to Townsville, Queensland, to help combat the tropical diseases which in New Guinea were causing more casualties among Australian troops than the fighting. He left behind a wife, Elizabeth (née Rowland) and a baby daughter, Elizabeth Anne. Mungo MacCallum aged 86 went back to the censorship part-time to read the Dutch letters. His only surviving child, Walter, in his second war against Germany, was evacuated from Greece, Crete, Egypt and Java before being appointed Deputy Director-General of Army Medical Services at Headquarters in Melbourne. War news from every theatre was gloomy for most of 1942. 'The whole situation calls for courage and for supreme effort,' wrote Wilson in August.[58]

Mungo MacCallum died in Sydney on 3 September 1942 aged 88, harrowed for the second time in his life by a war between the Empire and his 'spiritual home', and bereaved by the death of his daughter Isabella (Tibbie) Lightoller in 1940. Both of Wilson's 'fascinating pair of fellow passengers' on the RMS *Orient* in 1887 had predeceased their parents. Standish Lightoller wrote Wilson an account of his old friend's last days and E R Holme requested a biographical article for a memorial volume of *Southerly.* Over the next several months, intermittently – gone were the days of long concentration – Wilson put together the impressions of a friend of 55 years and an intimate associate of 33 years in Sydney.

He sketched the vigour and versatility of MacCallum's accomplishments as scholar, lecturer, dean, elder statesman and citizen, giving testimony, wrote an appreciative Holme, to 'the spirit of friendship & sense of the soul there was in that little bit of a body'. Wilson was discreet. He alluded only in general terms to MacCallum's failings and his antipathies with quondam opponents or, in Wilson's characteristic pro-and-con style, balanced them against endearing qualities. He had a compulsion to find the good in people and circumstances. Interesting were Wilson's observations on MacCallum's intellectual capacities. MacCallum's academic policy was 'sane and liberal ... mildly conservative in some matters, but certainly not unprogressive'. In debate he was a keen advocate and a formidable opponent with a 'power of rapier-like retort'. However, when circumstances of responsibility called for strictly judicial consideration, 'every trace of personal bias seemed to disappear, submerged in impartial judgement in which full recognition was given to arguments and points of view to which he was perhaps naturally unsympathetic or even hostile'. Wilson's best memories were of the early days of their friendship when he was a frequent weekend guest in the MacCallum household and they studied Idealist philosophy systematically. These were important years for Wilson's intellectual growth and, like an affectionate younger brother, he was grateful for them. But the benefits went both ways: MacCallum's major book, *Tennyson's Idylls of the King and Arthurian story from the XVIth century*, published in 1894, acknowledged only Wilson as a local helper. 'Do you remember the old Sundays at

Dulwich Hill when we read Green together?' MacCallum had enquired in a recent letter. 'Can I ever forget them!' replied Wilson.[59]

In the closing months of 1942 the fortunes of war favoured the Allies. In New Guinea the Australians pushed the Japanese back along the Kokoda track and into the sea at Buna by January 1943, and turned their attention to evicting them from other footholds in new Guinea; the Russians mounted a counter-attack at Stalingrad which by March 1943 had cleared the invaders off most of occupied Russian soil; in October in Egypt British and Australian troops under Montgomery broke the German front at El Alamein and by May 1943 had swept Rommel's army out of North Africa. Alamein marked the turning of the 'Hinge of Fate', said Churchill but, he cautioned, it was only 'the end of the beginning'. Wilson warned of the 'flurry': the final dangerous phase of whale hunting when the monster, mortally wounded, flails its hunters.[60]

In the course of 1943 the Allies won back the rule of the seas, a necessary pre-condition for a European second front. A combination of improved radar, full air support for North Atlantic convoys and an amazing acceleration in American shipbuilding made the 'bridge of ships' much safer. Losses of merchant shipping declined sharply as the Allied toll of U-Boats climbed. From June there was little impediment to the massive movement of men and materials from the United States to Britain. By August 1943 Americans were swarming over Cambridge, Matthew's Café being a focus for their entertainment. In the Mediterranean the U-Boat threat to convoys to the Middle East ended. Convoys to Russia were prey to the German navy in Norwegian waters until September when the battleship *Tirpitz* was put out of action by British midget submarines. With the sinking of the *Scharnhorst,* the last of Germany's battleships, on Boxing Day 1943 the British Home Fleet took complete control of the North Sea.[61] Confidence in ultimate victory lifted but the burden of anxiety on families continued. The fighting went on, bombs continued to fall and people were still dying. Thyne Reid's brother George and Anne Wilson's brother, George Colvin, were killed in action in late 1943.[62]

But in the summer of 1943 the Wilsons had cause for celebration. On 5 June in Cambridge, after 11 years of marriage, Douglas's wife Hazel gave birth to a son, James Angus Glover Wilson. He was the first 'Wilson grandson' and his grandfather was jubilant. The charm of this new 'wrastlin' Jamie', his weight gains and his exploits were catalogued in letters to family and friends. He was christened at St Columba's Presbyterian Church, Cambridge, on

25 July and afterwards Wilson photographed Jamie and the other participants in various combinations. The occasion was also marked by 'an intimate talk' between Wilson and Douglas about God and Man, the Past and the Future. 'We both share our faith in God and eternal life in Him', recorded Wilson. The following November when Douglas had another brief leave they read together the 90th Psalm (Prayer of Moses, man of God) and Wilson presented Douglas with his silver-backed brushes, 'which may', he noted in his diary, 'ultimately fall to Jamie (James Angus Glover Wilson!)'.

Wilson's commitment to Christianity grew stronger in his last years and his philosophical reservations about the supernatural less real. The utilitarian view that society could not, without great loss, dispense with the values of organized religion had never been enough for him: ethical social standards would not be maintained, he believed, without the spirit of the everlasting Christ. During the war he seemed to lean heavily on Old Testament texts, and he fulminated like an ancient prophet against the evil-doers who caused it. They would be struck down by the wrath of God. But much as he hated and berated the inhumanity of man to man, testimony to which was then abundant and spectacular, he still subscribed to the doctrine of progress in human affairs, a presupposition of Idealist philosophy antipathetic to the Christian creed. He had his own 'mix' of Christianity, Idealism and Science in which the fervent theology of the Free Church – the first religious imprint on his mind and soul – was strikingly resilient. It became very important to him that his children understand his convictions, especially his Idealist concept of Time with which he linked Heredity. A difficult concept to grasp, he put it most succinctly to Jeanie at the time of his 80th birthday.

> Time is a mysterious concept and, altho' inescapable as a form of apprehension, is not an absolute. 'Past' & 'Future' have equal validity & reality with the 'Present' ... your life & mine are bound up together for good & all, now & always. And we are both bound up with our forebears and our successors in the great stream of life.[63]

After a year in a shore job Douglas was posted in July 1943 to a cruiser of the Dido class, the *Royalist*, which saw action in the North sea and Norwegian waters – it was involved in the *Tirpitz* operation – and in home waters, in the Mediterranean in support of the Italian campaign, and in the Aegean when an operation in Turkey was mooted, but not in the Normandy invasion. Maxwell's outfit was.

After two years in Nigeria with the 36th General Hospital caring for native troops training for overseas service, and feeling sidelined from action, Maxwell transferred to the newly-forming 6th Airborne Division as Deputy Director of Medical Services with the rank of Major. He dropped rank to join the 225th Para Field Ambulance and was in the first wave dropped on Normandy during the night before D-Day. He 'wouldn't have missed the experience for worlds' he reported to the family; by 19 June he was attending to casualties all through the night. John, who had risen from private to captain in the Royal Artillery, was engaged in staff work at the War Office.[64]

The Normandy landing was a vast enterprise, elaborately planned. On 6 June in an endless stream, 6,000 ships of all sizes left the Channel ports supported by 11,000 first-line aircraft to land 156,000 troops and equipment on five Normandy beaches: 'the greatest armada that ever left our shores', said Churchill. Headlines over the next several days reported excellent progress. Difficulties of weather, supplies and German resistance at Caen in France and Arnhem in the Netherlands delayed the offensive but General Eisenhower's headquarters reported on 26 August that the end of the war was 'within sight, almost within reach'. Then a lack of supplies prevented a rapid advance across France and gave the Germans time to regroup and counter-attack. By mid-September it was clear the war would not be over by Christmas. The Allied lines were threatened in December by an all-out German offensive through the Ardennes, but they held firm and on Christmas Day the Allies could celebrate, if not the end of the war, the end of a major crisis.[65]

Morale on the home front was becoming critical. For a people who at the end of 1943 had expected final victory in 1944, the second front had been a long time coming. Between mid-January and mid-April the 'little Blitz' of 13 heavy bombing raids on London increased the malaise: in March and April industrial absenteeism reached serious proportions. A week after D-Day the Germans launched on the people of London a new kind of torment, the V-1 or 'flying bomb' with a motor which stopped at a prescribed range. The pregnant silence before their massive detonations had a powerful psychological impact on the whole population. On the night of June 15–16, 73 of these bombs fell on London. Alerts came day and night, and once again evacuees streamed out of London, including once again Anne and her two small daughters, to Cambridge. They arrived on 19 June. And once again 24 Millington Road had a full house: in early April Hazel and Jamie had sought refuge there after

Jamie went down with broncho-pneumonia in Okehampton. On 15 July Anne and her daughters left to stay for three months with the Cuthberts in Stirling. In Cambridge September was a difficult month for the Wilsons: illness kept Hazel in bed for a fortnight, Wilson almost every day was having radiation treatment for his throat which made him feel 'seedy' and tired, and Mabel had a few giddy turns and was under doctor's orders to rest. Meanwhile Jamie had to be looked after. The household's reserves of strength were fully stretched. It was most fortunate, Wilson remarked, that Maud and May were very amiable and that Jamie was well-behaved and attractive. In October, while Hazel took a ten-day holiday with friends in London, Jamie was cared for by Cambridge friends Millicent and Ralph Noble and the Wilson household had a respite.[66]

Wilson now accompanied Mabel almost everywhere she went, which by 1944 was not far and not often. Her sense of balance was uncertain and she feared falling. They went to church on Sundays except in bad weather, to meetings of her Christian Universities in China committee, to the occasional cinema show, occasional visits to friends, and regularly on Wednesdays to town, to the fishmonger, the butcher, the bank, the bookshop, the lending library – they were still voracious readers – and Matthews Café for coffee with Edith Martin. Constant companions, Wilson regretted his conversational limitations, which for Mabel, who enjoyed talking, was rather a trial. 'I wish I was different', he wrote in 1942. 'She is dearer to me than ever'. They usually travelled now by bus or taxi, and walked even less after one morning in August 1944 when Mabel reached home only with difficulty, due to her heart, Wilson thought. He was alarmed, but she recovered quickly. She had periodic bouts of faintness and giddiness, the worst of them on 11 October as they walked to the bus stop, where she collapsed on the bench and lost consciousness. She awoke, she explained to one of her daughters, 'to find myself uncomfortably lying on the bench with Dad kneeling down by my side. What brought me back was hearing Dad calling me, Darling, Darling. I fear I gave him a great fright'.[67] By the time the doctor arrived she was her normal self again. She was told to rest more. On Maxwell's suggestion a second opinion was sought, and an overhaul. The verdict was reassuring: her heart was in quite fair condition and the main cause of her trouble was a vascular spasm of the blood vessels in the cranial area, not uncommon in elderly folk. It could be triggered by nervous tension and she should take things quietly. More likely, Maxwell later considered, this episode was 'one of a series of so-called ischaemic attacks caused by small blood clots carried to the brain'.

A few weeks later, in similar circumstances, Mabel died in Wilson's arms in Millington Road at about noon on Saturday 18 November. 'My beloved darling died suddenly today', he wrote in his diary. The cause was one massive stroke and death was immediate. Fortunately Douglas was at home on leave and he attended to the funeral and cremation arrangements. All the family in Britain congregated for the funeral except Dorette who was ill, and Maxwell who was in the middle of an important field exercise. In the early afternoon of Tuesday 21 November, as the service was being conducted at St Columba's Church, Maxwell was flying overhead. J P Hill with his daughter Katie and Martin with Lady Edith were among many Cambridge dignitaries at the funeral service. The occasion had at least got Charlie Martin into a church, Wilson afterwards observed with a chuckle.

Christmas 1945 was a quiet affair at 24 Millington Road, with only three at the table – Wilson, Hazel and 18-month-old Jamie – but they had the traditional dinner. Wilson's charm had secured them a turkey from the fishmonger according to Hazel, and Australian gifts of dried fruits made a pre-war plum pudding. Douglas, Maxwell and Dorette telephoned their greetings and Wilson was showered with letters, cards and a good supply of books. Reading was now his main occupation. He had replied to all the bereavement messages and begun again to turn out family photographs. Mending Jamie's cot became a repetitive job in the workshop. A very attractive infant, merry, friendly and 'no trouble' during the day, at night he was given to 'jigging' rather violently. 'Jamie managed to smash up his cot again & poor Hazel had a disturbed night in consequence' was Wilson's first entry in his diary for Christmas day.

Hazel was devoted to Wilson, and a good housekeeper. Taking care of him was her 'greatest pleasure' and Wilson had a genuine affection for her. They were good companions. 'I love being with Father', she wrote to Jeanie in February 1945:

> we have the fiercest arguments on all manner of subjects & pull one another's legs (he pulls hardest by the way) & it's sheer delight to me to see him laugh & look pink & genial.

In Jamie they had a great bond. This 'little imp' not only gratified Wilson's patriarchal pride; he also gave his grandfather an absorbing interest in his feats, his sense of fun and the expressions that flitted across his face: 'when he bends his eyebrows, he looks like Jeanie at the same age', he observed.

Father finds all this enchanting, [wrote Hazel] & will sit & watch
him by the hour – with a most lovely expression on his own face of
which he is, of course quite unconscious.

Visits by other members of the family livened things up: a week
with Anne, John and their daughters just after Christmas; Dorette
and one of her daughters after that; and Douglas and Maxwell
whenever they had a few days leave. He was sustained too by the
flow of letters from family and old friends like Lady MacCallum,
Cecil Purser, H S Carslaw and Alexander MacCormick who revived
memories of the zest and hilarity of the old days, with which Wilson
then regaled Hazel. Almroth Wright engaged him in philosophy; in
February came an urgent request for Wilson to send him 'what Kant
said about being impressed by the starry Heavens and the categorical
Imperative in his breast. I can't find it in Caird's Kant that you got
me to buy in Sydney and what has been with me ever since'.[68]

But of course nothing could relieve Wilson of the burdens of
bereavement and infirmity. There were acute 'stabs & jolts' of grief
and periods of utter desolation. He was afflicted with fibrositis of
the neck and shoulder, as well as the nausea consequent on more
intensive and more frequent radiation treatments. He spent more
time reading in or on his bed. Depression was beginning to settle on
him. Douglas prescribed a daily walk which had the desired effect,
but the forces against were greater than the forces in favour of it.
Then their excellent cook, May, left and Hazel took over that
service, leaving her less time for other things. A visit to Stirling,
proposed for the summer, Wilson vehemently opposed: he was most
reluctant to face the ordeals of travel and visiting. But, for the sake
of others – Dorette who was eager for it, Maud who needed a rest,
Hazel and Jamie who should have a holiday near to Douglas's
station – he agreed. Ralph Noble and his wife Millicent, who were
driving to Scotland on July 20, offered him a lift.

The war news was better in the new year but no one any longer
speculated on when it would end. Strategic bombing of German
cities and communications went on from February to mid-April, till
no oil was produced, no transport moved and industrial Germany
was destroyed. The Rhine was crossed in March, the Ruhr overrun
in April, and Berlin encircled by the end of April. Victory in Europe
came at last on 8 May, but the wild celebrations which rocked the
country would not for long hide the fact that the British people
were exhausted. Attention turned to the war in the Pacific. By VE
Day Lord Mountbatten's British forces had reclaimed Burma and his

sights were trained on Malaya and Singapore. General MacArthur with his American troops had returned triumphantly to the Philippines in February. Australian troops were evicting the Japanese from New Guinea and surrounding islands. The prospect was a long campaign of amphibious landings, with the Australians and Americans island-hopping all the way to Japan. No one expected victory until 1946.

The war in the Pacific ended suddenly on 14 August after atomic bombs were dropped on Hiroshima and Nagasaki. Wilson in Stirling was electrified by the news. While most were relieved that a long fight of attrition through Japanese-occupied Pacific Islands was supervened, and others were aghast at the destructive power of a split atom, Wilson's first thoughts were of the scientific significance. It was the biggest event since the Creation. This new source of energy could transform the world. 'He tried to explain it all to us', recalled Anne Wilson, 'but I only realised that he had the vision to see past the awful present to a future with the world transformed by atomic power'.[69]

The Stirling visit had its highs and lows for Wilson. Very tired on arrival, he felt well for a week or two and was down again by the last week, when his breathing developed a loud purring sound. The main problem he gave Dorette was maintaining a supply of books. On the journey south with the Nobles they stopped for a few hours at Moniaive. Back in Cambridge on Friday 24 August, Dr Walford inspected Wilson's throat and delivered his verdict to Douglas. A considerable swelling of the vocal cords was interfering with his breathing; it was probably a recrudescence of the growth and it had grown rapidly, but since it could be an inflammatory reaction to the radiation treatment it was thought best not to alarm Wilson with that suspicion; for the same reason a tracheotomy was not proposed. By the following evening Wilson himself realized that only a tracheotomy would relieve his breathing difficulty. He was admitted to a private room in Addenbrooke's Hospital on Sunday 26 August and a tracheotomy was performed under local anaesthetic. His breathing became easy but his general condition worsened. He was able to greet Dorette's two elder daughters, just returned from their wartime interlude in Australia, and he was very glad to see J P Hill whom Douglas had notified of his condition.

Time now dragged for him, Douglas suspected, his prayers answered and duties fulfilled. He had been blessed, he reflected, with a long, full and in the main, a very happy life. He was ready to go. On Sunday 2 September, with his sons in attendance, he died in his sleep.

Resolution

The funeral service was held at St Columba's Church on Tuesday afternoon, 4 September. Wilson's three uniformed sons saluted his coffin as it was carried into the church and, with Dorette, they followed it up the aisle. In a simple ceremony a distinguished company farewelled James Thomas Wilson. Afterwards the Martins and the Hills joined the family for a brief service at the Crematorium. St John's College held a memorial service on 10 November. Some time later another service was held at the Free Church, Moniaive, for the interment of Wilson's and Mabel's ashes in the family grave. To their names on the headstone were added these words, from Deuteronomy:

> The eternal God is thy refuge
> And underneath are the everlasting arms.

Notes

1. Transfer of reins: JTW to J, 6.6, 27.6, and 17.10.34. Professor Emeritus: JTW to J.
2. Harris regime: Fairfax-Fozzard, 71. 'I was summoned' and 'an expendable demonstrator': Arthur Fell to JMGW, 9.10.1985. Frank Goldby to JTW 1937. HLHH Green to JTW 1936.
3. AJE Cave to author 15.8.84, Fairfax-Fozzard, 79–87.
4. Harris regime: Fairfax-Fozzard, 73–5.
5. Retirement research: JTW to J, 24.10.34 and 27.2.35. JTW 1938b.
6. Family letters.
7. 'the feeling': JTW to LH, 30.12.36. 'lived her life': AW to author.
8. Patrick's career: JTW to J, 23.10.35 and 30.3.38. Bosch Professor: *Centenary Book*, 346.
9. Presentation to Louis: *Centenary Book*, 286–7. Quotes: JTW to Louis, 22.7.36 and Louis to JTW, 29.8.36.
10. Fifth Congress of Universities: JTW to J, 22.7.36; *Report of Proceedings*, Universities Bureau of the British Empire, 1936, 53–63. [Titled '.... British Commonwealth' for next congress, in 1948.]
11. Baldwin's speech: *Report of Proceedings* for 1936 Congress, 21–30. 'On the University Ideal': Baldwin 1937, 48–60.
12. Cockburn and Ellyard, 62.
13. 'Public affairs': JTW to J, 9.9.36. 'God help us': JTW to J (n.d. probably 22.9.37) 'the narrowest' and 'much less': JTW to J, 8.12.37. *Round Table*: JTW to J, 22.12.37. 'full-blown': JTW to J, 11.9.35.
14. House plans: JTW to LH, 24.12.35; JTW to J, 1.1.36. 'I could never' and 'a few selected': JTW to J, 24.12.35.
15. *Ibid.*

400

16. New house and garden: family recollections to author; JTW to J, 26.8.36. Heating: JTW to J, 17.11.37.
17. 'as an intelligent': JTW to GHS Lightoller, 11.8.43. 'There were a lot' and 'the genuine': JTW to J, 27.4.37. Eighteen interviews: JTW to J, 3.4.35. Quinquennial work: JTW to J, 18.10.38.
18. 'I feel very guilty': Lightoller to JTW, 23.6.37.
19. 'He looks': JTW to J, 8.5.1935.
20. GES' physical disabilities: JPH to JTW, 12.12.1932; Dawson 102–7; Le Gros Clark to JTW, 3.11.1933. News of death: Abbie, 1959.
21. GES' funeral: MMW to KR, 6.1.1937.
22. *J of A* article: JTW to Woollard, 15.9.36. No formative stage: Cave in Dawson, 186.
23. 'I can even': JTW, 1936. JTW research area: Dart, 1974. No American contributors: Woollard to JTW, 16.9.36.
24. 'his fundamental': JTW 1938, 328. Fierce criticism: Woollard to JTW, 28.7.37. 'The difficulty is': JTW to Woollard, 26.7.37.
25. JTW, *RSO* on GES, 330.
26. 'treated me': GES to JTW, 28.11.36. Not competent: JTW to Sir Squire Sprigge, 1.1.37. Duckmaloi photograph: Dawson, 118; JPH to JTW, 13.7.39. Ceremony at UC: JTW to J, 4.5.38.
27. 'You were': Kathleen Elliot Smith to JTW, 8.10.37.
28. 'I have only': SAS to JTW, 30.4.38.
29. 'Dr S A Smith': Abbie, U of S, 1959, 107.
30. Interest in obituary columns: JTW to J. JTW's health: family correspondence.
31. 'I ... thought': Broom, quoted in Watson, *RSO* 1961, 40. 'the only': Chisholm, 1944, 150. Keith as commentator: JTW to J, 26.8.38.
32. Taung controversy: Wheelhouse, 40–57. Wilson wrote 25.3.25 to Dart, acknowledging the importance of his discovery 'whether or not your view of the precise position of your specimen is finally established'. (Dart to author, 15.3.1980.)
33. 'another of': Keith, *An Autobiography*, 480. 'a good deal': JTW to J, 1.3.21. Challenge to doctrine: Dart and Shellshear, 'The Origin of Motor Neuroblasts of the Anterior Cornu of the Neural Tube', *J of A* 56: 77–95, Jan. 1922. Banishment: Dart, 1973, 420–1; also, according to Dart, (quoted Elkin & Macintosh, 169) Elliot Smith saw Dart & Shellshear rejection of His's doctrine as an embarrassment and that 'further confrontation could be deferred or avoided in post World-War-I Europe, by settling Joseph Shellshear in Hongkong and myself in Jo'burg'. Davidson Black: *RSO* 1932–5, by GES; *RSO* on GES by JTW, 332. 'the most human': JTW to J, 26.8.38.

34. All quotes: *Nature*, 27.8.38. Le Gros Clark: *RSO* by Zuckerman, 217. British Association meeting: JTW to J, 26.8.38.
35. 'triumph of technique': JTW in *J of A Proceedings*, Vol. 69, Oct. 1934 – July 1935.
36. 'Only those with': *Nature* 7.9.40, 339.
37. 'I've got', 'plodding thro' and 'I worked': JPH to JTW, 24.2.40, 17.4.40 and 16.7.40.
38. Hill's collection: JPH to JTW, 4.3.38 and 25.10.38.
39. Wartime moves: JPH to JTW, 21.9.39 and 24.2.40. Vandalism: JPH to JTW, 12.8.43. Collection to Utrecht: Dr C Kirkham-Jones (née Hill) to Mrs Hooper of the Basser Library, 8.12.66.
40. Hill's applications: JPH to JTW, 4.3.38, 25.10.38 and 28.11.38. Halley Stewart and Wellcome Trust: de Beer, *RSO* on JPH, 105.
41. '*direct* & *soon*' etc.: JPH to JTW, 14.4. 39 and 28.11.38.
42. 'Do please': JTW to JPH, 1.11.33.
43. 'delightful': DMS Watson, *RSO* on JPH, 114. Downgrade and 'in face of': JPH to JTW, 4.3.38.
44. 'whatever I have': JPH to JTW, 3.12.40.
45. Rabbit research: *RSO* on CJM, 184, 201–3. Schedvin, 358–9.
46. Martin's later work: *RSO* on CJM, 184–6, 199–200.
47. Pneumonia: JPH to JTW, 24.2.40. 'He is terribly': JTW to J, 22.7.36. 'a tough': Chick in *RSO* on CJM, 200. 'got on to': JTW to KR, 10.11.41.
48. Mabel and Edith: AW Recollections.
49. Family information. 'I had hardly': JTW to J, 14.8.38. Prof. Bartlett: JTW to J, 11.10.38. Vilma Mehner: JMGW to author, 12.7.94.
50. Havighurst, 271–8. 'An incendiary' and 'We are': JTW to J, 3.6.40.
51. Changes: JTW to A B Ramsay, 10.11.39. 'neither fish': JTW to J, 20.10.40. 'We always' etc.: JTW to J, 2.9.40.
52. 'bridge of ships'; Havighurst, quoting Roosevelt, 312. Douglas: TDGW to J, 25.9.40. 'useless log' etc.: JTW to KR, 17.1.42. 'triumph of truth': JTW to JPH, 31.8.43.
53. 'Nestor of British anatomists': AJE Cave to JTW, 28.4.41. Confession by Hill: JPH to JTW, 23.12.41. MacCallum, *SMH*, 5.6.1920.
54. Blair to JTW, 18.12.41. Professiorial Board to JTW, 23.7.41. Purser to JTW, 11.10.42. MacCormick to JTW, 26.12.41. Carslaw to John Read, 26.10.42. 'Oh you mean': HLHH Green, *Nature* 29.12.45, 773.
55. '*now* – at this': Notes of JTW's speech, 27.12.1941. HMAS *Kuttabul*: Hermon Gill. War details: Grey, 171; Hoyt, 317.
56. '... invasion, in the sense': JTW to DC, 19.3.42. Official assessment: Grey, 172–4.

57. Havighurst, 314–16. Grey, 167–80.
58. Sydney: MacCallum to JTW, 15.12.42. Patrick de Burgh: *Centenary Book*, 346. Tropical diseases: Grey, 179. Allan Clunies-Ross: JTW to J, 9.3 and 30.8.42. Censorship: MacCallum to JTW, 21.11.39. Walter's movements: *MJA* 30.7.1960; MacCallum to JTW, 15.6.42. 'The whole situation': JTW to J, n.d. (?10.8.42).
59. MacCallum: JTW 1944, 'Memories of MacCallum' and *ADB* entry by K J Cable. 'the spirit of': E R Holme to JTW, 29.6.43.
60. Havighurst, 320–1. 'flurry': JTW to Holme, 12.8.43.
61. Havighurst, 331–2. Matthews Café: JTW to J, 27.8.43.
62. Anne's brother: JTW diary, 2.10.43.
63. JTW to J, 29.5.41.
64. JTW to J, 6.7.44 and 26.7.44.
65. Havighurst, 346. D-Day landing of 156,000 (175,000 by 8 June): AJP Taylor, 195; Chandler, 68.
66. JTW Diary and family correspondence. Also for remaining paragraphs.
67. 'to find myself': MMW to KR, 16.10.44.
68. 'we have': Hazel to J, 13.2.45. 'when he bends' and 'Father finds': Hazel to J, 26.2.45. 'what Kant': Wright to JTW, 20.2.45.
69. Wilson's response: AW Recollections.

16

Epilogue

J T Wilson was one of a multitude of practical, high-minded, constructive, combative and chauvinist Scots who manned the British Empire. They could identify with the Empire if not with England. Their heritage, in Wilson's estimation, was 'a wonderful mixture of nobility, faithfulness, narrowness & obstinacy – but heroic and a great contribution to the struggle for freedom'; they practised their 'perfervid religion', he noted particularly, with 'genuine piety'.[1]

Not the least of their imperial endeavours went into education, which the Scots place above most things. Their ideals were distinctive: broad, democratic and attentive to the development of moral and civic virtue. They transformed public education in New South Wales. Radical and comprehensive reform of the 'formal and lifeless' colonial school system was inaugurated in 1901 by a scathing public attack on it by the Glasgow-trained professor of philosophy, Francis Anderson, and carried into effect by the driving force of an Australian-born Scot, Peter Board, under-secretary and director of public instruction in New South Wales from 1905 to 1922 who, according to his biographer, 'approached his task with the zeal and logic of his Scottish forefathers'.[2] Board was assisted by the young import, Edinburgh-trained Alexander Mackie, principal of Sydney Teachers' College from 1906 and professor of education at the University of Sydney from 1910 to 1940.

A glance at Sydney University professorial appointments between 1880 and 1910, years of considerable expansion, shows a preponderance of Scots: out of 22 appointed 11 were Scots (8 from Edinburgh and 3 from Glasgow), while 6 were from Oxford and 2 from Cambridge; the remaining 3 were Sydney graduates. Seven of

404

these Scots chaired scientific professional schools. Edinburgh's dominance of the medical school was scandalous in the opinion of some. Till 1910 all of its professors were Edinburgh-trained Scots (Stuart, Wilson and Welsh) and so also, in the early years, were most of the clinical teachers. The Chancellor of the University from 1896 to 1914 was another Edinburgh-trained medical Scot, H N MacLaurin. The Edinburgh background ensured no concordance of principles or policies among the three professors of the medical school, but it did lead to growing resentment of the 'Edinburgh clique' as native-born students grew to maturity in their profession.[3]

Wilson's origins were modest, disciplined and secure, also intellectually lively and community-minded. An early enthusiasm for natural history, along with the need for a decent living, determined his choice of medicine. Science was his forté, anatomy his subject and William Turner his revered 'Chief' and exemplar. Unlike Anderson Stuart his academic record was not brilliant. Wilson felt secure enough and inquisitive enough in the university milieu to explore wider interests – philosophy not the least of them – and become firm friends with John Haldane and James Lorrain Smith along the way. Anderson Stuart was not so comfortable; he pursued a lonely prize-winning pathway to intellectual and social acceptance. He was Edinburgh's most decorated student. Wilson was Turner's 'soundest' product, a broad, thorough and systematic scientist, highly competent in histological techniques, passionate yet critical in the search for truth. Anderson Stuart was to build a grand physical structure for the medical school in Sydney; Wilson was to furnish it with a reputation.

Wilson's decision to accept the junior opening of demonstrator of anatomy in Sydney was a bold move, with only a distant prospect of a chair, and it was taken with some misgivings. But it was providential. In 1887 New South Wales was riding an economic boom and the expanding university brought together a group of keen young scientists and scholars who for some years to come would have light teaching loads: a rare opportunity for original research. Scientists were organizing for themselves a national forum, the Australasian Association for the Advancement of Science. Biologists were moving out of the 'collecting' phase of their Australian history and into the interpretive phase, asserting their competence as fully-trained professionals to wrest significance from Australia's indigenous materials without help from abroad. In keeping with the political mood of the time these Australia-based scientists were flying a national flag – or rather an Australian

[margin note: John Haldane / James Lorrain Smith]

federation flag for, like the general public, they had no thought of breaking loose from the Empire.

The Fraternity of Duckmaloi took its origin from the close friendship of Wilson, a comparative anatomist concerned as an evolutionist with ultimate causes, and C J Martin, an experimental physiologist concerned with proximate causes. At a time when the two great arms of biology were becoming increasingly separated a bond was forged between them at Sydney's medical school by these two men. Wilson represented 'learning' in Martin's view while Martin, according to Wilson, was 'the embodiment of common sense'. Both had 'the genuine itch for research' to use Wilson's phrase and in Martin's they 'meant business'. In early 1892, as the great depression of the 1890s engulfed Australia, they led a self-supporting and informal interdisciplinary team of researchers – including the young J P Hill and Grafton Elliot Smith – in the first sustained and authoritative studies of native fauna by Australia-based scientists. Martin's chief interests then were snake venoms and the heat-regulating mechanisms of monotremes; Wilson was drawn to comparative neurology (especially the peripheral nervous system) and embryology (especially of the monotremes); Hill specialized in the embryology and reproduction of marsupials and monotremes and Elliot Smith's focus was comparative neurology, especially of the brain. All four won Fellowships of the Royal Society. By 1906 they were dispersed but their subsequent careers interlaced and their sense of fraternity endured.

It was probably Martin, and the young American biologists whose opinions he read, who spurred Wilson to define his stance in the perennial debate on mechanism versus vitalism in biology. Inclined in 1888 toward the vitalist views of his friends John Haldane and James Lorrain Smith – vitalism dovetailed with monistic Idealism, a school to which they all subscribed – by 1898 Wilson as a scientist had pitched his tent with the mechanists: mechanism had to be pre-supposed he argued, if the scientist's work was to be made intelligible; on the greater spiritual aspect of reality science 'must be forever dumb'. He had become a dualist. Physically disconnected from his Edinburgh friends by coming to Australia, this debate estranged them ideologically. Wilson's urge to reconcile his religious and philosophical sensibilities with materialist science persisted, however, and he rejoiced when they seemed to merge, as for example when August Weismann's 'continuity of germ plasm' theory of heredity chimed with Idealist philosophy's 'Eternal Now' and Christianity's 'Life Everlasting'.[4]

406

Wilson was a 'practical Idealist' observed Mungo MacCallum *Mungo MacCallum*
who held that this philosophy was the source of Wilson's intellectual
power and moral ascendancy which from 1908, when he became
chairman of the Professorial Board, began to influence Sydney
University government. But it would also have come from the
intellectual stimulus, discipline and piety of his Scottish boyhood.
His received views and his acquired philosophy fitted reasonably
well, especially on ethics and citizenship. It is doubtful, however,
that 'the single spiritual principle' of the Idealists was for him an
adequate substitute for the personal God of the Christian faith. All
his life he followed Jesus Christ; in tribulation he found solace in
'the everlasting arms'; during both world wars he fulminated with all
the passion of the biblical prophets against the forces of evil; and at
the end he spoke of God as 'the Final Reality'.

Wilson was an exemplary citizen in the T H Green sense of *citizen*
realizing his 'best self' by serving the 'common good'. He supported
philanthropic ventures like the University Boys' Club and the
Sydney Medical Mission; he participated in the university outreach
programmes like the University Board extension lectures and the
Workers' Educational Association; he addressed student, medical
and scientific assemblies; as an alert nationalist he campaigned with
the National Defence League for compulsory military training from
1906 until 1909 when the Defence Act provided for it; as a staunch
imperialist he supported the Victoria League and the Round Table;
he studied the military arts from drill, camping and manoeuvring to
organizing and commanding the New South Wales section of the
Australian Intelligence Service (1908–13) and establishing and
commanding the Censor's Office (NSW) for the first 16 months of
the war. Except when Censor he did all of these things while
running a rapidly-expanding department with heavy teaching
commitments, assisted by a small technical staff and teams of
demonstrators, also chairing the Professorial Board (1908–13,
1916–20) as the University extended its educational mission. In *1919*
1919 it was Wilson who designed a new and enlarged academic *designed*
structure and set down the basic principles for defining faculties, *academic*
staff positions and degrees. Faculties increased from four to ten, the *structure*
new McCaughey Bequest funded the largest expansion in staff
positions in the University's history, and over the following several
years Wilson had an important influence on the selection of new
staff. All of this widened Wilson's outlook and strengthened his
grasp of thought on complex issues. In debate he was formidable.
Foresight and even-handedness characterized his opinions and

vehemence the expression of them. He was a commanding figure driven by a spiritual passion for justice and truth. By 1920 university government had become reliant on his judgement. There was an expectation among his colleagues that he would become Sydney University's first executive Vice-Chancellor: he would be their William Turner.

But he did not become Dean of Medicine till March 1920, following the death of his 'senior colleague', even though from about 1902 when Anderson Stuart's interests moved away from the medical school, it was Wilson's authority that pervaded its walls. The two medical leaders had much in common but their differences were of much more significance for Australian medicine. Inevitably they collided. Stuart had little interest in teaching or research. His métier was organization and his objective power and influence. Wilson was an evolutionary morphologist who taught anatomy to medical students, few of whom were interested in the scientific puzzles which preoccupied him. Their main requirement as future medical practitioners was a thorough grounding in topographical anatomy, which for Wilson was strictly on all fours with Greek irregular verbs: both essential to a larger body of knowledge, and equally uninspiring. Wilson's topographical anatomy lectures were dull, unlike his lectures on the difficult new subject of neurology which engaged his strongest research interest. On the medical curriculum a division of opinion opened and grew with the years: Wilson believed that to justify its presence in a university the medical course had to do more than train for a trade; it had also to educate and to inspire. For this reason he defended the basic scientific foundation of the medical curriculum against the increasingly strident claims of proliferating clinical specialisms. Sydney's 'intensely practical community' was more favourably disposed toward the clinicians, as also was Anderson Stuart. Stuart stood for vocational medicine, Wilson for scholarship. Stuart's legacy was material: 'the cathedral' he built to house medicine at the university and a foundation for the quasi-aristocratic rank enjoyed in Australia by the medical profession. Wilson's legacy was intellectual: an internationally respected tradition of research during his own lifetime, and a foundation for neuroscience in Australia.[5]

Wilson's appointment to the Cambridge chair of anatomy was initiated and manoeuvred by Grafton Elliot Smith who by 1919 had become Britain's leading anatomist as well as a neuromorphologist and anthropologist of international standing. His ambition was to reinstate British anatomy as an autonomous biological science and

408

the seat of medicine, central to which was the reclamation of histology after 50 years from the physiologists. Elliot Smith achieved this feat at the University of Manchester and at University College London. Perhaps, with the power and authority he then enjoyed, he might have done so at Cambridge where Wilson could not. But it is unlikely: histology supplied the ground on which Cambridge physiologists had won fame and they were veteran defenders of their territory. Wilson won the esteem of his peers and developed the work of his department along lines appropriate to the scientific spirit of Cambridge. But vocationalism and academic politics threatened his regime. His final teaching years were years of strenuous combat in defence of his subject, and though his warrior qualities impressed his opponents and he achieved in his own words 'a reasonable compromise' for anatomy in a revised medical curriculum, he knew that the brave hopes of 1920 for a reinstated and reinvigorated anatomy were over. In 1935, privately, Wilson acknowledged that anatomy, much as he loved it as a biological science, no longer had 'vital appeal'; that power had passed to physiology and its offspring.

The Fraternity of Duckmaloi was a distinguished band of biologists whose long careers began in Sydney and the bush in the early nineties with studies of Australia's native fauna and concluded in London and Cambridge. Their association is little known, their names with one exception virtually forgotten in Australia and their individual achievements little appreciated. The exception is the only Australian-born member, Grafton Elliot Smith who left Australia in 1896 and never returned except for short visits. His star rose early and blazed brilliantly. Honours were showered on him in his lifetime: FRS (1907), knighthood (1934), chevalier of the Légion d'honneur (1936), besides many honorary degrees, British and foreign, and elections by his peers to leadership of professional organizations. Two books on his life and work have since been published, one in London in 1938[6] and another in Sydney in 1973[7], and his contributions to neuroscience have been recorded in an international history of that field. But Australian biologists today are hesitant to assess Elliot Smith's stature as a scientist; suspicions emanating from significant errors of judgement, headstrong polemics and the impression that his drive for power tended to overwhelm his instinct for scientific discovery, have dimmed his reputation. He was rivalrous and cavalier. Yet his insights were arresting and his discoveries fundamental, especially in neuromorphology, in the history of which his place seems assured, as Wilson predicted. It might have been larger. In anthropology he added considerable data to its annals and his theory of the diffusion of culture though now discounted was at least stimulating. He had the touch of genius.

Martin

Charles James Martin's long and productive labours in laboratory science and its application were prodigious. He too was handsomely honoured in his lifetime with the FRS (1901), CMG (1919), knighthood (1927), five honorary degrees and election by his peers to high professional offices, besides the honour he most cherished: two Sir Charles James Martin travelling fellowships in medical science created by the Australian National Health and Medical Research Council in 1951 to commemorate 'the Martin spirit' which had a distinct influence on the development of Australian medical and biological sciences. He was purposeful, pragmatic, imaginative, ingenious in the improvisation of apparatus for precise measurements, and he was ever-responsive to calls for assistance from Australia where, but for his wife's homesickness, he might have stayed permanently. He was a touchstone of practical wisdom for Australian science as it grew, but his influence is now little appreciated because for the most part it was behind the scenes, and casual or unofficial. The influence of Martin's work and 'spirit' in Australia deserves thorough exploration.

Hill

James Peter Hill was the youngest of the Fraternity, only 19 and degreeless at the end of 1892 when he arrived in Sydney and joined the Wilson household for six years. Scots and disputatious, Wilson and Hill enjoyed a quite remarkable friendship for over 50 years. Their early collaboration in studies of the platypus brought international recognition for Sydney's medical school in 1905. When he left for a London chair the following year Hill took, besides a mass of monotreme and marsupial material, an impressive research record, an understanding of how to run a teaching department, train a technician, equip a modern laboratory and become fluent in German. His 14 years of 'intensive activity' in Australia determined his life work. His Australian material, with the Brazilian specimens he collected in 1913, occupied him for more than four decades. Painstaking and unhurriable, a master of the techniques for preparing rare and refractory material, Hill's work was detailed, accurate and unique. In the personal research chair Elliot Smith created for him in 1921 to expedite his research, characteristically he decided to teach anyway, and was rewarded by many of his students taking the DSc in embryology. Always esteemed by his peers and awarded several grants, fellowships and medals, he nevertheless could not find a

British home for his magnificent embryological collection which went to the Hubrecht Laboratory in Utrecht 12 years after his death. A paper on the history of British embryology published by Cambridge University Press in 1985[8] does not mention him. He is revered today by zoologists following in his footsteps but is otherwise virtually unknown. He might have stayed in Sydney in 1906 if the university had had a positive attitude to research – so Wilson argued at the time – and in 1919 Wilson had Hill's case in mind when he instituted the position of Associate Professor in Sydney's academic staff structure. But even a secure senior position, as with Martin, might not have been enough to withstand family pressures to return to Britain.

Wilson was the mentor of the Fraternity, the elder brother. He had the authority, expertise and enthusiasm to stimulate and sustain the appetite for research; he had also the critical acumen to keep research on track. Under Wilson's sponsorship Elliot Smith abandoned his ambition to be a surgeon for a life of anatomical research and teaching, and Hill deserted research in the Biology Department on abnormalities in vertebrates to join Wilson's more lively enterprise. Many anatomy students down the years were similarly drawn to the fascination of original investigation with Wilson. Research was essential to Wilson's sense of well-being, leading to his own solid achievements in embryology and neurology, but he pursued it, usually collaboratively, more as a teacher than a performer: 'the giving', said Raymond Dart, 'would be all his'. Dry lectures or not, Wilson was an inspiring teacher. Unfortunately, good teachers are all-too-often forgotten, because their product is intangible: it lives on in the spirit of their students. Wilson's great achievement lay in the intellectual, moral and practical leadership he gave to Sydney's medical school, university and community; in some matters his counsel reached into national affairs. This great influence was attained, as MacCallum observed, 'not ... by the ordinary methods of intrigue and wire-pulling, of "hustling" and push. He has modestly and silently made his way by the sheer momentum of his personality.'[9]

Wilson did not receive the highest personal honours, like Elliot Smith and Martin. He was elected FRS (1909), fellow of St John's College, Cambridge (1920), fellow of the Zoological Society of London, fellow of the Cambridge Philosophical Society and its president (1924–6), first overseas member of the Anatomical Society (1890) also its president (1922–4), which dedicated Volume 76 of its Journal to 'the Nestor of British anatomists' on his 80th birthday;

he also received the honorary LL.D of Edinburgh University (1926). But he received no essentially Australian honours. If he had stayed in Sydney, or not left so suddenly, or returned there as hoped in the mid-twenties, as the University's first executive Vice-Chancellor, he would have been knighted. His stature in 1920 was perhaps above any other in the government of the university and there was genuine grief in both colleagues and students when he left.

The remarkable thing is not that Wilson received no fitting Australian honours, but that over the next several decades his achievements and his reputation as a scientist and teacher were dismantled and distributed to his two most outstanding students. He had always had his detractors, for instance among Anderson Stuart's votaries and the clinicians, especially those who resented the 'Edinburgh clique'. The war created more of them – pacifists, anti-conscriptionists, and radical 'progressives' – though Wilson himself was respected by these opponents. But after the war, in a surge of national self-consciousness, both Anderson Stuart and Wilson in 1920 were demeaned as 'only [the] foster fathers' of the medical school which now passed into the hands of Professor Mills, 'one of us, one of our own kith and kin, the first chief of our race'. Johnny Hunter was the University's most precious 'home grown' deity. His death in December 1925 led to an extraordinary outpouring of grief which in the thirties during another outburst of chauvinism gave birth to a legend that exchanged roles in the relationship of Wilson and Hunter: in neurology even as a student Hunter had been Wilson's master, it was said in 1933; by 1939 Wilson was Hunter's satellite. Those who knew the truth remained silent, or were not heard; one of Wilson's successors lent his name to these falsehoods. Then came the recasting of the story of Wilson and his first outstanding student, Grafton Elliot Smith. Wilson's influence on Elliot Smith's career was, in 1938, 'of extreme importance' but by 1949 Elliot Smith had had 'no particular encouragement from his Sydney colleagues to study neurology', and by 1982 a Sydney anatomist believed that the youth who had left the country permanently in 1896 was the founder of neuroscience in Australia.[10]

The authors of the Sydney medical school's centenary history, published in 1984[11] do not commit themselves to these absurdities. They recount the facts, venture the occasional speculation and draw colour from a number of primary sources, relying rather too much at times on untested opinion. They are puzzled by the long adulation of Johnny Hunter, proud of the brilliant Grafton Elliot Smith and respectful (though not well-informed) of Wilson as a research scientist, teacher and departmental head. Their story of the medical school's first 37 years is the story of Anderson Stuart. Discord between the two founders is not registered, nor is the wrangle over histology. There is no appreciation of Wilson's work as a scientist, nor of his contribution to the building of the medical school. They deal only with the material. The authors of the first volume of Sydney University's history, published in 1991[12], also hold their focus on Anderson Stuart for their account of the medical school's foundation years. Wilson sinks deeper into obscurity. They record only odd details of fringe activities in Wilson's 33-years' service, giving no account of his contributions to science, the medical school or the university – and no inkling of the grandeur of his character.

Notes

1. 'a wonderful': JTW to J, 2.9.1938. 'perfervid' and 'genuine': JTW to J, 27.3.1935.
2. 'formal and' and 'approached his': Crane & Walker, 318 and 327 resp.
3. Professorial appointments: Turney *et al.*, Appendix 3, 639.
4. 'must be forever dumb': JTW 1898, 836.
5. Quasi-aristocratic rank: Dart, in *Nature* 27.1.23, 111.
6. Dawson W R.
7. Elkin & Macintosh.
8. Mark Ridley, *Embryology and Classical Zoology in Great Britain*, in Horder *et al.*
9. 'the giving would'; Dart to author, 15.3.1980. 'not ... by the': MWM, *SMH* 5.6.1920.
10. 'only [the] foster' and 'one of us': *SUMJ*, Oct. 1920. Sydney anatomist: M J Blunt to author, Jan. 1982.
11. Young, J A *et al.*
12. Turney, *et al.*

Bibliography

The Wilson Papers

J T Wilson's papers were deposited in the Basser Library in 1968 by his daughter Mrs Jane Clunies Ross who wrote a biographical sketch of her father, included with them. The collection is mainly manuscript material: correspondence, testimonials, drafts of speeches and public lectures. There are also family photographs, newspaper cuttings and official documents mainly relating to military service.

Supplementary papers from other members of the Wilson family were deposited in the Sydney University Archives in the 1980s and the Basser collection transferred to consolidate all of the Wilson papers at the institution where he spent most of his working life.

Principal correspondents include: Grafton Elliot Smith (1896–1936); the Haldanes (1883–1925); H S Carslaw (1924–44); T W Edgeworth David (1918–33); J P Hill (1897–1944); C J Martin (1895–1933); H E Barff; A N Burkitt; A E Mills; John Read; Louis Schaeffer (1924–42); Almroth Wright (1891–1945).

Archival Material

Australian Archives, Victoria
Department of Defence Accessions: MP 84/1 Australian Defence 1909–13; MP 95/1 Military Intelligence Reports; MP 367 Censor, POWs, aliens; MP 390/8 Deputy Chief Censor Diaries; MP 707/1 SS *Cumberland;* MP 1049/1/0 shipping, cables, Naval Intelligence.
Commonwealth Record Series: B 197/0 Intelligence; B 543 Censorship.

Australian Museum, Sydney
Board of Trustees: Minutes of meetings, 1890–5.
Correspondence in, by writer's name: 1890–1920.

Australian War Memorial, Canberra
Bean Papers [editor-in-chief and author, *Official History of Australia in the War of 1914–18*]
Butler Papers [author, medical vol. of *Official History of Australia in the War of 1914–18*]
Jose papers [author, naval vol. of *Official History of Australia in the War of 1914–18*]

414

Basser Library (Australian Academy of Science, Canberra)
C J Martin Papers
J P Hill Papers
R Scot Skirving Papers
G Elliot Smith Papers (microfilm of originals in Adelaide)

National Library of Scotland
Board of Education for Scotland, Reports for 1870s
HM Inspector's Reports, 1850s

National Library of Australia, Canberra
Novar Papers (Munro Ferguson, Australia's Governor-General, May 1914 to
Sept. 1920)

University of Sydney Archives
Board of Studies, Minutes, 1883–9
Holme Papers
Professorial Board, Minutes, 1886–1916
Peden Papers
Senate Minutes, 1878–1920
Wilson Papers

Writings by Wilson

(i) Published Papers

1888   Observations on the innervation of axillary muscular arches
        (Achselbogen) in man, with remarks on their homology suggested
        by comparative considerations. *J of A*, Vol. 22, 294–9.

1889   Abnormal distribution of the nerve to the *quadratus femoris* in man,
        with remarks on its significance. *J of A*, Vol. 23, 354–7.

1890a   Two cases of variation in the nerve supply of the first lumbrical
        muscle in the hand. *J of A*, Vol. 24, 22–6.

1890b   Further observations on the innervation of axillary muscles in man.
        J of A, Vol. 24, 52–60.

1893a   On the closure of the central canal of the spinal chord in the
        foetal lamb. *Trans Intercolonial Med Congress of Australasia*. 706–8.

1893b   On a series of varieties in human anatomy. *ibid.*, 709–12.

1893c   (with C J Martin) Observations upon the anatomy of the muzzle of
        Ornithorynchus. *Macleay Memorial Volume*, Linnean Society NSW,
        179–89.

1893d   (with C J Martin) On the peculiar rod-like tactile organs in the
        integument and mucous membrane of the muzzle of

Ornithorynchus. ibid., 190–200.

1894a   On the myology of *Notoryctes typhlops*, with comparative notes. *Trans Roy Soc of South Aust*, Vol. 18, 3–74.

1894b   (with W J S McKay) On the homologies of the borders and surfaces of the scapula in monotremes. *Proceedings, Linnean Soc. of NSW,* Vol. 8 (series 2), 377–88.

1894c   Preliminary note on the anatomy of the 'dumb-bell-shaped' bone in *Ornithorynchus*, with a new view of its homology. *ibid.*, Vol. 9, 44–5.

1894d   Observations upon the anatomy and relations of the 'dumb-bell-shaped' bone in *Ornithorynchus*, with a new theory of its homology; and on the character of the nasal septum in monotremes. *ibid.*, Vol. 9, 129–50.

1895a   (with C J Martin) Further observations on the anatomy of integumentary structures in the muzzle of *Ornithorynchus. ibid.*, Vol. 9, 660–81.

1895b   Description of a young specimen of *Ornithorynchus anatinus* from the collection of the Australian Museum, Sydney. *ibid.*, Vol. 9, 682–90.

1895c   On the dentition of Mammalia. *Hermes,* New Issue I, Nos 4 & 6, Med Supp, 1–2, 7–8, 31–3.

1897a   Notes on the innervation of the *musculus sternalis*, with remarks on its morphology. *Trans Intercolonial Med Congress of Australasia.* Dunedin 1896, 358–62.

1897b   Notes on the stephanion and on various descriptions of the temporal lines of the skull. *ibid.*, 362–6.

1897c   (with J P Hill) Observations upon the development and succession of the teeth in *Perameles*, with a contribution to discussion of the homologies of the teeth in marsupial animals. *Quarterly Journal of Microscopical Science*, Vol. 39, 427–588.

1898   Presidential address. *Proceedings, Linnean Society of NSW*, Vol. 22, 812–46.

1899   Presidential address. *Proceedings, Linnean Society of NSW*, Vol. 24, 1–29.

1900a   A new system of obtaining direction marks in microscopical sections for purposes of reconstruction by wax plate modelling. *Zeitschrift für wissenschaftliche Mikroscopie*, Band 17, 169–77.

1900b   On the skeleton of the snout and *os carunculae* of the mammary foetus of monotremes. *Proceedings, Linnean Soc. of NSW,* Vol. 25, 58–9.

1901   Ideals in medical education. *Intercolonial Medical Journal of Aust*, Vol. vi, No. 9, 405–31.

1902a   The medical curriculum. *The Australasian Medical Gazette.* 20 Feb. 1902, 62–6.

1902b On the skeleton of the snout of the mammary foetus of monotremes. *Proceedings, Linnean Soc of NSW,* Vol. 26, 717–37.

1902c Presidential address. *The Union Book,* 65–98, Sydney.

1903a (with J P Hill) Primitive knot and early gastrulation cavity co-existing with independent primitive streak in *Ornithorynchus. Proceedings of the Royal Society,* Vol. 71, 314–22.

1903b Are there Two Worlds – Nature and Spirit ? *The Australian Christian World,* 6 Feb. 1903.

1905a Demonstration of stereophotographs of wax plate models of the skull of a young mammary foetus of *Ornithorynchus. Proceedings, Anatomical Society,* 5–6.

1905b (with J P Hill) Demonstration of lantern diapositives and photomicrographs illustrative of various stages in the development of monotremes and marsupials. *ibid.,* 6. (title only).

1905c Two cases of fourth molar teeth in the skulls of an Australian aboriginal and a New Caledonian. *Journal of Anatomy and Physiology,* Vol. 39, 119–34.

1905d (with J B Nash) Absence of ascending, transverse and descending colon, and of the sigmoid flexure. *Australasian Medical Gazette,* Vol. 24, 210–11.

1906a On the fate of the 'taenia clino-orbitalis' (Gaupp) in *Echidna* and in *Ornithorynchus* respectively; with demonstration of specimens and stereophotographs. *J of Anat and Physiol,* Vol. 40, 85–90.

1906b On the anatomy of the calamus region in the human bulb; with an account of a hitherto undescribed 'nucleus postremus'. *J of Anat and Physiol,* Vol. 40, Part I, 210–41, Part II, 357–86.

1906c (with J P Hill) Observations on the development of *Ornithorynchus. Proceedings, Royal Society,* Vol. 78, 313–15.

1906d The historical development of the problem of the circulation of the blood. *J of the U of S Med Soc.* Vol. 8, 39–50.

1906e The urgency of the defence problem. *The Call.* Nov 1906, Sydney.

1907a (with J P Hill) Observations on tooth development in *Ornithorynchus. Quarterly Journal of Microscopical Science,* Vol. 51, 137–65.

1907b (with J P Hill) Observations on the development of *Ornithorynchus. Philosophical Transactions, of the Royal Society,* Vol. 199, 31–168.

1910a Improved methods of utilising organised structures as directing marks for plastic reconstruction, & other notes on microscopical technique. *Zeitschrift für Wissenschaftliche Mikroscopie,* Band 27, 227–34.

1910b Note on a new expedient for improving the colour injection of dissection cadavera. *J of Anat and Physiol,* Vol. 45, 1–2.

1910c   On a method of mounting and exhibiting frozen sections of the cadaver in the Anatomical Museum: *ibid.*, 3–6.

1911   The Influence of the University on the Community. *Report of the Inaugural Ceremony of the University of Queeensland, 1.6.1911,* 38–9.

1912   The innervation of the Achselbogen muscle. *ibid.*, Vol. 47, 8–17.

1913   On the Achselbogen muscle. *Trans, Australasian Medical Congress,* (Sydney), 1–16.

1914a   Observations upon young embryos. *J of Anat and Physiol,* Vol. 48, 315–51.

1914b   (with T W E David) Preliminary communication on an Australian cranium of probable pleistocene age. *Brit Ass Rep.* (Aust), 531. On the Talgai skull. *Sci Aust.* Vol. 20, 4–5.

1915   (with J P Hill) The embryonic area and so-called 'primitive knot' in the early monotreme egg. *Quarterly Journal of Microscopical Science,* Vol. 61, 15–25.

1916   On the neurones of the sensory ganglia. *J of the U of S Med Soc.,* 2 No. 8, 102–9.

1916a   Inaugural Address, Our General Attitude Towards the Problem, *Proceedings,* U of S Society for Combating Venereal Diseases, 6–11. Sydney, Dec. 1916.

1917   The War Records of the University of Sydney. *Hermes,* 291–2, Nov. 1917.

1918   The 'social inheritance' and the undergraduate's share in it. *J of the U of S M Soc,* 1 No. 20.

1920   The Medical School of the University of Sydney. *The Medical Journal of Australia.* Educ. No., Vol. 1 No. 13, 273–94.

1921a   The institution of a Sabbatical year for professors. *Report of Proceedings,* Congress of Univs of the Empire 1921, 393–8.

1921b   The double innervation of striated muscle. *Brain,* Vol. 44, 234–47.

1922   The ductless glands, in *Cunningham's Text-Book of Anatomy.* Fifth & Sixth Eds, 1922, 1931.

1924   On the application of the Spalteholtz clearing method to the study of thick serial sections of embryos, with demonstration of specimens. *J of Anat and Physiol,* Vol. 58, 101–4.

1925a   In memoriam: John Irvine Hunter, MD. *J of Anat and Physiol,* Vol. 59, 340–4.

1925b   Multiple hypoglossal ganglia in the calf. *ibid.*, 345–9.

1928a   Description of a convenient table for microscopy. *J Roy Microscopical Soc,* Vol. 48, 46–8.

1928b   On the question of the interpretation of the structural features of the early blastocyst of the guinea pig. *J of Anat and Physiol,* Vol. 62, 346–58.

1932   (1) Nature of the ligamentum nuchae. (2) A method of
       demonstrating thick serial sections of embryos. (3) The growth of
       the caudal end of the Mullerian duct and its relation to the
       Wolffian duct. *Proceedings, Anatomical Society,.* 1932, 208, in *J of
       Anat and Physiol,* Vol. 67 (titles only).
1936   Sir Grafton Elliot Smith: A biographical sketch of his earlier career.
       J of Anat and Physiol, 1–6.
1937a Obituary: Grafton Elliot Smith. *The Eagle,* Vol. 50, 64–70.
1937b On the nature and mode of origin of the foramen of Majendie. *J of
       Anat and Physiol,* Vol. 71, 423–8.
1938   Sir Grafton Elliot Smith. *RSO,* Vol. 2, 323–33.
1944   Memories of MacCallum. *Southerly: The Magazine of the Australian
       English Association, Sydney.* MacCallum Memorial Number, Vol. V,
       No. 2 1944. Angus & Robertson.

(ii) Unpublished Articles and Addresses (Selected items from Wilson Papers)
Address on traditional doctrines of the church and the newer teachings of
science. Presbyterian Church, Burwood, 1890.
Address on the function of science in general education. St Andrews
College, Univ. of Syd., 1891–2.
Address on chief end and purpose of university work. Opening, 1894
Session of Students Med. Soc.
Address on the teaching of science in the first year in Arts. The Senate,
Univ. of Sydney, early 1890s.
Address on character, culture and craftsmanship. Undergraduates, Univ. of
Sydney, Lent Term, 1904.
Ideas on children's education. Opening of Laboratory & Kitchen, Shirley
School, Woollahra, Sept. 1906.
Address on the Victoria League and the Empire. The Victoria League,
Sydney, 1906.
Address on Australia in the Commonwealth. Women's Political League,
Sydney School of Arts, 1906.
Address on Medical Education. Medical Students Society, Melbourne
University, 1907.
Address on Advances in Neurology. Australasian Medical Congress,
Melbourne, Oct. 1908.
Notes for address during first conscription campaign. Women students,
Sydney Univ., 1916.
Notes for opening address at inaugural meeting of Directorate of War
Propaganda, 1918.
Address at Sydney University celebration of Armistice. 14 Nov. 1918.
Speech notes, unveiling of Roll of Honour at University of Sydney, 11 Oct. 1919.

Bibliography

Notes for speech at Censorship Reunion Dinner, 16 Oct. 1919.
The university and the community, the study of science, its practical application and the role of government. Address to the Millions Club, 1920.
Teaching in the community, and contemporary political, economic and social questions. Conference of Workers Education Association lecturers, Sydney, 1920.
Inaugural Lecture. Cambridge University. 26 Jan. 1921.
The conviction that the world is not ultimately unintelligible. 'The Heretics', Cambridge, March 1922.
On the theory of evolution. Cambridge University Philosophical Society, May 1925.
The infringement of science on philosophy. Philosophical Soc dinner, St John's College, Dec. 1925.

Writings on Wilson

Burkitt, A N, 'Obituary. James Thomas Wilson'. 512–16, *The Medical Journal of Australia*, 29 Dec. 1945.

———— 'James Thomas Wilson, 1861–1945', *The Union Recorder*, Thurs. 22 Nov. 1945. Sydney Univ.

Cambridge University Medical Society, 'Professor J T Wilson, F.R.S.', 145–6, 1934 ?

Clunies Ross, J, Biographical Sketch of James Thomas Wilson, (unpub.), Wilson Papers.

Daily Telegraph, 'The Last Lecture: Professor Wilson's Farewell'. 30 July 1920.

Green, H L H H, 'James Thomas Wilson, M.A. (Cantab), M.B., C.M.(Edin), LL.D.(Edin), F.Z.S., F.R.S., 1861–1945', 84–5, *The Cambridge Review*, 10 Nov. 1945.

———— 'Obituaries: Prof. J T Wilson, F.R.S.', 772–3, *Nature*, Vol. 156, 29 Dec. 1945.

Hermes, 'Professor J T Wilson, M.B., Ch.M.', 2–3, 29 Oct. 1898, New Issue iv No. 5.

Hill, J P, 'J T Wilson, A Biographical Sketch of his Career', 3–8, *Journal of Anatomy*, Vol. LXXVI, Dedicated to J T Wilson, Oct. 1941–July 1942.

———— 'James Thomas Wilson, 1861–1945', 643–60, *RSO*, No. 18 Vol. 6, Nov. 1949.

Journal of Anatomy, 'Emeritus Professor J T Wilson, MA, MB, LLD, FRS.', 53, Vol. 80, 1946.

MacCallum, Prof. M W, 'Professor Wilson', *Sydney Morning Herald*, 5.6.1920.

M H, 'James Thomas Wilson', 390–1, *The Eagle*, (St John's College Magazine), Vol. LII, 1941–6.

Mills, A E Valedictory speech, 'Professor Wilson', 5–8, (with article, 'Farewell Dinner to Professor Wilson' 17–18), *Journal of the Sydney Univ. Medical Society*, Vol. XV, Oct. 1920.

Morison, Patricia 'Wilson, James Thomas', 525–7, *Australian Dictionary of Biography*, Vol. 12 1891–1939. MUP, 1990.

The Lancet, 'James Thomas Wilson', 354, 15 Sept. 1945.

The Times. 'Prof. J.T.Wilson, F.R.S.', and 'Anatomy at Sydney and Cambridge', Tues. 4 Sept. 1945.

Smith, S A Annual Post-Graduate Oration 'The Life and Work of James Thomas Wilson', 1–12, *Bulletin of the Post-Graduate Committee in Medicine*, Univ. of Sydney, Vol. 6 No. 1, April 1950.

Journals, Periodicals and Annuals (with abbreviations where used)
Australasian Medical Gazette (AMG)
British Medical Journal (BMJ)
Bulletin of the Post-Graduate Committee in Medicine, University of Sydney
Calendar, University of Sydney
Dumfries & Galloway Standard & Advertiser (D&GS&A)
The Call (Sydney)
Cambridge University Recorder (CUR)
Hermes, University of Sydney Undergraduates
Intercolonial Medical Journal of Australasia
Journal of the University of Sydney Medical Society (SUMJ)
Journal of Anatomy and Physiology, London (J of A)
Journal of the Royal Society of New South Wales (JRS NSW)
Medical Journal of Australia (MJA)
The Lancet
Philosophical Transactions of the Royal Society London
Proceedings of the Linnean Society of NSW (PLS)
Quarterly Journal of Microscopical Science (QJMS)
Royal Society Obituaries, or *Biographical Memoirs of Fellows of the Royal Society (RSO)*
Transactions, Intercolonial Congress of Australasia
The Scotsman
The Sydney Morning Herald (SMH)
The Union Recorder
The Union Book, University of Sydney
The University Review, Journal of the Melbourne Graduate Association

Books, Articles and Theses

Abbie, A A 'Sir Grafton Elliot Smith', *Bulletin of the Post-Graduate Committee in Medicine*, University of Sydney, Vol. 15, June 1959

Abercrombie, M 'Ross Granville Harrison 1870–1959', *RSO* 1961, Vol. 7

Alisma. (Pseud for G S Stephenson) *Reminiscences of a Student's Life at Edinburgh in the Seventies.* Oliver & Boyd, Edinburgh, 1918.

Allen, Garland E *Life Science in the Twentieth Century.* Wiley, New York, 1975.

———— *Thomas Hunt Morgan: The Man and His Science.* Princeton Univ. Press, 1978.

Allen, Gay Wilson. *William James – A Biography.* Rupert Hart-Davis, London, 1967.

Anderson, Francis. *Tendencies of Modern Education.* Angus & Robertson, Sydney, 1909.

———— *The Public School System of New South Wales.* Angus & Robertson, Sydney, 1901.

———— 'The University and National Education', *Hermes* Jubilee Number, 1902.

Arey, L B *Developmental Anatomy.* W B Saunders, Philadelphia, 1947.

Armstrong, W G 'An Eminent Epidemiologist', *Health,* July 1925, Vol. 3 No. 4.

Ashby, Eric *Community of Universities: An Informal Portrait of the Association of Universities of the British Commonwealth.* Cambridge University Press, 1963.

————& Anderson, Mary *Portrait of Haldane at Work on Education.* Macmillan, London, 1974.

Atkinson, Leon 'Australian Defence Policy: a Study of Empire and Nation (1897–1910)', Ph.D. Thesis, Aust. Nat. Univ., 1964.

Australasian Medical Congress *Transactions of the Eighth Session.* Victoria, 1909. *Australia's First.* See Turney

Baldwin, Stanley. *Service of Our Lives: Last Speeches as Prime Minister.* Hodder & Stoughton, London, 1937.

Barber, William. *The Sustentation Fund,* Glencairn Free Church. Dumfries, 1893.

Barclay Smith, Edward. *The First Fifty Years of the Anatomical Society of Great Britain and Ireland: A Retrospect.* Cambridge University Press, London, 1937.

Barff, H.E. *A Short Historical Account of the University of Sydney.* Angus & Robertson, Sydney, 1902.

Barrett, John. 'Gerald Campbell', *ADB.*

————*Falling In: Australians and 'Boy Conscription' 1911–1915.* Hale & Iremonger, Sydney, 1979.

Barrie, J M *An Edinburgh Eleven: Pencil Portraits from College Life.* Office of the British Weekly, London, 1889.

Barron, G H 'The Aims and Objectives of a Medical Society', *JUSMS,* Nov. 1910.

Bateson, Beatrice *William Bateson FRS: Naturalist, His Essays and Addresses.* Cambridge University Press, 1928.

Bateson, William *Materials for the Study of Variation.* Macmillan & Co., London, 1894.

Baumel, Howard B *Biology: Its Historical Development.* New York, 1975.

Bean, C E W *Two Men I Knew: William Bridges and Brudenell White.* Angus & Robertson, Sydney, 1957.

————*The Official History of Australia in the War of 1914–1918.* Vols I–VI. Angus & Robertson, Sydney.

Bennett, J M 'Sir Julian Salomons – Fifth Chief Justice of New South Wales', *Journal of Royal Austalian Historical Society,* June 1972.

Berlin, Isaiah *The Crooked Timber of Humanity.* Fontana Press, London, 1991.

Billings, Susan 'Concepts of Nerve Fibre Development 1839–1930', *Journal of the History of Biology,* 1971.

Binney, E H 'Looking Backwards', *SUMJ,* Vol. XVI Jan. & Aug. 1923.

Binding, Paul Editor's Introduction to *Weir of Hermiston and Other Stories by Robert Louis Stevenson.* Penguin, 1979.

Bishop, P O 'Synaptic and Neuromuscular Transmission', *Bulletin of the Post-Graduate Committee in Medicine University of Sydney,* March 1955.

————'Grafton Elliot Smith's Contribution to Visual Neurology and the Influence of Thomas Henry Huxley', in Elkin & Macintosh (eds).

Blackburn, Sir C B 'The Life and work of Sir Thomas Anderson Stuart', *Bulletin of the Post Graduate Committee in Medicine University of Sydney,* Vol. 4, No. 4, July 1948.

Blunt, Michael J *John Irvine Hunter of the Sydney Medical School, 1918–1924.* SUP 1985.

Boterenbrood, E C (ed.) *Concise Catalogue of the Central Embryological Collection of the Hubrecht Laboratory.* Universiteitscentum 'de Uithof'. Utrecht, 1977.

Bowers, J Z & Purcell, Elizabeth F (eds) *The University and Medicine: The Past, The Present and Tomorrow – Report of an Anglo-American Bicentennial Conference.* New York 1977.

Bracegirdle, Brian *A History of Micro-Technique: The Evolution of the Microtome and the Development of Tissue Preparation.* Cornell University Press, New York, 1978.

Bradley, O Charnock 'Two Cases of Supernumerary Molars', *Anat. Anzeiger,* Bd XXIV, S112, 1903.

Branagan, David & Holland, Graham (eds) *Ever Reaping Something New: A Science Centenary.* University of Sydney, 1985.

Brash, J C & Cave, A J E 'In Piam Memoriam, Sir Arthur Keith, F.R.S.', *Journal of Anatomy* Vol. 89, 404–18.

Brasher, N H & Reynolds, E E *Britain in the Twentieth Century.* Cambridge University Press, 1966.

Brazier, Mary A B 'The Historical Development of Neurophysiology', *Handbook of Physiology,* Vol. 1, eds Field and Magoon, American Physiological Society. Washington, 1959.

Brennan, C J 'The University and Australian Literature: A Centenary Retrospect' *Hermes,* Jubilee Number. Sydney, 1902.

Brett, John *Professor John Irvine Hunter.* Albury High School P & C Assoc., 1983.

British Association for the Advancement of Science, 1914. *Handbook NSW.* Sydney, 1914.

———— (1) *Narrative and Itinerary of the Australian Meeting.* London, 1915.

———— (2) *Report of the 84th Meeting in Australia 1914.* London, 1915.

British Parliamentary Papers. *Annual Report of Board of Education for*

Bibliography

Scotland 1876 G.D. 342/78/45 Vol. 3, *Schools in Glencairn.*

————— *H.M. Inspectors Reports for Glencairn Free Church School, 1854.* Vol. 52.

Brittain, Frederick *Arthur Quiller-Couch: A Biographical Study of Q.* Cambridge University Press, 1947.

————— *It's a Don's Life. Autobiography.* Heinemann Educational, London, 1972.

Brodsky, I I 'Unofficial History', *SUMJ.* Jubilee Issue. September, 1933.

Brooks, C McC, & Cranefield, Paul F (eds) *The Historical Development of Physiological Thought.* Symposium. New York, 1959.

Brownridge, W *Dumfries and Galloway Standard and Advertiser,* 11.1.1888.

Buchan, J *Memory Hold the Door.* Hodder & Stoughton, London, 1940.

Buckley, Martin J *Scarlet and Tartan.* Red Hackle Association, Sydney, 1986.

Burrell, H *The Platypus: Its Discovery, Zoological Position, Form and Characteristics, Habits, Life History.* Angus & Robertson, Sydney, 1927.

Butler, A G *Official History of the Australian Army Medical Corps.* AWM, Melbourne, 1930.

Cain, Frank *The Origin of Political Surveillance in Australia.* Angus & Robertson, 1983.

————— *The Wobblies at War: A History of the IWW and the Great War in Australia.* Spectrum, 1993.

Caird, Edward *Hegel.* William Blackwood, London, 1883.

Cajal, Ramon y (trans. A D Loewy) 'Ramon y Cajal and Methods of Neuroanatomical Research', Ed-trans from Chap 2, Cajal's monograph of 1901–11, *Perspectives in Biology and Medicine.* Autumn 1971, 7–35.

Calaby, J H see Mulvaney

Caldwell, W H 'The Embryology of Monotremata and Marsupialia – Part I', *Phil. Trans. Roy. Soc. 1887,* Vol. 178.

Cannon, Dorothy F *Explorer of the Human Brain: The Life of Santiago Ramon Y Cajal (1852–1934).* Life of Science Library, Henry Schuman, New York, 1949.

Carslaw, H S 'The University and Education in NSW', *Hermes,* Dec. 1909.

———— 'Sydney University and the "University (Amendment) Act 1912"', *The University Review,* Vol. I, No. I June 1913. Melbourne 1913.

Centenary Book of the University of Sydney Faculty of Medicine. (see Young)

Chandler, David G *Battles & Battlescenes of World War Two.* Arms & Armour Press, 1989.

Chick, Harriette 'Charles James Martin 1866–1955', *RSO,* 1956.

Chick, H, Hume, M, MacFarlane, M *War on Disease: A History of the Lister Institute.* André Deutsch, London 1971.

Chisholm, A R *The Incredible Year.* Angus & Robertson, Sydney 1944.

———— *Men Were My Milestones.* Melbourne University Press, 1958.

Churchill, F B 'The Modern Evolutionary Synthesis & the Biogenetic Law', Mayr & Provine. Harv.

———— 'Weismann, Hydromedusae, and the biogenetic imperative: a reconsideration', in Horder *et al.,* 7–33, 1986. (see Horder)

Clark, Axel *Christopher Brennan, A Critical Biography.* Melbourne University Press, 1980.

Clark, Ronald *JBS, The Life & Work of J B S Haldane.* Oxford University Press, 1984.

Clark, S L (see Ranson)

Clark, Wilfrid Edward Le Gros. see Le Gros Clark

Clark-Kennedy, A E *London Pride: The Story of a Voluntary Hospital.* Hutchinson Benham, London, 1979.

Clarke, E & O'Malley, C D *The Human Brain & Spinal Cord: A Historical Study Illustrated by Writings from Antiquity to the Twentieth Century.* University of California, 1968.

Cockburn, Stewart & Ellyard, David *Oliphant.* Axiom Books, Adelaide, 1981.

Cohen of Birkenhead, Lord 'Medical Education in Great Britain and Northern Ireland, 1858–1967', *British J of Medical Education,* 1968, 2, 87–97.

Cole, Leslie 'Cambridge Medicine and the Medical School in the Twentieth Century', Rook (ed.) *Cambridge & its Contributions to Medicine.* London, 1971.

Colebrook, Leonard *Almwroth Wright: Provocative Doctor and Thinker.* Heinemann, London, 1954.

———— 'Almwroth Edward Wright 1861–1947', *RSO.*

Coleman, W 'Bateson & Chromosomes : Conservative Thought in Science', *Centaurus.* 1970 Vol. 15.

Committee of the Privy Council on Education in Scotland, *Minutes and Reports 1839–1939.* HMSO.

Comrie, J D *History of Scottish Medicine.* Vol. II. Bailliere for Wellcome Hist. Med. Mus., London 1932.

Congress of Universities of the Empire, 1912. *Report of Proceedings.* (ed.) Alex Hill. London, 1912.

————, 1921 *Report of Proceedings.* (ed.) Alex Hill. London, 1921.

————, 1926 *Report of Proceedings.* (ed.) Alex Hill, London, 1926.

————, 1931 *Report of Proceedings.* London, 1931.

————, 1936 *Report of Proceedings.* London, 1936.

Copleston, Frederick *A History of Philosophy: Vol. 8 Part I. British Empiricism and the Idealist Movement in Great Britain.* Image Books, New York, 1967.

Cormack, Alexander A *William Cramond 1844–1907.* (see Scotland)

Corrie, John *Dumfries and Galloway Standard and Advertiser*, 11.1.1888.

Coulthard-Clark, C D *The Citizen General Staff: The Australian Intelligence Corps 1907–1914.* Military Historical Assoc. of Aust., Canberra, 1976.

———— *Heritage of Spirit: A Biography of Major-General Sir William Throsby Bridges.* Melbourne University Press, 1979.

———— *Duntroon: The Royal Military College of Australia 1911–1986.* Allen & Unwin, Sydney, 1986.

———— *No Australian Need Apply.* Allen & Unwin, Sydney, 1988.

Crane, A R & Walker, W G *Peter Board: His Contribution to the Development of Education in NSW.* Aust. Council for Educ. Research, Melbourne 1957.

Cravens, Hamilton *The Triumph of Evolution: American Scientists and the Heredity-Environment Controversy, 1900–1941.* University of Pennsylvania Press, 1978.

Crawford, R M *A Bit of a Rebel: The Life and Work of George Arnold Wood.* Sydney University Press, 1975.

Crew, B H 'Mansbridge and His Mission to Australia', *The Australian Highway.* Dec. 1969.

Crowther, J G *British Scientists of the Twentieth Century.* Routledge & Kegan Paul, London, 1952.

Cunneen, Christopher *King's Men: Australia's Governors-General from Hopetoun to Isaacs.* Allen & Unwin, Sydney 1983

Cunningham, D J 'The Relation of Nerve-Supply to Muscle-Homology', *J of A.* Vol. XVI, 1–9.

———— 'The Value of Nerve-Supply in the Determination of Muscular Homologies and Anomalies', *J of A.* Vol. 25 (1891), 31–9.

Curtis, Lionel *The Problem of the Commonwealth.* Macmillan, London 1915.

Cushing, Harvey *The Life of Sir William Osler.* Clarendon Press, Oxford, 1925.

Dart, R A 'Anderson Stuart: his Relation to medicine and to the Empire', *Nature,* 27 Jan. 1923, 111.

———— *Adventures with the Missing Link.* Harper, New York, 1959.

———— 'Recollections of a Reluctant Anthropologist', *Journal of Human Evolution,* Vol. 2. 1973.

———— 'Cultural Diffusion from, in and to Africa', in Elkin & Macintosh.

David, M E *Professor David.* Edward Arnold, London, 1937.

David, T W E 'Anniversary Address', *Journal of the Royal Society of NSW.* Sydney, 1896.

———— Address on 'University Science Teaching', 3.10.02, 93–121, *Record of the Jubilee Celebrations.* Sydney, 1903.

———— 'The Science Departments', p101–4, *Hermes* Jubilee Number. Sydney, 1902.

Davie, G E *The Democratic Intellect.* Edin. University Press, 1961.

Davies, R 'From Gay to Grave 1893–1953', *Sydney University Medical Journal* Jubilee Issue, Sept. 1933.

Dawes, J N I & Robson, L L *Citizen to Soldier: Australia Before the Great War, Recollections of Members of the First A.I.F.* Melbourne Univ. Press, 1977.

Dawson, W R *Sir Grafton Elliot Smith.* Jonathan Cape, London, 1938.

Deane, Henry 'Anniversary Address', *Journal of the Royal Society of NSW,* Vol. 32. Sydney, 1898.

de Beer, Gavin. 'Glimpses At Some Historic Figures of Modern Zoology', *Science, Medicine and History,* Vol. II. Oxford, 1953.

———— (ed.) *Autobiographies: Thomas Henry Huxley; Charles Darwin.* Oxford, 1974.

Detweiler, S R *Neuroembryology: An Experimental Study.* Hagner Publishing Co., New York, 1964.

Douglas, C G 'John Scott Haldane 1869–1936', *RSO* London, 1936.

Drummond, A L & Bulloch, J *The Church in Victorian Scotland, 1843–1874.* St Andrew Press, Edinburgh, 1975.

Eldridge, C C *Victorian Imperialism.* Hodder & Stoughton, London, 1978.

Elkin, A P & Macintosh, N W G (eds) *Grafton Elliot Smith: The Man and His Work.* Sydney University Press, 1974.

Elliott-Bateman, Michael (ed.) *The Fourth Dimension of Warfare*, Vol. 1. Manchester, 1970.

Epps, W *Life of Sir T P Anderson Stuart.* Angus & Robertson, Sydney, 1922.

Evans, M A & Evans, H E *William Morton Wheeler, Biologist.* Harvard, 1970.

Ewing, Rev. William (ed.) *Annals of the Free Church of Scotland*, Vol. 1. Edinburgh, 1914.

Fairbrother, W H *The Philosophy of T H Green.* Methuen, London, 1896.

Fenner, Frank *History of Microbiology in Australia.* Brolga Press, Canberra, 1990.

Ferguson, William *Scotland – 1689 to the Present.* Oliver & Boyd, Edin., 1968.

Fewster, K J. 'Expression and Suppression: Aspects of Military Censorship in Australia During the Great War'. Ph.D. Thesis, UNSW, 1980.

Field, L M *The Forgotten War.* Melbourne University Press, 1979.

Fischer, G L *The University of Sydney 1850–1975.* University of Sydney, 1975.

Fisher, H A L *An Unfinished Autobiography.* London, 1940.

Fitzhardinge, L F *The Little Digger 1914–1952, William Morris Hughes, A Political Biography.* Angus & Robertson, Sydney, 1979.

Forward, Roy & Reece, Bob (eds) *Conscription in Australia.* Queensland University Press, 1968.

Foster, Leonie *High Hopes: The Men and Motives of the Australian Round Table.* MUP, 1986.

Fozzard, J A Fairfax. *Professors of Anatomy in the University of Cambridge: The First two hundred and sixty-one years of the Cambridge University Department of Anatomy, 1707–1968,* Fosslia, 1983.

Freeden, Michael *The New Liberalism: An Ideology of Social Reform.* Clarendon Press, Oxford, 1978.

Fyffe, David *The History of Glencairn Free Church.* Dumfries, 1893.

Geison, Gerald L *Michael Foster and the Cambridge School of Physiology: The Scientific Enterprise in late Victorian Society.* Princeton University Press, 1978.

Gill, G Hermon *Royal Australian Navy 1942–1945.* Aust. War Memorial, Canberra, 1968.

Goldschmidt, Bertrand *The Atomic Complex: A Worldwide Political History of Nuclear Energy.* American Nuclear Society, Illinois, 1982.

Gollwitzer, Heinz *Europe in the Age of Imperialism 1880–1914.* Thames & Hudson, London, 1969.

Gordon, Peter & White, John *Philosophers as Educational Reformers.* Routledge & Kegan Paul, London, 1979.

Gosse, Edmund 'The Matriarch', *Leaves and Fruit.* Heinemann, London, 1927.

Gould, Stephen Jay *Ontogeny and Phylogeny.* Belknap Press, Harvard, 1977.

———— *Ever Since Darwin: Reflections in Natural History.* Penguin, 1980

———— (a) *The Panda's Thumb: More Reflections in Natural History.* Penguin, 1980

———— (b) *The Flamingo's Smile: Reflections in Natural History.* Penguin, London, 1986.

———— *An Urchin in the Storm.* Penguin, London, 1987.

———— *Bully for Brontosaurus: Reflections in Natural History.* Hutchinson, London, 1991.

Granit, Ragnar *Charles Scott Sherrington: An Appraisal.* Nelson, London, 1966.

Gray, John *History of the Royal Medical Society 1737–1937.* Edinburgh, 1952.

Green, T H (ed. A C Bradley)..*Prolegomina to Ethics.* Oxford, 1924.

Greenwood, G and Grimshaw, C (eds) *Documents on Australian International Affairs, 1901–1918.* Nelson, Melbourne, 1977.

Grey, Jeffrey. *A Military History of Australia.* Cambridge University Press, Sydney, 1990.

Griffiths, Mervyn *The Biology of the Monotremes.* Academic Press, London, 1978.

Guthrie, D *A History of Medicine.* Revised Ed. Nelson, London, 1958.

Haldane, J S 'Life and Mechanism', *Mind,* 27–47, Vol. 9, 1884.

———— (Pseudonym – A Medical Student). *A Letter to Edinburgh Professors.* London, 1890.

———— 'Vitalism', *The Nineteenth Century*, Vol. XLIV, July–Dec. 1898, London, 1898.

———— *The Philosophy of a Biologist.* Clarendon Press, Oxford, 1936.

Haldane, R B *Education and Empire: Addresses on Certain Topics of the Day.* London, 1902.

———— (chair). *Royal Comm. on University Education in London, Final Report.* HMSO, London 1913.

———— (a) *Selected Addresses and Essays.* London, 1928.

———— (b) *An Autobiography.* Hodder & Stoughton, London, 1928.

———— & Seth, A (eds) *Essays in Philosophical Criticism.* London, 1883.

Hamburger, Victor 'S Ramon y Cajal, R G Harrison and the Beginnings of Neuroembryology', *Perspectives on Biology and Medicine*, Summer 1980.

Hancock, W K *Perspective in History.* Aust. Nat. University, Dept Economic Hist., Canberra, 1982.

Harrison, J F C *Society and Politics in England 1780–1960.* Harper & Row, New York, 1965.

Haswell, W Presidential Address, Linnean Society of NSW *Proceedings,* Vol. 16. 1891.

————— Presidential Address, Linnean Society of NSW *Proceedings,* Vol. 17. 1892.

————— 'Recent Biological Theories', Section D, *Rep of Aust'asian Assn for the Adv of Sc,* 1891.

Havighurst, Alfred F *Twentieth Century Britain.* Harper & Row, New York, 1962.

Haymaker, W & Schiller, F (eds) *The Founders of Neurology.* Illinois, 1970.

Heseltine, Michael *Medical Press and Circular, 1949.* (in Newman)

Hetherington, H J W *The Life and Letters of Sir Henry Jones, Prof of Moral Philosophy in the Univ of Glasgow.* Hodder & Stoughton, London 1925.

Hill, A V *The Ethical Dilemma of Science.* The Scientific Book Guild, Beaverbrook Newspapers Ltd, London, 1962.

Hill, J P 'James Thomas Wilson 1861–1945', (see writings on Wilson.)

————— & Martin, C J 'On a Platypus Embryo from the Inter-Uterine Egg', *Proceedings,* Linnean Society of NSW, Vol. 19, 43–69, 1895.

————— 'Preliminary Note on the Occurrence of a Placental Connection in Perameles Obesula and on the Foetal Membranes of Certain Macropods', *Proceedings, Linnean Soc. of NSW* 10 (2nd Series), 578–81, 1895.

————— 'The Placentation of Perameles' (Contributions to the Embryology of Marsupialia, I). *Quarterly Journal of Microscopical Science,* 1898.

————— & Wilson, J T see Wilson Bibliography, 1897 to 1915.

————— 'The Developmental History of the Primates', *Philosophical Transactions of the Royal Society of London.* Series B, Vol. 221. London 1932.

Home, R W (ed.) *Australian Science in the Making.* Cambridge University Press, Sydney 1988.

Horder, T J, Witkowski, J A & Wylie, C C (eds) *A History of Embryology:*

Bibliography

The Eighth Symposium of the British Society for Developmental Biology, Cambridge 1986.

Horn, D B *A Short History of the University of Edinburgh*. Edin. UP, 1967.

Houston, George (ed.) *The Second Statistical Account of Scotland*. HMSO, 1835.

Howarth, T E B *Cambridge Between Two Wars*. Collins, London, 1978.

Hoyt, Edwin P *Japan's War: The Great Pacific Conflict*. Da Capo, 1986.

Huettner, A F *Fundamentals of Comparative Embryology of the Vertebrates*. New York, 1964.

Hughes, W M *Crusts and Crusades: Tales of Bygone Days*. Angus & Robertson, Sydney 1947.

Hyam, Ronald *Britain's Imperial Century 1815–1914: A Study of Empire and Expansion*. Batsford, New York, 1976.

Hyman, Libbie Henrietta *Comparative Vertebrate Anatomy*. University of Chicago, 1942.

Jones, Frederic Wood *Life and Living*. Kegan Paul, London, 1939.

Jones, Henry *Idealism as a Practical Creed*. James Maclehose, Glasgow, 1909.

———— *The Principles of Citizenship*. Macmillan, London, 1919.

Jose, Arthur W *The Official History of Australia in the War of 1914–1918, Vol. IX: The Royal Australian Navy*. Angus & Robertson, Sydney, 1978.

Judd, Denis *Balfour and the British Empire: A Study in Imperial Evolution 1874–1932*. St Martin's Press, New York, 1968.

Judson, Horace Freeland *The Eighth Day of Creation*. Jonathan Cape, London 1979.

Keith, Sir Arthur 'Anatomy in Scotland During the Lifetime of Sir John Struthers (1823–1899)', 7–33, *Edinburgh Medical Journal*, 1912.

———— 'Sir William Turner as anatomist and anthropologist', *BMJ*, 26.2.16.

———— 'The Progress of Anatomy', *J of A*. Vol. 62, 1927/8.

———— *An Autobiography*. Watts & Co., London, 1950.

433

Kendle, John E *The Round Table Movement and Imperial Union.* University of Toronto, 1975.

Knibbs, G H Presidential Address, *JRS NSW 1899*, Vol. 33. Sydney, 1899.

Kohler, Robert E *From Medical Chemistry to Biochemistry: The Making of a Biomedical Discipline.* Cambridge University Press, 1982.

La Nauze, J A *Alfred Deakin.* 2 vols. Melbourne University Press, 1965.

Langdon-Brown, Walter *Some Chapters in Cambridge Medical History.* Cambridge University Press, 1946.

Le Gros Clark, Wilfrid *Chant of Pleasant Exploration.* E & S Livingstone, London, 1968.

———— 'Arthur Keith 1866–1955', *RSO*, 19.

Lewis, Brian, *Our War: A View of World War I from inside an Australian family.* Melbourne University Press, 1980.

Lilley, F R *The Woods Hole Marine Biological Laboratory.* Chicago, 1944.

Little, Bryan *Cambridge Discovered.* W Heffer, Cambridge, 1960.

Liversidge, Archibald 'Presidential Address', *JRS NSW,* 1901 Vol. 35.

Luckett, W P 'Ontogeny of Amniote Fetal Membranes and their Application to Phylogeny', *Major Patterns in Vertebrate Evolution.* Hecht, Goody & Hecht, (eds). New York, 1976.

Luqueer, Frederick-Ludlow *Hegel as Educator.* New York, 1967.

MacAlister, Edith *Sir Donald MacAlister of Tarbert.* London, 1935.

MacCallum, M W Address, 'University Influence', 1.10.1902, *Record of the Jubilee Celebrations of the University of Sydney.* Sydney, 1903.

McCarthy, John (ed.) *Dependency? Essays in the History of Australian Defence & Foreign Policy.* ADFA, Defence Studies Publication No 1.

McHenry, Lawrence C *Garrison's History of Neurology.* Springfield Illinois, 1969.

McIntyre, A K 'Origins of Australasian Neuroscience: a personal view', *Proc. Aust. Physiol. Pharmacol. Soc.* 1983.

McKay, W J S 'The Morphology of the Muscles of the Shoulder Girdle in Monotremes', *Proceedings,* Linnean Society of NSW, Vol. 19, 1894.

Bibliography

Mackerras, C B 'Sir Henry Normand MacLaurin: 1835–1914', *Journal of the Royal Australian Historical Society* Vol. 54, Sept. 1968.

———— *Divided Heart: The Memoirs of Catherine B Mackerras*. Little Hills Press, Sydney, 1991.

Mackenzie, Donald 'Sociobiologies in Competition: The Biometrician – Mendelian Debate', Webster C (ed.) *Biology, Medicine and Society 1840–1940*. Cambridge University Press, 1981.

Mackenzie, J S 'Edward Caird as a Philosophical Teacher', *Mind* 1909.

Mackintosh, Ann (ed.) *Memoirs of Dr Robert Scot Skirving, 1859–1956*. Foreland, Sydney, 1988.

Mackintosh, N W G 'The Talgai Cranium: The Value of Archives', *Aust. Natural History*. June 1969.

McLaren, Moray *The Scots*. Penguin, 1951.

MacLeod, Roy (ed.) *The Commonwealth of Science: ANZAAS and the Scientific Enterprise in Australasia, 1888–1988*. Oxford University Press, 1988.

———— & Collins, Peter (eds) *The Parliament of Science: The British Assoc for the Adv. of Science 1831–1981*. Science Reviews, Midx, 1981.

MacMillan, David 'Seventy Five Years of the Faculty of Medicine' *Sydney University Medical Journal*, 1958.

Maddox, Kempson *Schlink of Prince Alfred*. Royal Prince Alfred Hospital, Sydney, 1978.

Magner, Lois N *A History of the Life Sciences*. M Dekker, New York, 1979.

Maienschein, Jane 'Preformation or New Formation – or neither or both', 73–108, in Horder *et al.*, 1968.

Mair, Alex *Sir James Mackenzie, M.D.: 1853–1925 General Practitioner*. Churchill Livingstone, Edinburgh, 1973.

Mandle, W F *Going It Alone: Australia's National Identity in the Twentieth Century*. A Lane, Melbourne, 1977.

Mann, Horace (See Scotland J.)

Manning, Sir William Chancellor's Address. 1886. University of Sydney, 1887.

Martin, C J 'The History of the Relations Between Morphology and Physiology During the Last Fifty years', Presidential Address, Section D,

Biology, *Report of 7th Meeting Australasian Assoc. for Advancement of Science.*
Sydney, 1898.

———— & Tidswell, Frank 'Observations on the Femoral Gland of
Ornithorynchus and its Secretion; together with an Experimental Enquiry
concerning its Supposed Toxic Action', Linnean Society of NSW
Proceedings Vol. 19. 1894.

———— & Hill J P (see Hill).

———— & Wilson, J T (See Wilson Bibliography)

———— 'Ernest Henry Starling, C M G, M D , FRS, Life and Work',
900–06, *BMJ*, 14 May 1927.

Masson, D *British Novelists and their Styles.* Macmillan, Edinburgh, 1859.

Mayr, Ernst *The Growth of Biological Thought.* The Belknap Press, Harvard,
1982.

———— 'Charles Otis Whitman', *DSB.*

———— & Provine, W B *The Evolutionary Synthesis: Perspectives on the
Unification of Biology.* Harvard University Press, Camb. Mass. 1980.

Meadows, A J *Science and Controversy: A Biography of Sir Norman Lockyer,
Founder Editor of Nature.* MIT Press, 1972.

Meaney, Neville *A History of Australian Defence and Foreign Policy 1901–23,
Vol. 1 Search for Security in the Pacific (1901–14).* Sydney University Press,
1976.

———— *Under New Heavens: Cultural Transmission and the Making of
Australia.* Heinemann EA, 1989.

Medlicott, W N *Contemporary England, 1914–1964.* Longmans, London, 1967.

Miller, Sir Douglas 'Alexander MacCormick, Man and Surgeon', *The
Australian and New Zealand Journal of Surgeons*, Vol. 38 ,1969.

Miller, J D B *The Commonwealth in the World.* London, 1958.

Mills, A E 'Professor Wilson', *Sydney University Medical Journal*, Vol. XV,
Pt 1, October 1920.

Mitchison, Naomi 'The Haldanes: Personal Notes and Historical Lessons',
'*Friday Evening Discourse*, 19 October 1973,.......'

Moll, W 'History of American Medical Education', *British Journal of
Medical Education*, 1968, 2, pp 173–81.

Monteith, John *The Parish of Glencairn*. Glasgow, 1876.

Moran, Herbert *Viewless Winds: The Recollections and Digressions of a Surgeon*. Peter Davies, London 1939.

———— *Beyond The Hill Lies China: Scenes from a Medical Life in Australia*. Peter Davies, London 1945.

Morris, James *Farewell the Trumpets: An Imperial Retreat*. Penguin, 1980.

Mosher, K G 'Sydney University Regiment', *The Gazette*, University of Sydney Vol. 1, No. 15. May 1958.

Moyal, A M 'Sir Richard Owen and his influence on Australian Zoological and Palaeontological Science', *Records of Australian Academy of Science*, Vol. 3, No. 2, Nov. 1975.

———— *Scientists in Nineteenth Century Australia, A Documentary History*. Cassell, Melbourne, 1976.

———— *'a bright and savage land': Scientists in Colonial Australia*. Collins, Sydney, 1986.

Muir, Edwin *Scottish Journey*. Wm Heinemann, London, 1935.

Muirhead, J H *The Platonic Tradition in Anglo-Saxon Philosophy: Studies in the History of Idealism in England and America*. Allen & Unwin, London, 1931.

———— *Reflections by a Journeyman in Philosophy*. London 1942.

Mulvaney, D J & Calaby, J H *'So Much That is New': Baldwin Spencer 1860–1929*. MUP, 1985.

Munro-Ferguson (Novar Papers, Aust. Nat. Lib.)

Munro, May (compiler) *Shirley, The Story of a School in Sydney*. Old Girls Union, Sydney, 1967.

Nadel, George *Australia's Colonial Culture: Ideas, Men and Institutions in Mid-Nineteenth Century Eastern Australia*. F W Cheshire, Melbourne, 1957.

Nature (on Flexner Report) 'A Criticism of Modern Methods of Medical Education', 21 Aug. 1913.

———— 'First International Congress of Anatomists', 24 Aug, 1905 London.

————'The Ninth International Congress of Zoology at Monaco', 17 April 1913.

437

Neill, Thomas P *The Rise and Decline of Liberalism*. Bruce, Milwaukee, 1953.

Nettleship, R L (ed.) *Works of Thomas Hill Green*, Vols I, II. Longmans & Co., London, 1899 and 1900.

Newman, Charles E *The Evolution of Medical Education in the Nineteenth Century*. Oxford University Press, London, 1957.

Nordenskiold, Erik *The History of Biology*. Tudor, New York, 1928.

Numbers, Ronald L (ed.) *The Education of American Physicians*. Berkeley, 1980.

Oppenheimer, Jane M 'Ross Harrison's Contributions to Experimental Embryology', *Bulletin of the History of Medicine,* Vol. 40. Johns Hopkins, 1966.

———— *Essays in the History of Embryology and Biology*. MIT, 1967.

Osborn, H F 'A Student's Reminiscences of Huxley', in Lilley.

O'Malley, C D (ed.) *The History of Medical Education*. UCLA Forum in Med. Sci. No. 12, University of California, 1970.

Orwin, C S 'Mansbridge, Albert (1876–1952)', *DNB.*

Paisley, Peter *Aust Broadcasting Commission*. 'Insight' 29.1.75.

Parker, W K *On Mammalian Descent: the Hunterian lectures for 1884*. Griffin & Co., London, 1885.

Passmore, John *A Hundred Years of Philosophy*. Pelican, 1975.

Pedersen, P A *Monash as Military Commander*. MUP, 1992.

Prebble, John *The Lion in the North*. Penguin, 1973.

Pockley, F Antill 'Some Reminiscences', *Sydney University Medical Journal,* Vol. XVI, Jan. 1923.

Portus, G V *Happy Highways*. Melbourne University Press, 1953.

Power, D'Arcy (ed.) *British Medical Societies*. Medical Press & Circular: London, 1939.

Purser, Cecil 'Early Days of the Medical School', *Sydney University Medical Journal*, Jubilee Issue, Sept. 1933.

Quiller-Couch, Arthur *Cambridge Lectures.* J M Dent, London, 1943.

Ranson, S W 'The Architectural Relations of the Afferent Elements Entering into the Formation of the Spinal Nerves', *J of Comparative Neurology and Psychology*, Vol. XVIII, April 1908, No. 2, 101–17.

———— & Clark, S L *The Anatomy of the Nervous System.* Philadelphia, 1959.

Raven, P (trans L de Ruiter) *An Outline of Developmental Physiology.* Pergamon, London, 1961.

Reeve, F A *Cambridge.* B T Batsford, London, 1964.

Richie, D G 'The Rationality of History', in Seth & Haldane, Ch. V.

Richter, Melvin *The Politics of Conscience: T.H. Green and His Age.* Weidenfeld & Nicholson, London, 1964.

Ridley, M 'Embryology & Classical Zoology in Great Britain', 35–68 Horder *et al.* 1986.

Riese, Walter & Hoff, E C 'A History of the Doctrine of Cerebral Localisation', 439–70, *Journal of the History of Medicine and Allied Sciences* Vol. vi, Connecticut, 1951.

Roberts, Ffrangcon. *Medical Education.* Lewis, London, 1948.

Robinson, F W 'The Great Hall and Voices from the Past', *The Union Book*, 1952, Sydney University Union, 1952.

Roe, Michael. *Quest for Authority in Eastern Australia, 1835–1851.* Melbourne University Press, 1965.

Rolleston, Prof. H D *Cambridge University Reporter*, 7.11.1932.

Rook, Arthur (ed.) *The Origins and Growth of Biology.* Penguin, 1964.

———— (ed.) *Cambridge & its Contributions to Medicine. Proceedings of the 7th British Congress on the History of Medicine.* Wellcome Institute for the History of Medicine, London, 1971.

Rothblatt, Sheldon *The Revolution of the Dons: Cambridge and Society in Victorian England.* London, 1968.

Rowse, A L *Memories and Glimpses.* Methuen, London, 1986.

Royal Sanitary Institute 'Obituary, J. Ashburton Thompson', *Journal of the Royal Sanitary Institute*, Vol. 36. London, 1916.

Russell, H C 'Anniversary Address', *JRS NSW*, Vol. 26 1892. Sydney, 1892.

Russell, K F *British Anatomy 1528–1800*. MUP, 1963.

————— *The Melbourne Medical School 1862–1962*. MUP, 1977.

Rutledge, Martha 'Sir William Montagu Manning', *ADB 1851–1890*.

Sanderson, Michael (ed.) *The Universities in the Nineteenth Century.* Routledge & Kegan Paul, London, 1975.

Schedvin, C B *Shaping Science and Industry: A History of Australia's Council for Scientific and Industrial Research, 1926–49*. Allen & Unwin, Sydney, 1987.

Scotland, James *The History of Scottish Education*, Vol. 1, University of London Press, London, 1969.

Scott, Ernest *Official History of Australia in the War of 1914–1918, Vol. XI: Australia During the War*. Angus & Robertson, Sydney, 1936.

Searle, G R *The Quest for National Efficiency : A Study in British Politics and Political Thought, 1899-1914*. Blackwell, Oxford, 1971.

————— *John Monash, A Biography.* Melbourne University Press, 1982.

Serle, Percival *Dictionary of Australian Biography,* Vol. II, L–Z.

Singer, Charles *A History of Biology to About the Year 1900*. Abelard Schuman, London, 1959.

Sissons, D C S 'Attitudes to Japan and Defence, 1890–1923', MA Thesis, Melbourne University 1956.

Slobodin, Richard *W.H.R. Rivers*. Columbia University Press, New York, 1978.

Smith, F B *The Conscription Plebiscites in Australia 1916–1917*. Revised edn 1974, Victoria.

Smith G Elliot 'The Teaching of Anatomy', *Edinburgh Medical Journal*, March 1918.

Smith, John Maynard *The Theory of Evolution*. Penguin, 1985.

Smith, S A 'The Life and Work of James Thomas Wilson', *Bulletin of the Post-Graduate Committee on Medicine*, University of Sydney, Vol. 6, No. 1, April 1950.

Sollas, W J *Obituary Notices 1936–8*. Royal Society, London.

Sommer, Dudley *Haldane of Cloan: His Life and Times, 1856–1928*. Allen & Unwin, London, 1960.

Sourkes, T L *Nobel Prize Winners in Medicine and Physiology 1901–1965*. Life of Science Library, New York, 1966.

Souter, Gavin *Lion and Kangaroo. Australia 1901–1919: The Rise of a Nation*. Fontana, 1978.

Sprigge, Sir Squire 'Medical Education in the United states and Canada', *The Lancet* (Special Supplement), 5 Jan. 1929.

Stevens, L A *Explorers of the Brain*. Angus & Robertson, London, 1973.

Stevenson, Robert Louis *Edinburgh: Picturesque Notes*. Seeley & Co., London, 1905.

————— *Weir of Hermiston and Other Stories*. (see Binding)

Strahan, Ronald *Rare and Curious Specimens. An Illustrated History of the Australian Museum 1827–1979*. Australian Museum, Sydney, 1979.

Stuart, T P Anderson 'The Majority of the Medical School', *Record of the Jubilee Celebrations of the University of Sydney 1902*: 61–91, University of Sydney, 1903.

Sydney University Undergrads Assoc'n. *Students' Festival Programme of Songs*. Sydney, 1910, 1911.

Sydney University Union. *The Union Book of 1952*. Aust'asian Med Publishing Co., Sydney, 1952.

Tait, P G *Lectures on Some Recent Advances in Physical Science*. London, 1876.

Taylor, A J P *The Second World War: An Illustrated History*. Penguin, 1976.

Thompson, J Ashburton 'The Medical Officer of Health', *Transactions of Eighth Session of Australasian Medical Congress, Melb. Oct 1908*. Melbourne, 1909.

Thompson, J R 'The Australian High Comm in London: Its Origins & Early History'. M.A. Thesis, *ANU* 1973.

The Times History of the War, Vol. XII, Ch. CLXXXVIII 'The War Government of the British Peoples'. *The Times*. London.

Thompson, John *On Lips of Living Men*. Lansdowne Press, Melbourne, 1962.

Troughton, E *Furred Animals of Australia.* Sydney, 1946.

Turner, A Logan *Sir William Turner, KCB, FRS: A Chapter in Medical History.* Blackwood, Edinburgh 1919.

Turney, Bygott & Chippendale *Australia's First: A History of the University of Sydney, Vol. I 1850–1939.* Sydney University Press, 1991.

University of Sydney. *Record of the Jubilee Celebrations of the University of Sydney.* Sydney, 1903.

——— *Book of Remembrance.* Sydney, 1929.

——— *Calendars* (see Annuals).

——— *Centenary Celebrations,* Sydney, 1952.

——— *Centenary Book of the University of Sydney Faculty of Medicine.* Sydney, 1984.

University of Sydney Union, (See Sydney University Union).

Wade-Ferrell, T F *In All Things Faithful.* Ure Smith, Sydney, 1985.

Walker, E P (*et al.*) *Mammals of the World.* Johns Hopkins Press, Baltimore, 1964.

Walkom, A B *The Linnean Society of New South Wales: Historical Notices of Its First Fifty Years.* Australasian Medical Publishing Co., Sydney, 1925.

Wallace, H 'Regeneration' 331–46 in Horder *et al.* 1986.

Walshe, F M R *Critical Studies in Neurology.* E & S Livingstone, Edinburgh, 1948.

Watson, D M S 'The Monotreme Skull: A Contribution to Mammalian Morphogenesis', in *Royal Society Philosophical Transactions*, Series B. 1916.

——— 'James Peter Hill, 1873–1954', *RSO*, 1955.

——— 'Robert Broom 1866–1961', *RSO*, 1952.

Waugh, Joseph Laing *Thornhill and Its Worthies.* Hunter Watson & Co., Dumfries, 1923.

——— 'The Late Dr Grierson', *D&GS&A*, 28.9.1889.

Bibliography

Webster, Charles (ed.) *Biology, Medicine and Society 1840–1940.* Cambridge University Press, 1981.

Wheelhouse, Frances *Raymond Arthur Dart: A pictorial Profile.* Transpareon Press, Sydney 1983.

Whitman, C O 'Biological Instruction in Universities', 507–19, *The American Naturalist* Vol. XXI, Philadelphia, 1887.

———— 'General Physiology and its Relation to Morphology', 802–7, *ibid.,* Vol. XXVII, Phil., 1893.

Wilkinson, Herbert J 'Experimental Studies in the Innervation of Striated Muscle', *Journal of Comparative Neurology,* V51, 1930.

Willey, Basil *Cambridge and Other Memories, 1920–1953.* Chatto & Windus, London, 1968.

Willier, Benjamin H & Oppenheimer, Jane M (eds) *Foundations of Experimental Embryology.* New Jersey, 1964.

Wilson, Edmund B 'The Mosaic Theory of Development', *Biological Lectures (1893).* Marine Biol. Lab., Woods Hole, 1896.

———— 'The Embryological Criterion of Homology', *Sixth Lecture (1884), Biological Lectures (1893).* Marine Biol. Lab., Woods Hole, 1896.

Wilson, J T (see Writings by Wilson).

Woollard, H *Recent Advances in Anatomy.* J & A Churchill, London, 1927.

———— 'An Outline of Elliot Smith's Contributions to Neurology', 280–94, *J of A,* V 72, 1937–8.

Young, J A , Sefton, A J Webb, N (eds) *Centenary Book of the University of Sydney Faculty of Medicine.* Sydney University Press, 1984.

Young, J Z *The Life of Mammals.* Clarendon Press, Oxford, 1957.

Select Biographical Notes on Scientists
Mentioned in Text

Allis, Edward Phelps, Jr (1851–1905), US benefactor of science, scientist. Law degree, University of Wisconsin 1903; zoology, Harvard 1911; MD Gröningen 1914. Established Allis Research Laboratory 1887, moved to Mentone, France 1890. Editor with C O Whitman of *Journal of Morphology*, and major supporter of US biological research. Produced many papers on the morphology of the head and skull of fishes.

Anderson, Hugh Kerr (1865–1928), English physiologist. Switched from classics to medicine Caius College Cambridge, natural science tripos; St Bart's Hospital; research at Foster's Physiological Laboratory 1892–1905 on the sympathetic nervous system (with Langley) and on sequential nature of neuron development. In 1905 moved to College administration, elected Master of Caius 1912. Member of Universities Commission from 1919. V-C Cambridge University. Knighted 1905; FRS 1907.

Anderson Stuart, Thomas Peter (1856–1920), Scottish-born physiologist, builder of Sydney Medical School. Prize-winning student Edinburgh University, MB & ChM 1880, MD 1882. Sydney University: professor of physiology and dean of medical school 1883–1920; chairman Royal Prince Alfred Hospital; member NSW Board of Health; founder of dentistry school. Compulsive organizer. Knighted 1914.

Assheton, Richard (1863–1915), English embryologist, zoologist. Trinity College Cambridge 1883, under Adam Sedgwick; Natural Sciences Tripos 1886; demonstrator Owens College Manchester 1889; laboratory research Cambridge 1893; lecturer Guy's Hospital and Imperial College of Science 1901; embryology lectureship created for him by Gardiner, Cambridge 1914. Researched early development of mammals and growth of vertebrate embryo; first in Britain to apply experimental methods. Textbook of Embryology (unfinished).

Baer, Karl Ernst von (1792–76), Estonian anatomist. Studied Vienna and Würzburg, theoretical science then research on evolutionary anatomy. Professor at Königsberg; academician at St Petersburg from 1834; travelled Russia; took up problems in anthropology, ethnography, archaeology. Discovered mammalian egg; propounded 'biogenetic law'; founder of modern embryology.

Balfour, Francis Maitland (1851–82), English embryologist. At Cambridge: Natural Science Scholar 1871; with Michael Foster 1872; lecturer in morphology and embryology 1873 then director of university's morphological laboratory where he attracted enthusiastic students. Studied embryology of elasmobranches at Naples Zoological Station and at Cambridge 1873–8. Published textbook, *Treatise on Comparative Embryology* 1880–1. FRS 1878, Royal Medal 1881.

Baldwin Spencer, Walter (1860–1929), English evolutionary biologist, anthropologist. Oxford University BA in science, 1884; demonstrator; University of Melbourne foundation chair of biology, 1887 to 1919. Researched central Australian Aboriginal culture; expeditions 1894–1903; publications 1904, 1912. An entrepreneur for natural science; FRS 1900, knighted 1916.

Bardeleben, Carl (Heinrich) von (1849–1918), German anatomist. University of Jena.

Bateson, William (1859–1926), English zoologist, geneticist. Cambridge University MB 1883; reader in zoology 1907; professor of biology Cambridge 1908; first director John Innes Horticultural Institute from 1910. Proponent of Mendelian genetics; opposed doctrine of natural selection and chromosome theory of inheritance. FRS 1894; Darwin Medal 1904.

Berry, Richard James Arthur (1867–1962), Scottish anatomist, neurologist and anthropologist. University of Edinburgh MB ChM, 1891. Lecturer in anatomy, school of medicine of the Royal Colleges Edinburgh 1896–1905; professor of anatomy University of Melbourne 1905–29. Research on topographical anatomy, physical anthropology and the brain.

Broom, Robert (1866–1951), Scottish-born anatomist, anthropologist. Glasgow University BSc 1887, MB CM 1889; practised medicine and researched monotremes in outback New South Wales. Professor of zoology and geology Stellenbosch University 1903–9; research in comparative anatomy and human anthropology; searched southern Africa for the origin of man. Croonian Lecturer 1913; FRS 1920.

Caldwell, W H (1859–1941), British embryologist. Studied at Cambridge; at Comparative Anatomy Laboratory 1882; awarded first studentship in memory of F M Balfour; expedition to Australia to collect monotreme, marsupial and lungfish material 1883–4; confirmed in August 1884 that

445

monotremes lay eggs. On return to UK wrote a few papers, but by 1887 had abandoned science for a career in paper manufacture.

Cunningham, Daniel John (1850–1909), Scottish anatomist. University of Edinburgh MD 1874, demonstrator under Turner 1876. Professorships in anatomy: School of Royal College of Surgeons of Ireland 1882–3; Trinity College Dublin 1883–1903; University of Edinburgh 1903–9. Research in comparative anatomy and anthropology. Wrote *Text Book of Anatomy*.

Dart, Raymond (1893–1988), Australian-born anatomist and anthropologist. University of Queensland BSc 1910; Sydney University MB, ChM 1917, MD 1927; demonstrator, University College London 1919–22; study year US 1921. Professor of anatomy Witwatersrand University 1923 to 1958. Described Taung part-skull in 1925, *Australopithecus africanus*; using southern African primate fossil material, developed theory that human bipedalism preceded brain expansion.

David, Tannant William Edgeworth (1856–1934), Welsh-born geologist, founder of geological science in Aust. Oxford BA 1881, MA 1926. Geological surveys NSW 1882–90, professor of geology Sydney 1891–1924. Study of Fanafuti atoll 1897–8 supported a theory by Darwin; FRS 1900. Studied glaciation in Australia; led first party to reach South Magnetic Pole 1908; Mining Battalion in France 1916–18. Knighted 1920. Published geological map of Australia 1932.

Dohrn, Felix Anton (1840–1909), German entomologist, morphologist, embryologist. Attended Universities of Königsberg, Bonn, Berlin; studied under Gegenbauer and Haeckel at Jena. Researched phylogeny of arthropods and origin of vertebrates. Planned and built the Zoological Station, Naples 1870–4.

Driesch, Hans Adolf Edvard (1867–1941), German experimental embryologist and philosopher. Studied under Weismann at University of Freiburg 1886; then Haeckel at University of Jena 1889. Experimental embryology at Zoological Station, Naples 1889–1909; showed that development is epigenetic; a mechanist till 1895, then a vitalist; professor of natural philosophy Heidelberg 1912; University of Cologne 1919; University of Leipzig 1921–33; visits to China, USA, South America, 1922–8.

du Bois-Reymond, Emil Heinrich (1818–96), German physiologist. Studied biology, University of Berlin under Müller, researched electric charges in fish; founded electrophysiology; demonstrated electrical nature of

446

nerve impulses. Succeeded Müller as professor of physiology at Berlin 1858. Important early supporter of Darwin's theory of evolution.

Duckworth, Wynfrid Lawrence Henry (1871–1956), English anatomist. Entered Jesus College Cambridge 1889, 'double first' in Natural Sciences Tripos 1893 and Cambridge University demonstrator in anatomy; lecturer 1899, reader 1921–36, then emeritus reader. Studied physical anthropology and primate anatomy; handbook for students 1904; important paper on early primate embryology 1907; *Prehistoric Man* 1912. Cautious and factual, not drawn to speculation. Master of Jesus College 1940–5.

Edinger, Ludwig (1855–1918), German neurologist, anatomist. Studied medicine in Heidelberg and Strasbourg, MD 1876; assistant to Kussmaul; practised in Frankfurt 1883–1914; professor of neurology Frankfurt 1914. First description of ventral and dorsal spino-cerebellar tracts.

Fielding, Una Lucy (1888–1969), Australian-born neuroanatomist. University of Sydney BA 1910, BSc 1919, MB, ChM 1922. University College London anatomy demonstrator 1925; lecturer 1928; reader 1935; acting head of evacuated dept in WWII. Co-discovered hypophyseal-portal system 1930, 1933; organized anatomy dept, Beirut 1930s.

Fletcher, Joseph James (1850?–1926), Australian biologist. University of Sydney BA 1870, MA 1876; University College London BSc 1879. Important contributor to natural science in Australia; among the first to research embryology of marsupials, 1881–4; studied flora of Sydney region 1919–26; guided the affairs of Linnaen Society of NSW from 1893 to 1926.

Flower, William Henry (1831–99), English surgeon, zoologist, museum conservator. London University medicine/surgery 1851, MRCS 1854, FRCS 1857; conservator Hunterian Museum, RCS 1861–84; succeeded Owen at British Museum 1884–98. Special interest in *Cetacea* and mammalian classification; papers on cerebral commissures in monotremes and marsupials (1865) and marsupial dentition (1867). FRS; knighted 1892.

Foster, Michael (1836–1907), English physiologist. London University BA 1854, MB 1858, MD 1859. Praelector of Physiology, Trinity College Cambridge 1870–83; first professor of physiology, Cambridge 1883–1903; founder of celebrated Cambridge Physiological Laboratory; founded and edited *Journal of Physiology* 1878–94. Published A *Textbook of Physiology* 1876. Baronet 1899; FRS 1900; MP 1900–6.

Gadow, Hans Friedrich (1855–1928), German-born zoologist. Moved to UK after graduation; curator and lecturer on morphology of vertebrates at Cambridge from 1884. Author of *A Classification of Vertebrates* 1898, *The Wandering of Animals* and other books. FRS.

Gardiner, Stanley (1872–1946), English zoologist. Cambridge University exhibition 1893; Demonstrator of animal morphology in Cambridge; Zoological Station, Naples 1905; various marine expeditions including to Fanafuti for coral reef boring 1906. Cambridge department of zoology: lecturer 1909; professor 1911–39. FRS 1908.

Gaskell, Walter Holbrook (1847–1914), English physiologist and morphologist. Trinity College Cambridge, BA 1869, MD 1878; disciple of Michael Foster; studied at Leipzig under Ludwig 1874–5; lecturer in physiology Cambridge 1883–1914. Researched action of the heart, autonomic nervous system. Croonian Lecturer 1881; FRS 1882.

Gaupp, Robert Eugen (1870–1953), German psychiatrist, neurologist. Studied medicine at Tübingen, Geneva, Strasbourg, MD 1894; practised psychiatry Breslau 1894–9, then neurology Breslau; lecturer under Kraepelin 1901 at University of Heidelberg, followed him to Munich 1904; professor of neurology Tübingen 1906–36. Researched progressive paralysis, paranoia, hysteria, depression, suicide, mass murder, homosexuality.

Goodsir, John (1814–67), Scottish anatomist. Universities of St Andrews and Edinburgh. Developed interest in marine biology; conservator in comparative anatomy at Edinburgh University Museum 1840; professor of anatomy 1846. Studied problems of living structures; special interest in cell theory.

Haldane, John Scott (1860–1936), Scottish-born physiologist. University of Edinburgh BA 1878; MB, ChM 1885; fellow of New College Oxford, 1901; reader in physiology 1907–13; director of mining research laboratory, Bentley Colliery, from 1912. From 1885 researched respiration and regulation of the blood; physiology applied to industry (medicine, mining, diving, engineering) and wartime defence against poison gas. FRS 1897.

Haldane, Richard Burdon (1856–1928), Scottish-born politician, lawyer, philosopher. Studied philosophy in Göttingen 1874 and later. Promoted German idea of 'civic universities', drafted university scheme for Ireland and helped establish Imperial College of Science & Technology, London. As

British War Minister reformed the army after Boer War. Created Viscount Haldane 1911; Lord Chancellor 1913–15 and in 1920s.

Harrison, Ross Granville (1870–1959), US pioneer in experimental embryology. Johns Hopkins University PhD in zoology 1894; University of Bonn MD 1899; Bronson Professor of comparative anatomy, Yale 1907; Sterling Professor of biology 1927; professor emeritus 1938. Developed technique of tissue culture to demonstrate growth of nerve fibres.

Haswell, William Aitcheson (1854–1925), Scottish-born marine zoologist. Studied under Wyville Thomson and Huxley at Edinburgh University: MA 1876, BSc 1878, DSc 1887. Challis Professor of Biology, University of Sydney 1889–1917. Marine zoological research on collections from *Chevert* expedition to New Guinea and marine fauna of Port Jackson, Sydney. Joint author, *A Text-book of Zoology* 1898. FRS 1897.

Head, Henry (1861–1940), English neurologist, clinician, teacher, experimental physiologist. Research on respiration Prague 1884–6. Worked under Foster, Gaskell and Langley at Cambridge and University College London; MD1890, MRCP 1894, FRCP 1900. Editor of *Brain* 1910–25. Did fundamental work on many aspects of sensory system; published *Studies in Neurology* 1920. FRS 1899, Croonian Lecturer 1921.

Herrick, Charles Judson (1868–1960), US comparative neurologist and psychobiologist. University of Cincinnati BSc 1891, Columbia University PhD 1900. Professor of natural history Kansas 1892–3; professor of neurology University of Chicago 1907–34. Correlated nervous structure with function in vertebrates and published extensively on neurology and animal behaviour.

Hill, Archibald Vivian (1886–1977), British physiologist. Trinity College Cambridge, under Morley Fletcher graduated in medicine 1907, MD 1920. From 1913 researched heat production and consumption of oxygen in muscles; served WWI. Professor of physiology at Manchester 1920; staff of University College London 1923; professorship of Royal Society 1926–51. Secretary to RS 1935–46; War Cabinet Scientific Advisory C'ttee in WWII. Nobel Prize 1922.

Hill, James Peter (1873–1954), Scottish-born embryologist. Edinburgh University BSc 1898. London 1890–1 with Howes; biology demonstrator Sydney 1892–1906; Jodrell Chair at University College London 1906; new University College London chair of embryology and histology 1921–38.

Definitive developmental studies of monotremes, and the marsupials of Australia and South America, as evidence of the evolutionary stages of higher mammals. FRS 1913; Darwin Medallist 1940.

Hines-Loeb, Marion (1889–1982), US neuroanatomist. Smith College graduate 1913; Chicago PhD 1917, post-doctoral research Cambridge and University College London. Johns Hopkins University 1925–47. Pioneer in neurological studies of the brain's control of movement.

His, Wilhelm (1831–1904), Swiss anatomist, histologist, embryologist. Studied at Universities of Bonn, Berlin and Würzburg, influenced by teachings of Virchow, von Kölliker and Leydig. Graduated 1855. Professor of anatomy and physiology Basel 1857–65, and of anatomy from 1872. Co-founder of German Anatomical Society. Invented microtome 1866. Strong proponent of mechanism.

Hopkins, Frederick Gowland (1861–1947), English biochemist. Guy's Hospital (University of London Gold Medal in chemistry); lecturer in chemical biology Cambridge 1897; professor 1914; Sir Wm Dunn Professor 1921–43. Studied biological oxidation, lactates and muscle contraction; discovered vitamins. FRS 1905, knighted 1925, shared Nobel Prize for physiology 1929.

Howes, Thomas George Bond (1853–1905), English anatomist, zoologist. Private education; from 1874–9 assisted Huxley's practical instruction in biology at Royal School of Mines; demonstrator 1880; assistant professor 1885; succeeded Huxley as professor in 1895. Investigated the comparative anatomy of vertebrata; his work illustrated the *Atlas of Elementary Biology* (1885) and *Atlas of Elementary Zootomy* (1902). FRS 1897.

Hubrecht, Ambrosius Arnold Willem (1853–1915), Dutch zoologist and comparative embryologist. Studied zoology at Utrecht, and at Leiden under Selenka; doctorate 1874. Co-founded Dutch Zoology Station; professor of zoology and comp anat University of Utrecht 1882–1910; studied embryology of mammals from 1888 for phylogenetic links. Founded Institut International d'Embryologie 1911. Hubrecht Laboratory founded in his memory 1916.

Hunter, John Irvine (1898–1924), Australian anatomist and neurologist. Sydney University MB, ChM 1920 (Gold Medal); studied with Elliot Smith at University College London and with Ariens Kappers in Amsterdam. Sydney University associate professor of anatomy 1921–2, professor 1923–4. Joint researcher with Norman Royle of 'spinal shock' and influence of sympathetic nervous system on plastic tonus in muscle.

Huxley, Thomas Henry (1825–95), English biologist. Studied at Charing Cross Hospital; studied marine animals while assistant surgeon on HMS *Rattlesnake* 1846–50; professor of natural history, Royal School of Mines 1854–85. Major contributor to phylogeny, including knowledge of the relationship of birds and reptiles. Foremost supporter of Darwin's theory; rejected social Darwinism; coined the term 'agnostic'.

Jones, Frederic Wood (1897–1954), English anatomist, anthropologist. London University MB BS 1904, DSc 1910. Medical Officer Cocos-Keeling Is 1905–6; with Elliot Smith on archaeological Survey, Nubia 1907–8; anatomy lecturer; professor of anatomy Royal Free Hospital 1915; Adelaide University 1919; professor of anthropology Hawaii 1928; professor of anatomy Melbourne 1913, Manchester 1938; conservator RCSE Museum 1943–51. Prolific writer and lecturer, provocative, Lamarkian evolutionist; worked from field studies or macroscopic observation; a wanderer.

Keibel, Franz (1861–1929), German anatomist, embryologist. Studied medicine in Berlin and Strasburg, qualified 1887; prosector in comparative anatomy under Wiedersheim in Freiburg 1889, professor 1900; professor at Strasburg 1914–18; succeeded Oscar Hertwig in Berlin 1922–9. Precise, thorough and systematic, did comprehensive work on the development of vertebrates. Early opponent of Haeckel's biogenetic law.

Keith, Arthur (1866–1955), Scottish-born anatomist and anthropologist. Aberdeen University MB 1888, MD and FRCS 1894. Studied Malay apes 1889–92; demonstrator in anatomy London Hospital 1895; worked briefly with His in Leipzig and Thane in London. Kept links with clinical medicine but turned to human palaeontology and anthropology: conservator Hunterian Museum from 1908. FRS 1913; knighted 1921.

Koch, Heinrich Hermann Robert (1843–1910), German physician and pioneer bacteriologist. University of Göttingen degree 1866; practised medicine; demonstrated cause of septicaemia 1876; isolated TB bacillus 1882 and cholera bacillus 1883; professor at Berlin 1885 and first director of Berlin Institute for Infectious Diseases 1891. Established clinical bacteriology as a medical science in 1890s. Nobel Prize 1905.

Kölliker, Rudolf Albert von (1817–1905), Swiss biologist. Studied zoology in Berlin, prosector to Henle. Professor at Würzburg 1847–1902. Foremost teacher of his age; active researcher for 60 years. Microscopist: investigated spermatozoa 1841; egg division; embryo of *cephalopoda*; nerve fibres and ganglionic cells; wrote first book on modern histology, 1852.

451

Kulchitsky, Nicholas (1856–1925), Ukrainian anatomist. University of Kharkov degree; professor 1893. In England after Russian Revolution; lecturer in histology at University College London, where he studied and demonstrated nerve endings in muscles.

Langley, John Newport (1852–1925), English physiologist. Studied at Cambridge under Foster: Natural Science Tripos 1874, BA 1875, MA 1878, ScD 1896. Demonstrator 1876; Heidelberg 1877. Cambridge: lecturer in physiology 1883; deputy to Foster 1900; professor of physiology 1903–25. Research 1875–90 on glandular secretions, and from 1890 on involuntary nervous system.

Lankester, Edwin Ray (1847–1929), English zoologist. Oxford University, zoology/geology; studied at Vienna, Leipzig and the Zoological Station Naples. Professor of zoology University College London 1874–91; Linacre Professor of comparative anatomy Oxford from 1891. Research over all major groups of living and fossil animals; promoted foundation of Marine Biological Assn Plymouth; systematized the field of embryology. FRS 1875; knighted 1907.

Le-Gros Clark, Wilfrid Edward (1895–1971), English comparative anatomist. Studied at St Thomas's Hospital, MRCS 1916, FRCS 1919. Served in RAMC; primate field research in Sarawak. Chairs of anatomy: St Bartholomew's 1924; St Thomas's 1930; Oxford 1934–8; University College London 1940–62. Studied neuroanatomy of tree-shrews, primate phylogeny, and from 1946 the primate fossil record in Africa. FRS 1935; knighted 1955.

Lightoller, George Henry Standish (1881–1944), Australian physician, comparative anatomist. Sydney University MB, ChM 1906; MD 1925. Researched functioning of human facial musculature and comparative anatomy of facial muscle group.

Liversidge, Archibald (1846–1927), English-born chemist, mineralogist. Cambridge MA 1887. Instructor in chemistry, Royal School of Naval Archives 1867; reader in geology University of Sydney 1872; professor of geology and mineralogy 1874; first dean of science 1879–1907. Organizer of Australian science: re-established Royal Society of NSW; formed AAAS for Aust congress 1888; founded school of mines 1892. FRS 1882.

Lorrain Smith, James (1862–1931), Scottish pathologist, bacteriologist. Edinburgh University MA 1884, MB CM 1889, MD 1893. Research on respiration, with Haldane in Oxford to 1893; summer 1891 in Strasburg;

Copenhagen with Bohr 1893/4. Pathology lecturer Belfast 1894; professor from 1901. Chairs of pathology: Manchester 1904; Edinburgh 1912 and dean of medicine from 1919. Research on fats and lipoids from 1904; developed 'case' method of studying disease. FRS 1909.

Ludwig, Carl Friedrich Wilhelm (1816–95), German physiologist. Medical student, University of Marburg; graduated 1840; anatomy prosector 1841; associate professor Marburg 1846. Professor anatomy and physiology Zurich 1849; Vienna 1855. Professor of physiology Leipzig from 1865; created laboratory with physical, chemical and anatomical divisions; co-founder of modern physiology, with demonstration of mechanisms including salivary and renal secretions, blood circulation, respiration.

Macalister, Alexander (1844–1919), Irish-born comparative anatomist. Studied at Royal College of Surgeons Ireland; demonstrator of anatomy 1860; professor of zoology Trinity College Dublin; professor of anatomy and surgery 1877; professor of anatomy Cambridge 1883–1919. Studied variation in human anatomy; co-founded the Anatomical Society 1887, published *Textbook of Anatomy* 1889.

Magendie, François (1785–1855), French doctor and researcher. Prosector, Anatomical Institute; hospital doctor; professor of Collège de France. A sceptic, did not theorize, opposed vitalism, explored vital functions of human body. Worked on blood circulation, respiration, sensory and motor nerve system; created basis for later physiological research techniques.

Martin, Charles James (1866–1955), English physiologist and pathologist. London BSc 1886; Leipzig under Ludwig; demonstrator in biology and physiology, King's College London, MRCS, LSA 1889, MB 1890. Physiology demonstrator University of Sydney 1891; lecturer University of Melbourne 1897, professor 1900; director Lister Institute 1903–30. Research on Australian fauna, bubonic plague in India, typhoid, heat regulation, myxoma virus. Organized integration of Australian Army Pathology Services 1915–18; director CSIR division of animal nutrition, Adelaide 1930–3. FRS 1901; knighted 1927.

Masson, David Orme (1858–1937), Scottish-born chemist. Edinburgh MA 1877, BSc 1880. Göttingen 1879, Lecturer at Bristol 1880, doctoral research Edinburgh 1881–4. Chair of chemistry Melbourne 1886–1923; dean of science 1905–23. Research on ionic theory; Antarctic research from 1911; prime mover in founding (Royal) Australian Chemical Institute 1917, Aust. National Research Council 1921 and CSIR 1926. FRS 1903, knighted 1923.

Minot, Charles Sedgwick (1852–1914), US anatomist, embryologist, educationist. Graduated MIT 1872; Leipzig under Karl Ludwig 1873; Harvard DSc 1878. Joined Harvard histology and embryology dept 1883; professor 1892. Research on vertebrate embryos; invented rotary microtome 1886. *Human Embryology* published 1892. Prime mover in founding of Carnegie Laboratory of Embryology, Baltimore. Broadened US anatomy to include embryology, histology, physical anthropology.

Osborne, William Alexander (1873–1967), British-born physiologist. Queen's College Belfast graduate 1895; biochemistry and physics at Tübingen University, DSc 1899. Assistant professor of physiology University College London; professor University of Melbourne 1904–38; dean of Medicine 1929. Designed chlorine gas respirator 1915; adviser on dietetics to Australian Army, WWII.

Owen, Richard (1804–92), English zoologist and palaeontologist. Studied medicine Edinburgh and at St Bartholomew's Hospital, London. Curator of Royal College of Surgeons; supt. of natural history dept British Museum from 1857. Work on living and extinct specimens charted knowledge of changing nature of species; distinguished homology from analogy in structure of organisms; implacable opponent of Darwin. Knighted 1884.

Parker, William Kitchen (1823–90), English comparative anatomist. Articled to a surgeon in Rutland; medical assistant in London 1844, and studied under Owen; licentiate 1849. Hunterian professor of comp. anat. at RCS 1873; detailed studies with illustrations, especially the avian skull; practice till 1883. Lectures were published under title *Mammalian Descent*, 1885. FRS 1865. His eldest son was Professor Thomas Jeffery Parker FRS (1850–97), professor of zoology Otago University.

Poulton, Edward Bagnall (1856–1943), British zoologist. Graduate in zoology Jesus College Oxford 1876; demonstrator in comp. anat.; Burdett-Coutts scholarship in geology 1878; Hope Professor of zoology Oxford 1893–1933. Morphological studies of vertebrates to 1894, especially marsupials and monotremes; supporter of Darwin's theory of evolution; produced *The Colours of Animals* (1890). Entomological studies of variation and mimicry from 1884. FRS 1889, Darwin medallist 1914; knighted 1935.

Ramon Y Cajal, Santiago (1852–1934), Spanish anatomist, histologist. University of Zaragoza graduate 1873, doctorate 18.... Chairs: anatomy Valencia 1883; histology Barcelona 1887; histology and pathological anatomy Madrid 1892–1922. Royal Society Croonian Lecturer 1894;

elected foreign member 1909. His work from 1886 to 1906 reshaped scientific knowledge of cellular architecture of the nervous system with the neurone theory. Founded Spanish school of histology. Shared Nobel Prize for medicine 1906.

Ranson, Stephen Walter (1880–1942), US neurologist. University of Minnesota BA 1902; MS, PhD, MD by 1907; joined staff of Northwestern University Medical School 1909, professor of anatomy 1912; first director, Institute of Neurology at Northwestern 1928. Developed new technique (stereotaxis) to research central nervous system control of body function.

Retzius, Anders Adolf (1796–1860), Swedish biologist. Studied at Copenhagen; professor at veterinary institute, Stockholm; developed early factual account of nervous system; pioneered comparative anatomy in Sweden. Later work was on comparative anthropology of prehistoric Swedish human remains.

Rivers, William Halse Rivers (1864–1922), English physiologist and anthropologist. Founded Cambridge experimental school of psychology. Anthropological expeditions to Torres Straits 1898 and Melanesia 1908. Psychopathologist during and after WWI. Wrote *History of Melanesian Society* (1914).

Roux, Wilhelm (1850–1924), German experimental embryologist. University of Jena under Haeckel and Schalbe; University of Berlin under Virchow; medical degree 1878. Anatomical Institute in Breslau 1879–89; professor of anatomy Innsbruck 1889; director anatomical institute at University Halle 1895–1921. Proselytized the theory of developmental mechanics.

Royle, Norman Dawson (d.1944), Australian medical practitioner. Physical training instructor before taking Sydney University medical degree; demonstrator at medical school 1915–18. Clinical practice, concerned especially with war-wounded; as a result of surgery on the sympathetic nervous system he developed theory with J I Hunter of the dual innervation of muscle.

Russell, Henry Chamberlain (1836–1907), Australian astronomer and meteorologist. University of Sydney BA 1859. Joined Sydney Observatory; acting director 1862–4; government astronomer 1870; high quality observations of the transit of Venus (1874), Mercury (1881) and double star discoveries gave international recognition; pioneered global view of meteorology. V-C Sydney University 1891–2. Founder of technical education in NSW. FRS 1886.

Rutherford, William (1839–99), Scottish physiologist and histologist. Edinburgh MD 1863; studied in Berlin and Leipzig; published *Practical Histology* late 1860s and 'Lectures in Experimental Physiology' The *Lancet* 1871; one of Huxley's demonstrators (with Foster) of the new experimental biology, London early 1870s; professor of physiology University of Edinburgh 1874–99. Did not himself do much research. FRS.

Schwalbe Gustav (1844–1917), German anatomist and anthropologist. Studied in Leipzig, Jena, Königsberg in Germany and Kalininberg USSR. Research on *Pithecanthropus erectus* 1899, Neanderthal man 1901, and anthropological development of man, demonstrating the continuous development of hominids.

Semon, Richard Wolfgang (1859–1918), German zoologist, embryologist. Studied zoology at Jena under Haeckel from 1879, medicine at Heidelberg from 1881. PhD Jena 1883, medical degree 1886. Naples Zoological Station 1885–6; assistant at Jena anatomical institute 1886, lecturer 1887, extraordinary professor 1891. Expedition to Australia 1891–3. Private study in Munich from 1897 on concept of cell memory and inheritance of acquired characteristics.

Sharpey Schäfer, Edward Albert (1850–1935), English histologist and physiologist. Schäfer qualified in medicine, University College London 1874, under William Sharpey whose name he took in 1918. (Sharpey introduced teaching of histology in Britain as part of practical physiology.) Assistant professor of physiology University College London 1874; professor 1883–99; professor at University of Edinburgh to 1933. Extensive research, most notably in endocrinology. Edited *Textbook of Physiology*, founded *Quarterly Journal of Experimental Physiology* (editor 1908–33). FRS 1878; knighted 1913.

Shearer, Cresswell (1874–1941), Canadian-born zoologist, embryologist. Medical graduate McGill University 1901, widened interests while at Zoological Station Naples 1903–9. Lecturer experimental embryology in Dept of Zoology Cambridge 1910–14, 1918–22; wartime research on meningococcus, then on sea urchins from 1918; lecturer in embryology in Dept of Anatomy 1922–37, then Zoology Dept in retirement. FRS 1916.

Shellshear, Joseph Lexden (1885–1958), Australian anatomist and anthropologist. University of Sydney MB, ChM, 1909; general practice, Albury NSW; Aust. Army Medical Corps; demonstrator St Bartholomew's Hospital London; anatomy professor University College London; Rockefeller study grant to US, then to chair in Hong Kong 1925; Sydney University from early 1930s.

Sherrington, Charles Scott (1857–1952), English neuro-physiologist. RCS exam 1875, MRCS 1884, Cambridge MB 1885. Worked with Goltz in Strasbourg 1884–5; met Cajal in Spain 1885; studied in Italy 1886 (cholera), Germany 1887. Cambridge research on nerve supply to muscles with Langley and Gaskell worked out main patterns of spiral reflexes and their interaction. Demonstrator in anatomy Cambridge 1883; chairs of physiology Liverpool 1895–1913, Oxford 1913–36. FRS 1893, knighted 1924, Nobel Prize 1932.

Smith, Grafton Elliot (1871–1937), Australian-born neuroanatomist, anthropologist. Sydney University MB, ChM 1893, MD 1895. Anatomy demonstrator 1894; research on monotreme and marsupial brains 1894–6; Cambridge research on mammalian brain for BA 1898; completed descriptive catalogue of the mammalian and reptilian brains in RCS 1901. Anatomy chairs: Cairo 1900 (opened interest in anthropology); Manchester 1909; University College London 1919–36. Work in neuromorphology and localization of brain function of fundamental importance. FRS 1907; knighted 1934; Chevalier of Legion d'honneur, 1936.

Stirling, Edward Charles (1848–1919), Australian anatomist, anthropologist. Cambridge natural science graduate 1870, MB 1874, MD 1880, DSc 1910. Physiology lecturer Adelaide University 1882, professor 1900, director South Australia Museum 1889–1912, FRS 1893, knighted 1917.

Streeter, George Linius (1873–1948), US neuroanatomist, human embryologist. Columbia University MD 1899, studied with Edinger and His in Germany. Anatomy lecturer Johns Hopkins Medical School 1904; assistant professor of anatomy Wistar Institute Philadelphia 1906–7; professor University of Michigan 1914; director, dept of embryology of Carnegie Institution, Johns Hopkins University from 1917. Main work in embryology on development of human nervous system and human ear.

Symington, Johnson (1851–1924), Scottish topographical anatomist. Edinburgh MB, ChM 1877; demonstrator to Turner 1877; anatomy lecturer, medical school, Minto House 1879; professor of anatomy Queen's

College, Belfast, 1893–1918. Papers on cranio-cerebral topography and form of the viscera; editor *Quain's Anatomy*; published *Atlas of Topographical Anatomy*. FRS 1903.

Tidswell, Frank (1867–1941), Australian microbiologist. University of Sydney medical graduate 1892; trained in London; physiology demonstrator, Sydney 1897; medical officer and microbiologist, NSW Board of Health 1898; founding Director, Government Bureau of Microbiology 1908–13; private practice then Director of Pathology, Royal Alexandra Hospital for Children to 1941.

Thane, George D (1851–1930), English anatomist. Graduate of University College London; appointed demonstrator 1870; professor 1877; then emeritus professor 1919. Wide knowledge of the history and literature of anatomy, and a fine artist. Edited 9th and 10th editions of *Quain's Anatomy*. Knighted 1919.

Thomson, Arthur (1858–1935), Scottish-born anatomist. Demonstrator of anatomy Edinburgh; lecturer at Oxford 1885 then professor of anatomy 1895 to 1933. Also professor of anatomy at the Royal Academy of Arts for which he produced the illustrations for *Anatomy for Arts Students*.

Thompson, John Ashburton (1846–1915), English-born medical officer, epidemiologist. University College London, Guy's and Middesex Hospitals, LRCP, MRCS, LM, LSA, 1868; Brussels MD 1876; Cambridge dip. pub. health 1882. Established public health system in NSW; epidemiological studies of typhoid 1886, lead poisoning 1892–3, leprosy 1897, bubonic plague 1900.

Turner, William (1832–1916), English-born anatomist, academic administrator. St Bartholomew's Hospital, London, LRCP 1853, MB 1857. Edinburgh University: anatomy demonstrator under Goodsir 1854; chair of anatomy 1867; dean of medicine 1878–81; University principal 1903–16. General Medical Councillor 1873–1905. Factual studies in placentation, comp. anat. of mammals, craniology of man. Early follower of Darwin. Knighted 1886.

Virchow, Rudolf (1821–1902), German pathologist. Graduate in medicine, Berlin; professor of pathological anatomy, Würzburg 1849–56 and then of Berlin. Promoter of Schwann's cell theory and the technology for modern pathology; published *Cellularpathologie* 1858. Sceptical of Darwin's theory.

Waldeyer-Hartz, Wilhelm von (1836–1921), German anatomist, histologist, pathologist. Universitys of Göttingen, Berlin. Physiology assistant Königsberg 1862; physiology, histology, pathology lecturer Breslau 1864; professor of pathology 1868; studied cancers; professor of anatomy Strasbourg 1872, Berlin 1883–1916. Best work morphological; lucid and systematic presenter, coined terms 'neurone' and 'chromosome'.

Watson, David Meredith Seares (1886–1973), English palaeo-biologist. Manchester BSc 1907, MSc 1909 in geology. Demonstrator 1909 then lecturer at University College London from 1911 under J P Hill; professor of zoology 1921–51. Worldwide travel including Karroo 1911 and 1928, Sydney 1914, North America 1915, Canada 1924 to study fossil vertebrates and invertebrates. Silliman lecturer, Yale, 1937; FRS 1922.

Weismann, August (1834–1914), German biologist. Studied medicine, practised, did treatise on evolution of fleas. Professor at Freiburg till 1914. Research specialized on evolution of lower animals, including *Daphniidae*. Developed germ plasm theory of descent and inheritance of parental (not acquired) characteristics, supporting Darwin's theory of natural selection.

Weldon, Walter Frank Raphael (1860–1906), English embryologist, biometrician. Studied at University College London, Cambridge; Natural Sciences Tripos 1881; Naples Zoological Station 1881; demonstrator Cambridge 1882; dissertation on invertebrate morphology 1883; professor of zoology University College London 1890; Linacre Professor, Oxford 1900. Turned to statistics to study variation, associated with Karl Pearson from 1891. Bitter conflict with Bateson in controversy between Mendelians and biometricians. FRS 1890.

Whitman, Charles Otis (1842–1910), US biologist. Attended Agassiz summer school of natural history 1873–4, University Leipzig PhD 1877. Zoology chair Imperial University of Japan two years; Zoological Research Station Naples 6 months; Harvard University 1883; Allis Lake Laboratory 1886; Clark University 1889; zoology professor University of Chicago 1892–1910. Founding director Marine Biological Laboratory Woods Hole 1888–1908, editor of *Biological Lectures* 1890–9. Introduced European scientific zoology into America. Wide-ranging research, notably on evolution in pigeons.

Wilkinson, Herbert John (1891–1963), Australian anatomist. Adelaide BA 1914, Sydney MB 1925, MD 1930. Anatomy lecturer Sydney 1925; as Rockefeller Scholar studied in Europe and USA 1930; opposed Hunter and

Boeke on sympathetic innervation of muscle. Professor of anatomy and histology Adelaide 1930; professor of anatomy University of Queensland 1936–59.

Wilkinson, William Camac (1857–1946), Australian pathologist. Sydney University BA in classics and natural science 1877; University of London MB, BSc 1882, MD, MRCP 1884. Trained University College London Hospital, Strasburg and Vienna. Lecturer in pathology and bacteriology, Sydney University 1884; worked with Koch in Berlin; lecturer in medicine at Sydney 1901–9; then for 30 years in London as a leading authority on treatment of TB.

Wilson, Edmund Beecher (1856–1939), US biologist, experimental embryologist, cytologist. University of Chicago 1874–5, Yale PhB 1878, Johns Hopkins PhD 1881. Studied two years in Cambridge, Leipzig, and at Zoological Station Naples under Dohrn 1882–3. Taught at MIT 1884; biology professor at Bryn Mawr 1885, then Columbia University 1891. Research each summer at Woods Hole; main work in cell lineage, organization of the egg; relation of Mendelism to cytology. Published *The Cell in Development and Inheritance* 1896, and *The Cell* 1925.

Wright, Almroth Edward (1861–1947), Irish-born physiologist, pathologist. Trinity College Dublin BA 1882, MB, BCh 1883; Leipzig with Ludwig; research on coagulation of blood with Wooldridge. Demonstrator in pathology Cambridge 1887; in physiology Sydney 1889; professor of pathology Army Medical School Netley and pathologist to St Mary's Hospital from 1892; professor of experimental pathology University of London from 1908. Developed typhoid inoculations for Boer War, vaccinations against wound infections WW1. FRS and knighted 1906.

Woollard, Herbert Henry (1889–1939), Australian-born experimental anatomist. Melbourne University 1910, MD 1912. War service AAMC; study year Johns Hopkins 1921, then demonstrator University College London under Elliot Smith; assistant professor 1923–7. Chair of anatomy and histology Adelaide 1928; St Bartholomew's College 1930; University College London 1936–9. Early research on primate brains; after 1925 on peripheral innervation (including experiments on self). Synthesized anatomical and physiological aspects of biological studies. Published *Recent Advances in Anatomy*, 1927. FRS 1938.

Patricia Morison: Biographical Details

Raised in Kalgoorlie, Patricia Morison took a history major at the University of Western Australia and acquired her interest in the history of medicine through health research work in Canberra for the Australian Government and in London for the County Council. After a few domestic years, she took up postgraduate studies at the Australian National University and tutored for four years in its Hisoty Department before turning to writing.

Interested in biography as a way of presenting history, she has written articles on a number of people in medicine and science, including entries in the Australian Dictionary of Biography while working on this full-length biography.

Index

Australopithecus africanus 378 [handwritten]

Bayview 206 349 [handwritten]

Eurotas p205

Sheoks 206 170